# New Developments in Medical Research

nova
Medicine & Health
New York

# New Developments in Medical Research

**Leptin and its Role in Health and Disease**
Stephen E. Bradley (Editor)
2023. ISBN: 979-8-89113-274-0 (Softcover)
2023. ISBN: 979-8-89113-334-1 (eBook)

**Inflammation and Chronic Disorders: The Secret Connection**
Ashwani K. Dhingra, PhD (Editor)
Priyanka Kriplani, PhD (Editor)
Bhawna Chopra, PhD (Editor)
Ajmer Singh Grewal, PhD (Editor)
Geeta Deswal, PhD (Editor)
Peeyush Kaushik, M. Pharm (Editor)
2023. ISBN: 979-8-88697-980-0 (eBook)

**Antidiabetic Plants: Properties and Applications**
Arpita Roy, PhD (Editor)
2023. ISBN: 979-8-88697-957-2 (Hardcover)
2023. ISBN: 979-8-88697-982-4 (eBook)

**The Dangers of Psychoactive Substances**
Denise J. Burton (Editor)
2023. ISBN: 979-8-88697-705-9 (Softcover)
2023. ISBN: 979-8-88697-712-7 (eBook)

**An Innovative Program at Alfaisal Medicine: A Brief History and Guide to Success**
Paul Ganguly, MBBS, MD, FACA (Editor)
2023. ISBN: 979-8-88697-638-0 (Softcover)
2023. ISBN: 979-8-88697-703-5 (eBook)

More information about this series can be found at
https://novapublishers.com/product-category/series/new-developments-in-medical-research/

**Sushil Kumar Upadhyay**
**Manoj Singh**
**and Anil Kumar Sharma**
Editors

# Therapeutic Advances in Human Health and Diseases

nova
Medicine & Health
New York

## NOTICE TO THE READER



**Library of Congress Cataloging-in-Publication Data**

ISBN: 979-8-89113-304-4

Published by Nova Science Publishers, Inc. † New York

# Contents

# Preface

The book has imperative and up-to-date information on the basics to advanced therapeutic approaches against various life-threatening diseases including vector and parasite-borne diseases, COVID-19, Mucormycosis, and cancer as well. The book harbors extensive knowledge about the applications and effective utilization of advanced personalized medicines, target-based nanoencapsulated phytochemicals, and herbal nanomedicines against life-threatening diseases including cancer, thereby having implications in the cancer biology field encompassing pharmaceutical and life science sectors considerably. Moreover, the proposed book would provide a strong platform for delineating the complex mechanism underlying the disease therapeutics along with the potential therapies countering the existing menace of drug resistance, especially concerning cancer. More so the book will showcase the recent advances in the use of nanocomposite films and molecular-mediated drug delivery for therapeutic applications.

The uniqueness of this book is to provide all the possible information from basics to advanced nano-therapeutics at a single platform making it a valuable informative source to the graduates of various universities across the globe to understand multifaceted therapeutic applications against life-threatening diseases. The book is an outstanding compilation comprising comprehensive information on therapeutic advances at a single platform. The book is apt to the present needs and well aligned with the offered curricula in Universities across the globe for UG, PG, and Ph.D. programs encompassing life sciences, medical, paramedical, and pharmaceutical courses. The diversity of chapters in the book are going to covers various aspects of the parasites, pathophysiology, and pathogenesis along with the pivotal role of nanotechnology in drug discovery and nano-biosensors for the detection of coronavirus as well. Moreover, the book has interesting elements of futuristic personalized medicines in combating coronavirus along with remedial therapeutic measures against coronavirus-induced mucormycosis. Another chapter deals with multifaceted therapeutic advances in life-threatening human diseases from traditional, complementary, and integrative medicine to nano-based targeted drug delivery. In the end, the authors have shed light on understanding oncogenesis and cancer and finding an amicable therapeutic nanomedicine solution paving the way towards individualized medicine therapeutics against cancer.

With the advent of newer technologies such as combinatorial chemistry high-throughput screening, next generation sequencing, it is now possible to consider that nanotherapeutics and personalized medicines could be the sound death knell for a variety of dreadful diseases including cancer and also to deal with the growing menace of drug-resistance. Once again, our sincere thanks to all the contributing authors who worked like a team to let us complete this book. Special thanks to the Editorial team of the publishing house who were available all the time to impart their valuable input and assistance. Words of appreciation also go to the whole Production Team as well.

Sushil Kumar Upadhyay, PhD
Manoj Singh, PhD
Anil K. Sharma, PhD

## Chapter 1

# Parasites and Pathogenesis: Disease Etiology, Progression, Control Measures and Advancements in Therapeutic Strategies

**Sushil Kumar Upadhyay**[1,*]
**Manoj Singh**[1]
**Mukesh Yadav**[1]
**Nirmala Sehrawat**[1]
**Mayank Raj**[1]
**Siddhartha Dan**[2]
**Kiran Upadhyay**[3]
**Yogendra Prasad Pandey**[4]
**Vikas Kumar**[5]
**Sunil Kumar**[6]
**Prabhakar Mishra**[7]
**Mukesh Kumar**[1]
**Nisha Kashyap**[8]
**Raj Singh**[1]
**and Anil Kumar Sharma**[9]

[1]Department of Bio-Sciences and Technology, M. M. E. C., Maharishi Markandeshwar (Deemed to be University), Mullana-Ambala, Haryana, India
[2]Department of Biotechnology, Dr. B. R. Ambedkar, National Institute of Technology, Jalandhar, Punjab, India

---

[*] Corresponding Author's Email: upadhyay.k.sushil@gmail.com.

In: Therapeutic Advances in Human Health and Diseases
Editors: Sushil Kumar Upadhyay, Manoj Singh and Anil Kumar Sharma
ISBN: 979-8-89113-304-4

[3]Department of Zoology, K. P. Higher Education Institute, Jhalwa–Prayagraj, Uttar Pradesh, India
[4]Department of Zoology, Government Model Science College, Rewa, MP, India
[5]Department of Microbiology, International Medical School, UIB, Almaty, Kazakhstan
[6]Department of Microbiology, Faculty of Biomedical Sciences,
Kampala International University, Western Campus, Ishaka, Uganda
[7]Department of Biotechnology, School of Applied Sciences, REVA University, Bengaluru, Karnataka, India
[8]Department of Medical Microbiology, PGIMER, Chandigarh, India
[9]Department of Biotechnology, Amity University, Mohali, Punjab, India

## Abstract

Parasites and parasitism have long been a significant concern for human health and the sustainability of various ecosystems. This abstract highlights the evolving landscape of parasitic diseases and the emerging challenges they pose in the realms of health and sustainability. Additionally, it sheds light on the modern therapeutic strategies that have been developed to combat these challenges. Parasitic diseases affect billions of people worldwide, particularly those in impoverished regions with limited access to adequate healthcare and sanitation facilities. These diseases caused by various types of parasites such as protozoa, helminths, and arthropods, lead to a range of debilitating symptoms and can have severe consequences on individual and community well-being. Furthermore, parasites can also impact the sustainability of ecosystems by affecting the health and survival of animal and plant populations. Parasitic infections can disrupt food chains, alter biodiversity, and contribute to ecological imbalances. As a result, addressing parasitism is not only crucial for human health but also for the preservation of ecosystems and the sustainable development of communities. Fortunately, significant advancements have been made in the development of therapeutic strategies to combat parasitic diseases. These strategies encompass various approaches, including the discovery and development of new antiparasitic drugs, the improvement of diagnostic techniques for early detection, the implementation of preventive measures, and the integration of multidisciplinary approaches in research and healthcare systems.

**Keywords:** parasites, parasitism, disease etiology, helminths, mucormycosis, diagnosis, pathogenesis, therapy

# 1. Introduction

Parasites and parasitism have long been a topic of interest and concern in various fields, including biology, medicine, ecology, and public health. The relationship between parasites and their hosts is complex and often characterized by a delicate balance between survival and harm (Preston and Johnson, 2010). This introduction provides an overview of parasites and parasitism, highlighting their significance, diversity, and impact on both human and ecological systems. Parasites are organisms that rely on other organisms, known as hosts, for their survival and reproduction (Olano et al., 2011; Upadhyay, 2012). They encompass a wide range of organisms, including protozoa, helminths (worms), arthropods (such as ticks and fleas), and even certain fungi and bacteria (Upadhyay, 2020; Upadhyay, 2023a,b). Parasites have evolved a diverse array of strategies to exploit and inhabit their hosts, often at the expense of the host's health and well-being.

Parasitism is a unique ecological relationship in which the parasite benefits while the host suffers. Parasites can cause a variety of diseases and infections in their hosts, leading to symptoms ranging from mild discomfort to severe illness and even death. These diseases can affect humans, animals, and plants, impacting both individual organisms and entire populations (Wilkinson et al., 2011; Upadhyay, 2020a). In the context of human health, parasitic diseases are a significant global burden, particularly in regions with poor sanitation, inadequate healthcare infrastructure, and limited resources. Examples of parasitic diseases include malaria, caused by the *Plasmodium* parasite and transmitted by mosquitoes, and schistosomiasis, caused by blood flukes and contracted through contact with contaminated water (Sangweme et al., 2010; Moriyasu et al., 2018). These diseases can cause immense suffering, and financial losses, as well as hinder social and economic development.

Beyond human health, parasites play a crucial role in shaping ecological systems. They can influence the structure and dynamics of communities, regulate population sizes, and impact the evolution of hosts. Parasites are often involved in complex food webs and interact with multiple host species, exerting ecological pressures and shaping biodiversity (Lafferty et al., 2008; Roche and Guégan, 2011; Upadhyay, 2023a). Understanding parasites and parasitism is essential for multiple reasons. Firstly, it provides insights into the intricate dynamics of host-parasite interactions, shedding light on the co-evolutionary processes that have shaped these relationships over millions of years. Secondly, studying parasites can help identify and monitor emerging infectious diseases, enabling proactive measures for prevention, control, and treatment. Lastly, recognizing the ecological roles of parasites can contribute to the conservation and management of ecosystems, safeguarding biodiversity and ecosystem functioning (Dunn et al., 2013; Giari et al., 2020).

In recent years, the field of Parasitology has witnessed significant advancements in terms of research, diagnostics, and treatment strategies. Rapid diagnostic techniques, innovative therapeutic interventions, and integrated control measures have contributed to progress in combating parasitic diseases and minimizing their impact on human health and ecosystems (Hemingway et al., 2016; Bahk et al., 2018; Upadhyay, 2023b). Thus parasites and parasitism are of great significance in various disciplines, from medicine and biology to ecology and public health. Their diverse nature, impact on host organisms, and role in shaping ecosystems make them a subject of continuous study and concern. By deepening our understanding of parasites and developing effective strategies for their control, we can mitigate the challenges they pose and work towards a healthier, more sustainable future.

Addressing emerging challenges requires a multifaceted approach. This includes strengthening surveillance and early warning systems, investing in research and development for new drugs and vaccines, promoting responsible use of antiparasitic agents, implementing vector control measures, improving sanitation and hygiene practices, and raising awareness among communities (Upadhyay, 2020a, 2023a,b). Furthermore, building resilience and adaptive capacity in healthcare systems and ecosystems can help mitigate the impacts of emerging parasitic diseases on health and sustainability. The emerging parasitic challenges pose significant threats to human health and ecosystem sustainability (Horwitz and Wilcox, 2005; Chomicz et al., 2016; Sures et al., 2017). The dynamic nature of parasites, coupled with factors such as climate change, drug resistance, and global interconnectedness, necessitates proactive measures and collaborative approaches. By addressing these challenges head-on, we can enhance our ability to prevent, control, and manage parasitic diseases, protecting both human well-being and the long-term viability of ecosystems.

Cutting-edge technologies, such as genomics, proteomics, and bioinformatics, have significantly contributed to the understanding of parasite biology and the identification of potential targets for therapeutic interventions (Upadhyay, 2017a, 2018a,b; Upadhyay et al., 2019a, 2023a). Additionally, innovative drug delivery systems, including nanotechnology-based approaches, have enhanced the efficacy and targeted delivery of antiparasitic drugs, minimizing side effects and improving patient compliance. Moreover, community-based initiatives, education programs, and collaborations between governments, researchers, and non-governmental organizations have played a pivotal role in raising awareness about parasitic diseases and implementing sustainable control and prevention measures. These efforts encompass integrated approaches, such as improved sanitation facilities, access to clean water, vector control programs, and mass drug administration campaigns.

## 2. Parasitic Protozoa and Diseases

Protozoa are single-celled or unicellular eukaryotic organisms with worldwide occurrence in various habitats (Yaeger, 1996). Parasitic protozoa can invade the tissues and cells of humans as well as other animals (MacMillan, 1991). These parasitic protozoa may lead to a range of effects on human and other animal's health. Parasitic protozoa may result in non-threatening asymptomatic to serious life-threatening disease even death which depends on various factors related to parasite and host (Yaeger, 1996). These microorganisms can be acquired via fecal-oral transmission, through sexual contact, or from arthropod vectors such as ticks and mosquitoes.

The protozoa are responsible for various diseases throughout the world (Kumar et al., 2022). The diseases caused by protozoa are generally found associated with poor sanitation, lack of hygiene, food contamination, contaminated drinking water, lack of proper food storage, and related aspects. Some of the protozoa-mediated diseases have been discussed along with their diagnosis and potential treatment possibilities.

There are four classes of Protozoa including sporozoa, flagellate protozoa, ciliate protozoa, and amoebae. Ciliate protozoa are motile because the cell surface is covered in tiny hairs called cilia. Many protozoa are free living, but others cause serious infections. Protozoa can infect any human tissue and are the cause of a variety of diseases but there are no ciliate protozoa known to cause human disease (Yaeger, 1996). Parasitic protozoans can spread using a variety of strategies. Some produce cysts to survive outside the body, others are spread by insects, and yet others spread during human sexual contact. Infections caused by protozoa include, for example, toxoplasmosis, amoebic dysentery, malaria, trypanosomiasis, leishmaniasis (Kala-Azar), and amoebic meningitis caused by *Naeglaria fowleri* that colonizes natural hot water springs (Andrews et al., 2014). It is because of the presence of this amoeba that people are no longer allowed to swim in the Roman Baths at Bath.

A variety of protozoans are commonly observed on the external surfaces of farmed and feral fishes. Their significance to the fish is dependent upon the protozoan type, number, species complex, pathogenicity, and the attendant condition of the host. Their significance to an aquaculturist is dependent primarily on their economic impact. Economic impact is a multidimensional determination based on protozoan biology and population dynamics, host morphologic and physiologic conditions, host population dynamics, and environment (MacMillan, 1991). The difference between the perceived and actual economic impact also depends on fish production expectations. The economic impact of external protozoan infestations is difficult to assess and varies dramatically depending on fish culture conditions.

Many protozoan infestations occur simultaneously or as sequelae to a bacterial, viral, or environmentally mediated disease. However, protozoans are believed to be contributing factors in 65% of the fish kills associated with various bacterial, viral, or other parasitic (e.g., proliferative gill disease) diseases. Independently, external protozoans may cause an estimated $6 million loss to the commercial catfish industry. The aquaculturist, just as other animal producers, must be concerned with the allocation of scarce resources (capital, labor, equipment, and supplies) to determine the optimal control of diseases or to establish a cost-effective "herd" (fish school) health program. The disease is a poorly defined condition associated with morbidity and mortality, but also associated with losses due to decreased growth rate (weight gain) decreased reproductive success and fecundity increased costs associated with culling and replacement, salvage value or cost of dead fish disposal, loss from condemnations in the processing plant, loss of quality, shortening of shelf life and losses from consumer fear of disease and resultant loss of market. Fortunately, external fish protozoans have not been determined to present human health hazards.

## 2.1. *Entamoeba histolytica*

Amoebae move by pushing out pseudopodia (false feet). Human pathogens include *Entamoeba histolytica* a well-known protozoan infecting and adversely affecting a large human population worldwide. Recently, Kantor et al. (2018) have discussed the updates in the clinical manifestation, pathogenesis, and vaccine development of *E. histolytica.* Amoebiasis, also known as amoebic dysentery, is an infection caused by the protozoan *E. histolytica* (Haque et al., 2003; Kantor et al., 2018). Although the majority of *E. histolytica* infections are asymptomatic, but estimated around 50 million people become symptomatic (Chou and Austin, 2022). Most infections are asymptomatic, but invasive intestinal disease may occur manifesting with several weeks of cramping, abdominal pain, watery or bloody diarrhea, and weight loss (Haque et al., 2003). Several other associated health conditions have also been described including liver abscess, purulent pericarditis, pneumonia, and even cerebral amoebiasis (Haque et al., 2003; Cheepsattayakorn and Cheepsattayakorn, 2014; Kantor et al., 2018). The affected population is chiefly from developing countries. It is responsible for over 100,000 deaths a year (Chou and Austin, 2022). Transmission generally occurs by the ingestion of infected water or food due to fecal excretion of cysts, and even fecal-oral transmission within the household and during male homosexual activity (Haque et al., 2003; Salit et al., 2009; Cheepsattayakorn and Cheepsattayakorn, 2014).

## 2.2. *Giardia lamblia*

Flagellate protozoa are motile because they possess flagella (*singular*: flagellum). *Giardia lamblia* is a flagellate protozoan parasite. *G. lamblia* is also known as *G. intestinalis* and *G. duodenalis*. It is a unicellular eukaryotic microorganism known to cause diarrheal disease throughout the world (Adam, 2001; Kumar et al., 2022). The diarrheal illness caused by *G. lamblia* is generally known as giardiasis. It is among the common causes of waterborne outbreaks of diarrhea and it is also occasionally seen as a cause of food-borne diarrhea (Mintz et al., 1993; Barwick et al., 2000; Adam, 2001). Higher prevalence and incidence of infection have been reported in developing countries. It has been suggested from data that growth retardation can result from chronic giardiasis (Fraser et al., 2000; Adam, 2001). The infection ranges from asymptomatic to prolonged illness associated with diarrhea, malabsorption, and weight loss (Hanevik et al., 2009; Kumar et al., 2022). The infective stage is trophozoite which is rounded at the posterior end, tapered posteriorly, and flattened dorso-ventrally (Bogitsh et al., 2019; Kumar et al., 2022). In some parts of the world, water contaminated with *G. lamblia* cysts commonly results in travel-related giardiasis among tourists (Brodsky et al., 1974). Recently, Kumar et al. (2022) have discussed the symptoms of giardiasis which include diarrhea, weight loss, nausea, and abdominal distension. Trophozoite attachment resulted in inflammation in the intestine as well as lesions on mucosal cells (Lopez et al., 2015). Further, the infected person is unable to absorb vitamin B12, folate, and carotene due to malabsorption.

### 2.3. *Trichomonas vaginalis*

*Trichomonas vaginalis* is a parasitic protozoan. It is the etiologic agent of trichomoniasis i.e., a sexually transmitted disease (STD) that has attained worldwide attention (Petrin et al., 1998). *T. vaginalis* (TV) is likely among the most common non-viral sexually transmitted infections (STIs) in the world (Kissinger, 2015). Women with trichomoniasis generally have vaginal discharge, urinary tract infection symptoms, painful intercourse, vaginal itching, or pelvic pain. Men with trichomoniasis may be asymptomatic, or occasionally, develop symptoms including penile discharge, testicular pain, dysuria, urinary frequency, or cloudy urine (Schumann and Plasner, 2022). *T. vaginalis* is the most widely studied parasite of all the trichomonads. The disease shows a wide range of symptoms from a state of severe inflammation and irritation with a frothy malodorous discharge to a relatively asymptomatic carrier state (Brown, 1972; Catterall, 1972; Wisdom and Dunlop, 1965; Petrin et al., 1998). Also, it has been suggested that trichomoniasis may lead to increased transmission of HIV through local accumulations of HIV-infected or HIV-susceptible cells like lymphocytes and macrophages (Laga et al., 1991). *T. vaginalis*, a urogenital pathogen has been found to vary in size and shape, with the average length and width being 10 and 7 μm, respectively (Honigberg and King, 1964; 130; Petrin et al., 1998). It is a flagellated protozoan having five flagella. Four flagella are located at its anterior portion while the fifth flagellum is incorporated within the undulating membrane of the parasite (Arroyo et al., 1993; Warton and Honigberg, 1979). The flagella and the undulating membrane provide a characteristic quivering motility to this parasite (Honigberg and King, 1964). Further, it has been reported that under unfavorable growth conditions, *T. vaginalis* can round up and internalize the flagella (Fari et al., 1985; Honigberg and Brugerolle, 1990).

### 2.4. *Plasmodium* Species

Sporozoa include the intracellular parasites of the genus *Plasmodium*. These cause malaria, an illness characterized by recurrent bouts of fever and sweating. It is spread by mosquitoes of the genus *Anopheles*. Malaria is among the most destructive infectious diseases of humans. According to World Health Organization (WHO, 2023a) nearly half of the world's population was at risk of malaria in 2020. Further, most cases and deaths occur in sub-Saharan Africa. There were an estimated 247 million cases of malaria in 2021, and the estimated number of malaria deaths stood at 619,000 as per the WHO (2023a) official website (https://www.who.int/health-topics/malaria). The causative agents of malaria are unicellular protozoan parasites. These protozoa parasites belong to the genus *Plasmodium*. Not only humans, these parasites also infect other vertebrates, from reptiles and birds to mammals. Though, over 200 species of *Plasmodium* have been formally described five *Plasmodium* species are found to infect humans naturally and cause malaria (Sato, 2021). These are (i) *P. falciparum*, (ii) *P. vivax*, (iii) *P. malariae*, (iv) *P. ovale* and (v) *P. knowlesi*. Out of these five species, the first four are specific to humans (Sato, 2021). *P. falciparum* causes the most serious infection and remains high in economically poor countries, especially in Africa (Cibulskis et al., 2016; Sato, 2021).

Naturally, the uninucleate sporozoites in the salivary glands of infected mosquitoes are injected into a human host when the mosquito feeds (Crutcher and Hoffman, 1996). The sporozoites rapidly invade liver parenchymal cells, where they mature into liver-stage schizonts, which burst to release 2,000 to 40,000 uninucleate merozoites. In *P. vivax* and *P. ovale* infections, maturation of the schizont may be delayed for 1 to 2 years. Each merozoite can infect a red blood cell. Within the red cell, the merozoite matures either into an uninucleate gametocyte (the sexual stage), infectious for *Anopheles* mosquitoes, or, over 48-72 hours, into an erythrocytic stage schizont containing 10 to 36 merozoites. Rupture of the schizont releases these merozoites, which infect other red cells. If a vector mosquito ingests gametocytes, the gametocytes develop in the mosquito gut to gametes, which undergo fertilization and mature in 2 to 3 weeks to sporozoites (Crutcher and Hoffman, 1996).

At an earlier stage, the patients develop fever, chills, sweating, headache, weakness, and other symptoms similar to viral syndrome (Crutcher and Hoffman, 1996). Later, severe disease may develop, with an abnormal level of consciousness, severe anemia, renal failure, and multisystem failure. The fever and chills of malaria are associated with the rupture of erythrocytic-stage schizonts. In severe falciparum malaria, parasitized red cells may obstruct capillaries and postcapillary venules, leading to local hypoxia and the release of toxic cellular products. Obstruction of the microcirculation in the brain (cerebral malaria) and in other vital organs is thought to be responsible for severe complications (Crutcher and Hoffman, 1996).

### 2.5. *Leishmania* Species

Leishmaniasis is caused by a protozoa parasite from over 20 *Leishmania* species. It is endemic in Asia, Africa, the Americas, and the Mediterranean region (Torres-Guerrero et al., 2017). The occurrence of Leishmaniasis is found in parts of the tropics, subtropics, and southern Europe (CDC, 2023a). Over 90 sandfly species are known to transmit *Leishmania* parasites. There are 3 main forms of the disease including visceral leishmaniasis (VL), cutaneous leishmaniasis (CL), and mucocutaneous leishmaniasis (WHO, 2023b). Leishmaniasis has been classified as a neglected tropical disease (NTD). Leishmaniasis is spread by the bite of phlebotomine sand flies. Cutaneous leishmaniasis causes skin sores and visceral leishmaniasis affects several internal organs usually the spleen, liver, and bone marrow (CDC, 2023a). *Leishmania* parasites are transmitted through the bites of infected female phlebotomine sandflies, which feed on blood to produce eggs.

## 3. Diagnosis and Therapeutic Approaches for Protozoan Diseases

Various diagnostic techniques, procedures, and tools are available for the detection of parasitic protozoan and diseases caused by them. Currently, both conventional and advanced approaches are followed to diagnose the protozoan infection depending on the requirements.

### 3.1. *Entamoeba histolytica*

Various diagnostic tools exist for the diagnosis of *E. histolytica* including simple microscopy, serological analysis, antigen detection, relevant molecular techniques, and colonoscopy with histological examination (Kantor et al., 2018). Microscopy has been used for a long time to detect the parasite in stools but this method has some limitations including lack of accuracy. The identification of *E. histolytica* specific nucleic acids can be done with the help of PCR. The PCR-based method has been suggested as quick, accurate, and effective in detecting both forms of disease i.e., intestinal and extra-intestinal (Cheepsattayakorn and Cheepsattayakorn, 2014). Also, stool and serum antigen detection assays are available that are sensitive, specific (differentiating between strains), and easy to perform (Haque et al., 1993; Kantor et al., 2018). These assays can potentially diagnose early infection (Haque et al., 1993). ELISA, radioimmunoassay, or immunofluorescence can be performed for detection of antigen-specific to *E. histolytica.* For the diagnosis of *E. histolytica,* the indirect hemagglutination test (IHA) has been suggested as the most sensitive serology assay (Peterson et al., 2011; Kantor et al., 2018). Besides, above mentioned methods, direct visualization of the colon by colonoscopy has also been suggested to diagnose amoebiasis, particularly in cases where, non-specific gastrointestinal symptoms make the diagnosis difficult (Horiki et al., 2015; Kantor et al., 2018).

The amoebiasis can be prevented by following good hygiene practices. Awareness and education regarding the role of hand washing and hygiene is very important measure in preventing the spread of amoebiasis and other infectious diseases (Kantor et al., 2018). For clinical treatment, noninvasive colitis may be treated with only a luminal agent such as paromycin, to eliminate intraluminal cysts (Haque et al., 1993). For invasive amoebiasis and extra-intestinal disease, the uses of nitroimidazoles (e.g., metronidazole) are the main therapeutic candidates but are only active against the trophozoite stage (Haque et al., 1993; Simpson et al., 2015; Kantor et al., 2018). Nitroimidazoles with longer half-lives, such as tinidazole, secnidazole, and ornidazole, allow for shorter treatment periods. If fulminant amoebic colitis develops, broad-spectrum antibiotics should be added to the treatment due to the risk of bacterial translocation (Simpson et al., 2015; Kantor et al., 2018).

### 3.2. *Giardia lamblia*

Hooshyar et al. (2019) have reported an important review of current diagnostic strategies for *Giardia* app. The laboratory diagnosis of *Giardia* spp. is mainly based on observation of microscopic cysts or trophozoite in stool samples. The microscopic examination of fecal samples is considered the preferred routine diagnosis method for giardiasis. The sensitivity of the microscope-based technique depends on various methods including using direct or concentration methods, the number of examined fecal samples, and the employment of professionally trained persons (Hooshyar et al., 2019). Microscopy with direct fluorescent antibody testing (DFA) is considered the test of choice for diagnosis of giardiasis since it provides increased sensitivity over non-fluorescent microscopy techniques (CDC, 2023b). Besides, this basic method, several immunological-based assays and molecular methods are also available for giardiasis diagnosis. The direct examination method is also useful in diagnosis. Examination of direct wet saline preparation of a fresh stool specimen allows motile trophozoites to be seen (Hooshyar et al., 2019). Fecal concentration is another recommended and routine procedure that allows the detection of a small number of *Giardia* cysts (Hooshyar et al., 2019). The sedimentation procedures are the recommended methods as being the easiest to perform and less prone to technical errors (Smith and Mank, 2011). Straining, culture method, and String test (Entero-test) are also used to diagnose the infection. Immunodiagnostic tests based on antigen-antibody reactions have also been developed to diagnose giardiasis. PCR-based detection of giardiasis has also been developed but this molecular detection is not followed frequently for routine diagnosis. Various drugs can be used to treat the *Giardia* infection. The effective treatment options may include the use of metronidazole, tinidazole, and nitazoxanide (CDC, 2023b). Other medication that may be used includes paromomycin, quinacrine, and furazolidone (CDC, 2023b).

### 3.3. *Trichomonas vaginalis*

Garber (2005) has reported the laboratory diagnosis of *Trichomonas vaginalis*. According to the author, the diagnosis of trichomoniasis has traditionally depended on the microscopic observation of motile protozoa from vaginal or cervical samples and from urethral or prostatic secretions (Garber, 2005). The broth culture technique has been considered important for the diagnosis of *T. vaginalis* for the past 40 years. Cultivation on cell cultures has been suggested as more sensitive, enabling the observation of *T. vaginalis* from an inoculum containing even 3 organisms/mL. The cell culture-based method remains expensive, inconvenient, and even more prone to vaginal bacterial contamination (Garber, 2005). Though, the nucleic acid detection-based approach has also been experimented (Riley et al., 1992; Garber, 2005) still it is in its infant stage and needs to be developed more elaborately. Identification of *T. vaginalis* in men has been reported with the use of the urine-based polymerase chain reaction (PCR)-ELISA technique described (Kaydos-Daniels et al., 2003). Besides these techniques and methods, antibody-based techniques including complement fixation, hemagglutination, gel diffusion, fluorescent antibody, and ELISA, have been used to determine the presence of trichomonal antibodies have been reported (Garber et al., 1986; Krieger et al., 1985). Antimicrobial susceptibility testing has been set up but susceptibility testing is not performed routinely due to lack of standardized methods. Also, no proficiency testing is available for this method (Cudmore et al., 2004). As discussed by Schumann and Plasner (2023) the recommended drugs for the treatment of trichomoniasis include metronidazole and tinidazole.

## 3.4. *Plasmodium* Species

Malaria is a very serious and fatal disease caused by the protozoan parasites of the genus *Plasmodium*. Its diagnosis is very important for proper and effective management of malaria. Tangpukdee et al. (2009) have reviewed the diagnosis of malaria. The most widely practiced and least expensive method is clinical diagnosis. It is based on the signs and symptoms of the patient, and also on physical findings at examination. A clinical diagnosis of malaria is still challenging because of the non-specific nature of the signs and symptoms (Tangpukdee et al., 2009). Malaria is conventionally diagnosed by microscopic examination of stained blood films using Giemsa, Wright's, or Field's stains (Warhurst and Williams, 1996). The most important shortcoming of microscopic examination is its relatively low sensitivity, particularly at low parasite levels. Further, Microscopy is laborious and ill-suited for high-throughput use, and species determination at low parasite density is still challenging. The QBC (Quantitative buffy coat) technique has been designed to enhance the microscopic detection of parasites and simplify the malaria diagnosis (Clendennen et al., 1995). This method is based on the staining of parasitic deoxyribonucleic acid (DNA) in micro-hematocrit tubes with fluorescent dyes, i.e., acridine orange, followed by its detection by epi-fluorescent microscopy. Rapid diagnostic tests (RDTs) have been developed to diagnose malaria in a fast and accurate manner. The RDTs are generally based on the detection of malaria antigens in blood flowing along a membrane containing specific anti-malaria antibodies (Tangpukdee et al., 2009). Further, the RDTs do not require laboratory equipment. The malaria parasite can be detected by serological tests. These tests are based on the detection of antibodies against asexual blood-stage malaria parasites. Immunofluorescence antibody testing (IFA) has emerged as a reliable serologic test for malaria (She et al., 2007). Besides the mentioned techniques, new and emerging molecular diagnostic techniques have been experimented. These techniques play an important role in malaria research. According to authors (Tangpukdee et al., 2009), molecular biological-based techniques including PCR, microarray, loop-mediated isothermal amplification (LAMP), mass spectrometry (MS), and flow cytometric (FCM) assay techniques have permitted elaborated as well as extensive characterization of the malaria parasite.

The antimalarial drugs have been discussed by Sato (2021). Currently, five classes of antimalarial drugs are used in the clinical treatment of human malaria. These five classes are based on their structural backbone and apparent action (Ross and Fidock, 2019). These classes include (i) endoperoxides (e.g., artemisinin and its derivatives), (ii) 4-aminoquinolines (chloroquine), aryl-amino alcohols (quinine, mefloquine), (iii) antifolates (pyrimethamine, proguanil, sulfadoxine), (iv) naphthoquinones (atovaquone) and (v) 8-aminoquinolines (primaquine, tafenoquine).

### 3.5. *Leishmania* Species

Diagnosis of *Leishmania* parasite is based on the clinical and congruent epidemiological context (Torres-Guerrero et al., 2017). The protozoan may be found in the scraping of cutaneous or mucosal ulcerations. The protozoan may be present in the non-ulcerated lesions. A biopsy of the affected part may be taken for confirmation of infection. A smear may reveal the parasites in free form or inside macrophages or less frequently in polymorphonuclear leukocytes (Torres-Guerrero et al., 2017). According to Torres-Guerrero et al. (2017), the common and effective treatment with satisfactory clinical and microbiological results for all the clinical forms of leishmaniasis includes intravenous pentavalent antimonials in the form of sodium stibogluconate or meglumine antimoniate, except some cases (if the case of resistant microbe). Intralesional treatment has also been documented. Alternative drug options are also available and may be used accordingly (Torres-Guerrero et al., 2017).

## 4. Parasitic Helminthes and Diseases

Parasitic helminths, commonly known as worms, are a diverse group of multicellular parasites that infect humans and animals, causing a wide range of diseases (Pritchard and Wilson, 1997; Upadhyay, 2012). They can be classified into two main categories: Nemathelminthes/ Aschelminthes (nematodes or roundworms) and Platyhelminthes (flatworms include trematodes and cestodes) (Upadhyay, 2018b; Upadhyay, 2020a,b; 2023a,b; Upadhyay et al., 2023c).

## 4.1. Trematodes

Trematodes, commonly known as flukes, are a group of parasitic helminths that belong to the class Trematoda (Yamaguti, 1958). They have a flattened body shape and are characterized by complex life cycles involving multiple hosts. Trematodes can infect various animals, including humans, and cause a diverse range of diseases (Malhotra et al., 2009; Upadhyay, et al., 2013a,b; Jaiswal et al., 2014a,b; Upadhyay et al., 2015; Rani and Upadhyay, 2019). Liver flukes, such as *Fasciola hepatica* and *Opisthorchis viverrini*, infect humans through ingestion of contaminated raw or undercooked freshwater fish or aquatic plants (Upadhyay et al., 2023a). These parasites cause hepatobiliary diseases, including hepatomegaly, liver fibrosis, and cholangiocarcinoma. Schistosomes, also known as blood flukes, are trematode parasites that cause schistosomiasis (Baron, 1996). The main species responsible for human infection are *Schistosoma mansoni*, *S. haematobium*, and *S. japonicum* (Cox et al., 2007). Schistosomiasis is acquired through contact with fresh water contaminated by parasite-infected snails (Kali, 2015). The disease can lead to chronic inflammation, fibrosis, and organ damage, affecting the gastrointestinal tract (*S. mansoni*), urinary system (*S. haematobium*), or liver (*S. japonicum*).

### *4.1.1. Life Cycle and Transmission*

Trematodes have complex life cycles that often involve alternating between different hosts. They typically have an intermediate host, such as snails or freshwater crustaceans, where the parasite undergoes larval development (Upadhyay, 2017b; Upadhyay and Singh, 2018). Humans or other mammals serve as the definitive host, where the adult worms mature and produce eggs. Infections are acquired through the ingestion of contaminated water, food, or raw/undercooked intermediate hosts.

### *4.1.2. Tissue and Organ Involvement*

Trematodes can infect various tissues and organs in the human body, depending on the species. *Schistosoma* species infect the blood vessels surrounding the intestines or urinary system, while *Clonorchis sinensis* and *O. viverrini* mainly infect the bile ducts in the liver (IARC, 1994). The presence of adult worms and their eggs can lead to inflammation, fibrosis, and damage to the affected organs.

### *4.1.3. Clinical Manifestations*

Trematode infections can cause a range of symptoms and complications. In the early stages, infected individuals may experience fever, rash, fatigue, and gastrointestinal disturbances. Chronic infections can lead to more severe manifestations, such as hepatomegaly (enlarged liver), splenomegaly (enlarged spleen), hepatosplenomegaly (enlargement of both liver and spleen), anemia, bladder dysfunction, and increased susceptibility to other infections (PAHO, 2003; Talwani et al., 2011). Long-term consequences of untreated infections can include liver fibrosis, liver cirrhosis, and bladder cancer.

### *4.1.4. Prevention and Control*

Control measures for trematode infections involve a combination of strategies. These include the treatment of infected individuals with specific antiparasitic drugs, such as praziquantel, improvement of sanitation and hygiene practices to minimize contamination of water sources, and snail control measures to reduce the intermediate host population (Hedegaard Clausen et al., 2012; Madsen and Stauffer, 2022). Health education and community awareness programs are also important in promoting preventive measures, such as avoiding contact with contaminated water bodies and the consumption of raw or undercooked intermediate hosts.

Efforts to control and eliminate trematode infections are ongoing, with a focus on integrated control programs, surveillance, research, and community engagement. Access to safe water sources, improved sanitation, and education regarding proper hygiene practices are vital for the prevention of trematode infections (Upadhyay, 2020a; Paliwal et al., 2023; Upadhyay et al., 2023d). Thus in a nutshell trematodes are parasitic flukes that can cause significant diseases in humans and other animals. Understanding their life cycles, transmission dynamics, and clinical manifestations is crucial for effective control and prevention. Through a combination of treatment, sanitation, and education, the burden of trematode infections can be reduced, improving the health and well-being of affected populations.

## 4.2. Cestodes

Cestodes, commonly known as tapeworms, are a type of parasitic helminths that belong to the class Cestoda (Yamaguti, 1959). They are characterized by their long, flat, segmented bodies, which are composed of repetitive units called proglottids. Cestodes can infect various animals, including humans, and cause a range of diseases. Several species of cestodes can infect humans and cause diseases known as cestodiasis or tapeworm infections (Heyneman, 1996; Upadhyay et al., 2019a,b,c; Upadhyay et al., 2020; Babita et al., 2022; Upadhyay et al., 2023b). Examples include *Taenia saginata* (beef tapeworm), *T. solium* (pork tapeworm), and *Diphyllobothrium latum* (fish tapeworm) (Lesh and Brady, 2022). Tapeworm infections primarily occur through the ingestion of undercooked or raw meat-containing cysts with the larvae (cysticerci). *T. solium* (pork tapeworm) causes cysticercosis when the larvae form cysts in various tissues, including the brain, leading to neurocysticercosis. *T. saginata* (beef tapeworm) causes taeniasis, where adult worms reside in the human intestine and may cause mild gastrointestinal symptoms (Upadhyay, 2023a,b).

### *4.2.1. Life Cycle and Transmission*

Cestodes have complex life cycles that typically involve two hosts. The adult tapeworm resides in the intestines of the definitive host, which can be a human or other vertebrate (Heyneman, 1996; Lesh and Brady, 2022). The tapeworm releases eggs or gravid proglottids containing eggs, which are passed in the feces of the definitive host. These eggs can contaminate the environment and be ingested by intermediate hosts, such as cows, pigs, or fish. In the intermediate host, the eggs hatch, and the larvae form cysticerci in the muscle or other tissues. Human infection occurs when individuals consume the infected intermediate host (Upadhyay, 2020b; Upadhyay et al., 2021).

### *4.2.2. Tissue and Organ Involvement*

Cestodes primarily reside in the intestines of the definitive host, where they attach to the intestinal lining using specialized suckers or hooks. They absorb nutrients from the host's digestive system (McCoy, 1935). In humans, the presence of adult tapeworms may cause gastrointestinal symptoms such as abdominal pain, diarrhea, or weight loss (Heyneman, 1996). However, the symptoms can vary depending on the species of tapeworm and the location of infection.

### *4.2.3. Clinical Manifestations*

Cestode infections can lead to various clinical manifestations depending on the species and location of infection. Infections with *T. saginata* or *T. solium* can cause taeniasis, which may be asymptomatic or present with mild gastrointestinal symptoms (Heyneman, 1996; Lesh and Brady, 2022;

Upadhyay, 2023a,b). However, the larval form of *T. solium*, known as cysticercosis, can cause more severe symptoms and complications when the larvae form cysts in tissues such as the brain, muscles, or eyes.

#### *4.2.4. Prevention and Control*

Prevention of cestode infections involves various measures. These include proper cooking of meat to destroy any potential cysticerci, improved sanitation and hygiene practices to minimize fecal contamination of the environment, and proper disposal of human waste. Health education and community awareness are crucial in promoting preventive measures. Treatment of cestode infections typically involves the use of anthelmintic drugs, such as praziquantel or niclosamide, which can effectively eliminate adult tapeworms from the intestines (Chai, 2013; Lloyd et al., 2014).

Efforts to control cestode infections focus on education, surveillance, and treatment. Additionally, interventions such as meat inspection and meat hygiene practices can help reduce the risk of tapeworm transmission through contaminated meat. Thus in a nutshell, the cestodes, or tapeworms, are parasitic helminths that can infect humans and other animals. Understanding their life cycles, modes of transmission, and clinical manifestations is crucial for prevention, diagnosis, and treatment. Through proper sanitation, hygiene practices, and appropriate cooking of meat, the burden of cestode infections can be minimized, promoting better health and well-being for affected individuals and communities.

### 4.3. Nematodes

Nematodes, commonly referred to as roundworms, are a diverse group of parasitic helminths that infect humans, animals, and plants (Yamaguti, 1962). They are cylindrical and have a complete digestive system. Nematodes can cause a variety of diseases in their hosts, and their impact on global health and agriculture is significant (Upadhyay et al., 2009; Kumar et al., 2011; Upadhyay, 2017a; Upadhyay 2018a; Upadhyay and Nanware, 2020; Panwar et al., 2022). Filariasis is caused by filarial nematodes transmitted by various types of mosquitoes (Cross, 1996a; Erickson et al., 2009). Lymphatic filariasis, caused by *Wuchereria bancrofti*, *Brugia malayi*, and *B. timori*, leads to lymphedema, elephantiasis, and hydrocele (Chakraborty et al., 2013). Onchocerciasis, caused by *Onchocerca volvulus*, causes severe skin and eye lesions, leading to blindness (river blindness) (Gyasi et al., 2023). Loiasis, caused by *Loa loa*, can result in subcutaneous migration of adult worms and eye involvement (Rodriguez et al., 2021). Understanding nematode biology, improving diagnostics, and developing novel control strategies are important areas of ongoing research (Jaiswal et al., 2013; Babita et al., 2019; Upadhyay, 2020c). Additionally, education and awareness about proper hygiene practices, particularly in regions with a high prevalence of nematode infections, are crucial for prevention. Thus nematodes are a diverse group of parasitic roundworms that can infect humans, animals, and plants, causing a range of diseases and significant economic losses. Addressing nematode infections requires a multi-faceted approach involving research, diagnostics, drug development, and integrated pest management to mitigate their impact on human health and agricultural productivity.

#### *4.3.1. Human Nematode Infections*

Several nematodes infect humans and cause diseases. Examples include *Ascaris lumbricoides* (causing ascariasis), *Trichuris trichiura* (causing trichuriasis), *Enterobius vermicularis* (causing enterobiasis or pinworm infection), and *Strongyloides stercoralis* (causing strongyloidiasis) (Cross, 1996b; Hall et al., 2008; Upadhyay, 2020a, 2023a,b). These infections are prevalent in areas with poor sanitation and hygiene practices.

#### *4.3.2. Animal Nematode Infections*

Nematodes also infect various animal species, including livestock and pets. For instance, the filarial nematodes *Dirofilaria immitis* (causing heartworm disease) and *O. volvulus* (causing onchocerciasis or river blindness) affect dogs and humans, respectively (Morchón et al., 2012; Gyasi et al., 2023). Gastrointestinal nematodes, such as *Haemonchus contortus*, can cause severe health issues in livestock, leading to economic losses in the agricultural industry (Arsenopoulos et al., 2021; Flay et al., 2022).

#### *4.3.3. Soil-Transmitted Nematodes*

Soil-transmitted nematodes (STNs) include roundworms (*A. lumbricoides*), whipworms (*T. trichiura*), and hookworms (*Necator americanus* and *Ancylostoma duodenale*) (Incani et al., 2022; Ghodeif and Jain, 2023). STNs are transmitted through contact with soil contaminated with helminth eggs. They predominantly affect individuals in low-income, tropical regions with poor sanitation. STN infections can lead to malnutrition, anemia, stunted growth, cognitive impairment, and overall reduced physical fitness (Mascarini-Serra, 2011; Mbong et al., 2020; Ellwanger and Cavallero, 2023).

### *4.3.4. Plant-Parasitic Nematodes*

Plant-parasitic nematodes (PPNs) are a major concern in agriculture, causing significant damage to crops (Pulavarty et al., 2021; Bahadur, 2022). These nematodes feed on plant roots, affecting their growth, nutrient uptake, and overall health (Pires et al., 2022). Crop losses due to nematode infestations can result in reduced yields and economic losses. Important plant-parasitic nematodes include *Meloidogyne* spp. (root-knot nematodes) and *Heterodera* spp. (cyst nematodes) (Clapp et al., 2000; Bernard et al., 2017).

### *4.3.5. Entomopathogenic Nematodes*

Entomopathogenic Nematodes (EPNs) are the group of nematodes that are available in soil ecosystems in a free-living state. These nematodes of the family Heterorhabditidae and Steinemematidae are found to be associated symbiotically with the genus of bacteria *Photorhabdus* and *Xenorhabdus* (Bhat et al., 2016; Istkhar et al., 2016; Subramanian and Muthulakshmi, 2016; Dhiman et al., 2021). The name "entomopathogenic nematodes" originated from the Greek vocables "entomos," "insects," "pathê," "disease," and "guenos," "creating," and refers to a group of nematodes that can cause infection in insects through weakening their immune systems (Chauhan et al., 2023). Entomopathogenic nematodes must quickly kill their hosts with the help of bacterial partners, and they must pass on the associated bacteria to future generations." The Heterorhabditidae family holds an account of one genus, *Heterorhabditis* (Stock et al., 2002). The Steinernematidae family consists of two genera i.e., *Steinernema* Travassos, 1927 (George, 2018) and *Neosteinernema* (Nguyen and Hunt, 2007).

### *4.3.6. Life Cycle and Transmission*

Nematodes have a complex life cycle that often involves stages in both the host and the external environment. Depending on the species, nematodes may be transmitted through ingestion of contaminated food or water, contact with contaminated soil, or vector-borne transmission. Some nematodes have direct life cycles, while others involve intermediate hosts or vectors.

### *4.3.7. Prevention and Control*

Controlling nematode infections and their impact on health and agriculture is challenging. Strategies for control include the use of anthelmintic drugs, such as albendazole and ivermectin, to treat infected individuals or animals (Crump, 2017; Conterno et al., 2020). In agriculture, integrated pest management practices, crop rotation, resistant plant varieties, and soil management techniques are employed to reduce nematode populations (Frank et al., 2022). However, the development of resistance to anthelmintic drugs and the limited availability of effective control measures remain significant challenges.

Helminth parasites are highly antigenic and particularly adept at exerting a pro-allergic adjuvant effect, where Th-2 lymphocytes and their cytokines (particularly, IL3, 4, and 5) promote mastocytosis, IgE synthesis, and eosinophilia (Pritchard, 1993, 1997). An increase in our understanding of the mechanisms employed by parasites to support this potentially host-protective (Pritchard et al., 1995) or parasite-protective immune response - Th-1 responses seem to be successful in controlling invasive larval stages of some parasites (Pritchard and Wilson, 1997) - would serve the dual purpose of providing: (i) a sound basis for the development of anti-parasitic immuno-therapeutic strategies; (ii) an insight into the mechanisms responsible for the development of upsurge in allergic disease in parasite-free countries. This observation led to the hypothesis that parasite proteases might accelerate the natural proteolytic cleavage of CD23 from the leucocyte surface, leading to an upregulation of immediate-type hypersensitivity through the generation of soluble CD23 (a pro-allergic cytokine) and the removal of a negative feedback signal for IgE synthesis (Pritchard, 1997).

## 5. Parasitic Arthropods and Diseases

Parasitic arthropods impair animal production and welfare in various ways. They may be responsible for production losses due to (a) irritation such as that caused by non-biting flies; (b) ‘worry’, compounded of irritation, allergic responses, and blood losses from feeding, as by fleas, lice, keds, biting flies, mites and ticks; (c) deaths, or debilitating effects with possible damage to carcass, fleece or skin, such as result from the attacks of myiasis flies; (d) paralysis or toxicosis, as produced by the feeding of certain ticks; and (e) transmission of pathogenic organisms (Zeni et al., 2021). There are just a few examples of parasitic arthropods including mosquitoes, ticks, fleas, lice, bedbugs, botflies, etc. Each species has its own unique adaptations and life cycle to exploit their hosts. Parasitic arthropods can pose health risks to humans and animals, and their control and prevention often involve measures such as insecticide use, personal protection, and public health initiatives (Wharton and Norris, K.R 2010).

Mosquitoes are insects that require blood meals from animals, including humans, to nourish their eggs. Female mosquitoes are the ones that feed on blood, while males typically feed on nectar. Mosquitoes can transmit diseases such as malaria, dengue fever, Zika virus, and West Nile virus (Singh et al., 2022). However, the ticks are arachnids that attach themselves to the skin of animals, including humans, to feed on blood. They are known for transmitting diseases such as Lyme disease, babesiosis, anaplasmosis, and Rocky Mountain spotted fever.

Fleas are small wingless insects that infest the fur or feathers of mammals and birds. They feed on the blood of their hosts and can irritate, and allergic reactions, and transmit diseases like bubonic plague (Bitam et al., 2010). While lice are small, wingless insects that infest the hair, feathers, or clothing of mammals, and birds. They feed on the blood of their hosts and can cause itching, and skin irritation, and transmit diseases like trench fever and epidemic typhus.

Bedbugs are small insects that infest beds, furniture, and other areas where humans sleep. They feed on human blood and their bites can cause itching, skin rashes, and allergic reactions. On the other hand, botflies are a type of fly that lays their eggs on the skin of mammals. When the eggs hatch, the larvae burrow into the host's skin and develop. They can cause skin lesions and other health issues (Yan et al., 2019).

## 5.1. Parasitic Arthropods Borne Diseases

Parasitic arthropods can cause a variety of diseases in humans. Here are some examples of human diseases caused by parasitic arthropods. It's important to take preventive measures such as using insect repellents, wearing protective clothing, and avoiding known infested areas to reduce the risk of exposure to these diseases. If you suspect you have been infected with a parasitic arthropod or are experiencing symptoms, it is best to seek medical attention for proper diagnosis and treatment (Stejskal et al., 2018).

### *5.1.1. Malaria*

Malaria is a severe disease caused by parasites of the genus *Plasmodium*, which is transmitted to humans by a bite of an infected female mosquito of the species *Anopheles*. Malaria remains the leading cause of mortality around the world, and early diagnosis and fast-acting treatment prevent unwanted outcomes. It is the most common disease in Africa and some countries of Asia, while in the developed world malaria occurs as imported from endemic areas. The sweet sagewort plant was used as early as the second century BC to treat malaria fever in China. Much later, quinine started being used as an antimalarial drug (Singh et al., 2022).

### *5.1.2. Lyme Disease*

Lyme disease, caused by spirochete *Borrelia burgdorferi*, is the most common vector-borne disease in the United States. The clinical presentation varies depending on the stage of the illness and includes erythema migrans, carditis, central nervous system disease, and arthritis. Regardless of the clinical presentation, most patients with Lyme disease have resolution of their clinical symptoms when treated with appropriate antimicrobials. Persistent symptoms after therapy are most often due to misdiagnosis rather than treatment failure. Although Lyme disease is a public health concern, extensive publicity has resulted in a degree of anxiety about Lyme disease that is out of proportion to the actual morbidity that it causes (Steere, 2001).

### *5.1.3. Dengue Fever*

Dengue, caused by the dengue virus (DENV), is one of the most important re-emerging arboviral diseases in the tropical and subtropical regions of the world, including Southeast Asia. The virus is transmitted between humans primarily by the mosquitoes *Aedes aegypti*, and *A. albopictus* being a secondary vector (Sim et al., 2019). The disease is endemic in more than 100 countries, with more than 2.5 billion people at risk. There are an estimated 390 million DENV infections annually, of which 96 million are symptomatic, ranging from mild dengue fever, with or without warning signs, to severe dengue with plasma leakage that may lead to shock, bleeding, and/or organ impairment (Limkittikul et al., 2018). Increasing numbers of dengue cases, and the propagation of all four serotypes of DENV, are facilitated by uncontrolled urbanization, suboptimal management of water and solid waste, gaps in vector control, and rapid population movement, especially travel (WHO, 2009).

### *5.1.4. Chagas Disease*

Chagas disease, is one of the 17 neglected tropical diseases, which have persisted in the poorest, most marginalized societies. It is estimated that close to 6–8 million people worldwide are infected with *Trypanosoma cruzi* and that

65–100 million people are at risk of becoming infected (Kowalska et al., 2011). The majority are in Latin America, where the disease represents a major problem concerning the morbidity and mortality of the general population, and has become a burden that depletes the region's economic resources and affects the social and occupational environment of those suffering from it. International migration has led to the influx of infected subjects from Latin America to the rest of the world, thus rendering the disease a problem for health systems on a global scale (Haberland et al., 2013).

### *5.1.5. Scabies*

Scabies is a contagious skin infestation by the human itch mite (*Sarcoptes scabiei* var. *hominis*) that affects an estimated 300 million people around the world every year. While scabies can affect people at all socioeconomic levels, individuals who are young, elderly, immune-compromised, or developmentally delayed are at significantly higher risk for scabies and related complications. Community-wide and institutional outbreaks have occurred in childcare settings, long-term care facilities, and prisons. Because scabies are associated with poverty, overcrowding, malnutrition, and reduced access to health care, some indigenous and resource-poor communities are disproportionately impacted (Fuller, 2013).

### *5.1.6. Pediculosis*

Pediculosis (louse infestation) affects hundreds of millions of people worldwide each year and has been reported in all countries and within all socioeconomic classes. Lice are obligate, parasitic insects that have no free-living stage in their life cycle. They are transmitted by direct skin-to-skin or fomite-to-skin contact, and symptoms do not typically present for 3 to 4 weeks. The three varieties that are parasitic to humans are *Pediculus humanus capitis* (head louse), *Pthirus pubis* (pubic or crab louse), and *Pediculus humanus* (body louse). Head lice are the most common lice that cross all socioeconomic barriers, whereas body lice more commonly affect homeless and displaced populations and should be suspected in these groups when there are signs of scratching, poor hygiene, and in the colder months of the year (Bonilla et al., 2013).

## 5.2. Prevention and Control Measures of Arthropods Borne Diseases

The prevention and control of arthropod diseases combines tactics aimed at disease vectors, pathogens, and hosts. The recommended treatment of an arthropod disease depends upon the specific disease. Treatment often involves a course of antibiotics and, in some cases; a vaccine may be available for the specific disease. However, prevention measures are similar for all arthropod diseases. The most effective prevention method is to avoid being bitten by the arthropod vector in the first place. This can be achieved by wearing clothing that covers bare skin, using repellants to deter insects, avoiding outdoor activities at times when the arthropods are most active, and sleeping under mosquito netting (Sutherst, 2007). Travelers may want to avoid visiting tropical countries where certain arthropod-borne diseases are common, and anyone traveling to countries where these diseases are endemic certainly should take precautions to prevent being bitten. Vaccinations exist for some of these diseases to prevent the development of the disease if transmission occurs (Arlian, 2007). However, vaccinations are not available for all arthropod-borne diseases, and everyone does not have access to those vaccines that do exist. For mechanically transmitted infections, prevention measures include excluding insects from areas where food is prepared and served, washing or thoroughly cooking any food that may have come into contact with an arthropod, and avoiding water bodies inhabited by arthropods. If these precautions are taken, ingestion or absorption of possible pathogens is unlikely (Miglianico et al., 2018).

## 6. Parasitic Fungi, Pathogenicity and Control Measures

A fungus (Plural: Fungi) is a eukaryotic organism with a distinct separate kingdom (domain Eukarya) and is divided into three distinct groups i.e., molds, yeasts, and mushrooms. While some fungi are free-living in soil or water, others form parasitic or symbiotic associations with plants or animals. Fungi are indeed eukaryotic microorganisms that can exist in different forms such as yeasts or molds. Yeasts are single-celled fungi that reproduce through a process called budding, where a small bud grows off the parent cell and eventually detaches to become a new independent cell (Euker et al., 2001). On the other hand, molds are composed of long filaments called hyphae, which can grow by extending at their tips. Hyphae can be either sparsely septate (having few or no cross-walls) or regularly septate (divided into distinct segments by cross-walls), and they may contain multiple nuclei.

Fungi exhibit heterotrophic nutrition, meaning they obtain their nutrients by consuming organic matter from their environment. Unlike plants, which perform photosynthesis to produce their food, fungi lack chlorophyll and cannot generate energy from sunlight. Instead, fungi secrete hydrolytic enzymes into their surroundings, breaking down complex organic compounds into smaller molecules that can be absorbed by the fungus (Bartnicki, 1968). This external digestion allows fungi to obtain nutrients from a wide range of organic materials, including dead plants, animals, and other organic substances. In addition to their ecological roles as decomposers and recyclers in nature, some fungi can also cause various types of diseases in humans.

## 6.1. Common Pathogenic Fungal Species

Parasitic fungi are a group of fungi that can infect humans and cause a variety of diseases, known as fungal infections or mycoses. Fungi can cause a wide range of diseases in humans, collectively known as fungal infections or mycoses. These diseases can be superficial, affecting the skin or mucous membranes, or they can be deeper and systemic, affecting internal organs (Baron, 1996). These infections can affect various parts of the body and present with diverse clinical manifestations.

Fungal infections can also be allergic, triggering immune responses in individuals with specific sensitivities to fungal allergens. Four fungal species *Aspergillus, Mucor*, *Cryptococcus,* and *Candida* infect the human body, resulting in endangering diseased conditions namely aspergillosis, mucormycosis, cryptococcosis, and candidiasis, respectively. Numerous varieties of pathogenic fungi can make people sick.

### *6.1.1. Candida Species*

The human microbiome is frequently populated with fungi that resemble yeast and belong to the genus *Candida.* They can, however, overgrow in specific circumstances and result in diseases including oral thrush, vaginal yeast infections, and invasive candidiasis in those with impaired immune systems (Calderone and Clancy, 2011).

### *6.1.2. Aspergillus Species*

*Aspergillus* is a family of molds that can cause a variety of respiratory illnesses, including invasive aspergillosis and allergic bronchopulmonary aspergillosis (ABPA), which typically affects those with weaker immune systems (Bodey, 1989).

#### *6.1.3. Cryptococcus neoformans*

*Cryptococcus neoformans* is the fungus that causes cryptococcosis, a fungal infection that typically affects people with weakened immune systems, such as those with HIV/AIDS. It often affects the lungs, but it can potentially extend to the brain and spinal cord (Casadevall and Perfect, 1998).

#### *6.1.4. Histoplasma capsulatum*

A dimorphic fungus, *Histoplasma* is responsible for histoplasmosis, a respiratory ailment spread by inhaling fungal spores found in soil tainted with bird or bat droppings. Although it can spread to other organs, the lungs are its primary site of damage (Antinori, 2014).

#### *6.1.5. Coccidioides Species*

*Coccidioides* fungi are the source of coccidioidomycosis or Valley fever. Specific geographic areas, such as the southwestern United States, have soil that contains fungus spores that can be inhaled to contract this condition. When it's bad, it might spread to other organs and exhibit flu-like symptoms (Taylor and Barker, 2019).

#### *6.1.6. Dermatophytes*

A group of fungi known as dermatophytes cause diseases like ringworm (*Tinea corporis*), athlete's foot (*Tinea pedis*), and nail fungus (onychomycosis), which affect the skin, hair, and nails (Al-Janabi, 2014).

### 6.2. Fungal Infection and Treatment

These are only a few instances of pathogenic fungi that can harm humans and make them sick. It's crucial to remember that the type of fungus involved, the person's immune system and other factors can greatly affect the severity and presentation of a fungal infection. Effective management of fungal infections depends on a professional's accurate diagnosis and treatment. Depending on the fungus involved and the site of infection, the signs and symptoms of human pathogenic fungal infections might change. Infections caused by fungi frequently exhibit the following symptoms, along with standard treatments below:

#### *6.2.1. Skin Infections*

Itching, redness, rash, scaling, blisters, or raised, circular patches on the skin are the main symptoms. Such infections can be treated using antifungal creams/ointments. Creams with antifungal ingredients like clotrimazole, miconazole, or terbinafine that are available over the counter are successful in treating common fungal infections like ringworm. In some cases, oral antifungal medications may be prescribed for severe or recurrent infections. Some common examples of skin fungal infections in humans include:

##### *6.2.1.1. Superficial Infections*

These affect the outer layers of the skin, hair, and nails. Examples include tinea infections (ringworm), candidiasis (yeast infections), and pityriasis versicolor.

- *Tinea infections (Ringworm):* These are caused by different species of fungi belonging to the genera *Trichophyton, Microsporum*, and *Epidermophyton*. They result in skin lesions with a characteristic ring-shaped appearance, such as *Tinea corporis* (body), *Tinea pedis* (foot or athlete's foot), *Tinea cruris* (groin or jock itch), and *Tinea capitis* (scalp).
- *Candidiasis:* Caused by the yeast *Candida*, candidiasis can affect various mucosal surfaces, such as the mouth (oral thrush), genitals (vaginal yeast infection), and skin folds. It can also lead to invasive candidiasis in immunocompromised individuals, potentially affecting multiple organs.
- *Pityriasis versicolor:* This fungal infection, caused by *Malassezia* species, presents as patches of discolored skin, often on the chest, back, and arms.

##### *6.2.1.2. Cutaneous Infections*

These involve the deeper layers of the skin and can cause conditions such as dermatophytosis (deep fungal skin infection), sporotrichosis, and chromoblastomycosis.

- *Dermatophytosis:* Also known as ringworm, dermatophyte fungi invade the skin, hair, and nails, causing conditions like *Tinea corporis, T. pedis*, and *T. capitis*.
- *Sporotrichosis:* This chronic fungal infection, caused by the fungus *Sporothrix schenckii*, usually affects the skin and subcutaneous tissues, resulting in nodular lesions along the lymphatic channels.
- *Chromoblastomycosis:* Caused by several different fungi, chromoblastomycosis leads to slowly progressive skin lesions characterized by raised and wart-like nodules.

##### *6.2.1.3. Subcutaneous Infections*

These infections occur beneath the skin and can involve deeper tissues. Examples include mycetoma and subcutaneous zygomycosis.

#### ***6.2.2. Vaginal Yeast Infections***

Itching, burning sensation, abnormal vaginal discharge (thick, white, cottage-cheese-like), and redness or swelling of the vulva are the main symptoms. These infections can be treated by over-the-counter antifungal creams, suppositories, or oral medications that can be used to treat vaginal yeast infections. However, recurrent or severe cases may require prescription-strength antifungal medications. The doctors could advise oral antifungal drugs like fluconazole in cases of more severe or recurrent yeast infections.

#### ***6.2.3. Oral Infections***

Creamy white lesions on the tongue, inner cheeks, or roof of the mouth are the main symptoms which may be painful or bleed when scraped. These infections can be treated by antifungal mouthwashes, lozenges, or oral medications commonly prescribed to treat oral thrush. Good oral hygiene practices are also important. These are prescription pills that include antifungal medications like fluconazole and clotrimazole. Until symptoms subside, the lozenges are slowly dissolved in the mouth numerous times each day.

#### ***6.2.4. Respiratory Infections***

Persistent cough, shortness of breath, chest pain, fever, and fatigue are the main symptoms of respiratory fungal infections. These infections can be treated using antifungal medications, typically taken orally, are used to treat respiratory fungal infections. Severe cases may require hospitalization and intravenous antifungal therapy. Azoles: Fungal respiratory infections are frequently treated with azole antifungal drugs such as fluconazole, itraconazole, voriconazole, or posaconazole. Amphotericin B: For severe or systemic fungal infections, Amphotericin B is a broad-spectrum antifungal drug. Echinocandins: Some types of fungal infections are treated using echinocandin antifungal drugs, such as caspofungin, micafungin, or anidulafungin.

### *6.2.5. Systemic Infections*

These are more severe and can affect multiple organs and systems, including the bloodstream, lungs, central nervous system, and internal organs. Examples include aspergillosis, cryptococcosis, candidemia, and invasive mucormycosis. Fever, chills, headache, fatigue, muscle aches, joint pain, and organ-specific symptoms depending on the site of infection are the main symptoms. Parasitic fungi can cause localized or systemic infections in humans. Systemic fungal infections are often severe and require aggressive treatment with long courses of antifungal medications, usually administered intravenously. The nature and severity of the disease depend on various factors, including the virulence of the fungus, the immune status of the host, and the site of infection. Hospitalization and close monitoring may be necessary. The same common examples of systemic fungal infections include:

- *Aspergillosis:* It is caused by *Aspergillus* species, this infection can manifest as allergic bronchopulmonary aspergillosis (ABPA) or invasive aspergillosis, which primarily affects individuals with weakened immune systems.
- *Cryptococcosis:* This infection, caused by *Cryptococcus neoformans* or *Cryptococcus gattii*, primarily affects the lungs and can spread to the central nervous system, causing meningitis.
- *Histoplasmosis:* It is caused by the fungus *Histoplasma capsulatum*. The histoplasmosis is primarily a respiratory infection but can disseminate to other organs, particularly in immunocompromised individuals.
- *Coccidioidomycosis:* Commonly known as Valley fever, coccidioidomycosis is caused by the fungus *Coccidioides immitis* or *Coccidioides posadasii*, and primarily affects the lungs but can disseminate to other organs.

### *6.2.6. Opportunistic Infections*

These infections typically occur in individuals with weakened immune systems, such as those with HIV/AIDS, organ transplant recipients, or individuals on immunosuppressive therapy. Opportunistic fungal infections include invasive candidiasis, aspergillosis, cryptococcosis, and pneumocystis pneumonia. In immunocompromised individuals, candidiasis can be invasive, affecting the bloodstream, vital organs, and other body systems.

### *6.2.7. Mucormycosis*

Following aspergillosis and candidiasis, mucormycosis is the third most aggressive fungal illness (Eucker et al., 2001). *Mucor*, a member of the Mucorales order of fungi, is the source of mucormycosis or black fungus infection (Gandra et al., 2021). About 250 species and 150 genera make up the Mucorales order. They are saprophytic species that thrive on decaying organic matter, and only a few of them are parasitic. Because they produce black spores, these fungi are frequently referred to as "black molds." The aseptate mycelium is highly branched. Currently, mucormycosis is a pandemic that has spread widely over India and is harmful to people. There are several types of mucormycosis are known including (i) *Rhinocerebral mucormycosis, (ii) Disseminated mucormycosis, (iii) Pulmonary mucormycosis, (iv) Cutaneous mucormycosis, (v) Gastrointestinal mucormycosis (*Bhandari et al., 2021). For the treatment of mucormycosis, Liposomal Amphotericin B is given in doses of (2-4 mg kg-1 d-1) as a monotherapy for the treatment regime (Guo et al., 2019). Finally, flucytosine is a fluorinated, cytosine-5 analog (5-FC). Of all these drugs, the gold standard $1^{st}$ line antimycotics against mucormycosis are amphotericin B and with a high dose of intravenous isavuconazole delayed-release tablet and posaconazole de-escalation maintainers, therapy is generally in use against mucormycosis.

## 6.3. Control Measures of Fungal Infections

Controlling parasitic fungal infections involves several approaches.

### *6.3.1. Antifungal Medications*

Treatment typically involves the use of antifungal medications, which can be administered topically, orally, or intravenously depending on the severity and location of the infection. The choice of antifungal drug depends on the specific fungus causing the infection.

### *6.3.2. Prevention and Hygiene*

Practicing good hygiene is important in preventing fungal infections. This includes regular handwashing, keeping the skin clean and dry, avoiding sharing personal items, and maintaining proper sanitation in healthcare settings.

### *6.3.3. Environmental Control*

Some fungal infections are acquired through exposure to fungal spores present in the environment. For example, respiratory fungal infections can be prevented by reducing exposure to contaminated soil, dust, or bird droppings. In specific settings like hospitals or immunocompromised patient care units, strict infection control measures and air filtration systems may be implemented.

### *6.3.4. Immunization*

Vaccines are available for some fungal infections, such as the pneumococcal vaccine, which can help prevent certain invasive fungal infections in susceptible individuals.

### *6.3.5. Education and Awareness*

Increasing awareness about fungal infections, their risk factors, and preventive measures is essential. This includes educating healthcare professionals, individuals with compromised immune systems, and the general public about the importance of early diagnosis and treatment.

It's worth noting that the specific control measures may vary depending on the type of fungal infection, the mode of transmission, and the individual's risk factors. Therefore, it is crucial to consult healthcare professionals for accurate diagnosis, appropriate treatment, and guidance on prevention and control strategies tailored to the specific fungal infection and individual circumstances. Overall, controlling parasitic fungal infections in humans requires a multidimensional approach involving medical interventions, hygiene practices, environmental management, and education to minimize the impact of invasive fungal infections.

## 7. Emerging Parasites-Based Challenges for Health and Sustainability

Emerging parasites-based challenges present significant threats to both human health and the sustainability of ecosystems. These challenges arise from the emergence of new parasitic species, changes in parasite distribution and behavior, the development of drug resistance, and environmental factors that facilitate the spread of parasites. This section discusses some key emerging challenges in the context of health and sustainability.

### 7.1. Emerging Infectious Diseases

New parasitic diseases are continuously being discovered, posing challenges for healthcare systems and public health. For instance, the emergence of novel coronaviruses, such as SARS-CoV-2, has highlighted the potential for zoonotic spillover events, where parasites or pathogens transfer from animals to humans. Other examples include the re-emergence of neglected tropical diseases like Chagas disease, leishmaniasis, and dengue fever in previously unaffected regions.

### 7.2. Climate Change and Parasite Distribution

Climate change alters temperature and precipitation patterns, affecting the geographic distribution and transmission dynamics of parasites. Rising temperatures can expand the ranges of disease vectors, such as mosquitoes and ticks, facilitating the spread of diseases like malaria, dengue fever, and Lyme disease to new areas. Changes in rainfall patterns can also influence parasite life cycles and increase the risk of waterborne diseases.

### 7.3. Drug Resistance

The emergence and spread of drug-resistant parasites pose a significant challenge to effective treatment and control strategies. Overuse and misuse of antiparasitic drugs in humans, livestock, and agriculture have contributed to the development of resistance. Parasites such as *Plasmodium* (malaria),

*Trypanosoma* (sleeping sickness), and helminths (worms) have shown resistance to multiple drugs, limiting treatment options and increasing the burden of disease.

### 7.4. Vector-Borne Diseases

Parasitic diseases transmitted by vectors, such as mosquitoes, ticks, and sandflies, continue to be a major concern. The expansion of vector habitats, facilitated by factors like deforestation and urbanization, increases the potential for disease transmission. Vector-borne diseases like malaria, Zika virus, and Lyme disease have experienced outbreaks and geographical expansion, posing significant challenges for disease control and prevention.

### 7.5. One Health Approach

The interconnectedness of human, animal, and environmental health is crucial in addressing emerging parasite-based challenges. The One Health approach recognizes the interdependence of these domains and emphasizes collaborative efforts between disciplines to combat parasitic diseases. It involves integrating surveillance, research, and control strategies across human and veterinary medicine, ecology, and environmental sciences to achieve comprehensive and sustainable solutions.

## 8. Advances in Disease Therapeutic Strategies

### 8.1. Conventional or Traditional Medicine System

Millions of individuals worldwide are afflicted with parasitic infections, which significantly increase morbidity and mortality. Treatment for parasite infections has come a long way in both conventional medicine and traditional medicine systems. Traditional medical systems make use of herbal medicines and local knowledge, while Western medicine depends on synthetic pharmaceuticals and contemporary technology (Serban, 2019). This article examines the therapeutic developments in these two healthcare systems for the treatment of parasitic illnesses. The creation of antiparasitic medications has advanced significantly in conventional medicine. One of the worst parasite diseases, malaria, was treated in a completely new way after the discovery of artemisinin and its derivatives. As the go-to medication for treating uncomplicated malaria, artemisinin-based combination treatments (ACTs) have significantly decreased the number of people dying from malaria worldwide (Su and Miller, 2015).

Conventional medicine has created efficient medications for diseases caused by various parasites in addition to malaria. For instance, the treatment of intestinal helminth infections like hookworm, roundworm, and whipworm is frequently carried out using albendazole and mebendazole. Lymphatic filariasis and onchocerciasis, two parasite illnesses, have both been successfully treated with ivermectin (Chai et al., 2021). The accuracy and speed of diagnosing parasite diseases have also increased because to developments in molecular diagnostics. Next-generation sequencing (NGS) and polymerase chain reaction (PCR) methods, for example, allow for the highly sensitive and specific identification of parasites. This makes early detection, suitable therapy, and treatment outcome monitoring easier (Liu et al., 2023).

Plant-based treatments for parasite infections have a long history in traditional medical systems that are strongly anchored in indigenous cultures. The development of antiparasitic treatments has benefited greatly from these systems. Numerous plants have been used to treat various parasite illnesses because they naturally have antiparasitic qualities (Yuan et al., 2016). For instance, quinine, which is powerful against *Plasmodium* parasites, is present in the bark of the cinchona tree, which is a traditional treatment for malaria. Other healing herbs, like neem, garlic, and *Artemisia annua*, have shown antiparasitic effects against various parasites. For their antiparasitic effects, traditional medical systems also use additional natural compounds (Odugbemi et al., 2006). Propolis and royal jelly, for instance, are bee products that have demonstrated potential against specific parasites. In addition, conventional techniques like moxibustion, acupuncture, and herbal baths have been used to assist the body's natural defense mechanisms and relieve symptoms (Olas, 2022).

An effort has been made to combine traditional and mainstream medical systems because of their potential advantages. To provide comprehensive and all-encompassing care, integrative medicine blends evidence-based procedures from the two systems. Promising findings have come from collaborative studies between practitioners of conventional medicine. Studies, for instance, have looked at the synergistic effects of mixing standard antiparasitic medications with conventional herbal therapies. This comprehensive strategy might improve therapeutic effectiveness, lower medication resistance, and lessen negative effects. Additionally, conventional medical practices offer a wealth of drug discovery prospects (Yuan et al., 2016). Many naturally occurring substances originating from medicinal plants have been used as models for the creation of traditional antiparasitic medications. Scientists can find new therapeutic targets and create cutting-edge treatment plans by combining knowledge from traditional medicine. Both conventional and traditional medical systems have made therapeutic improvements for parasite infections. In the creation of molecular diagnostics and antiparasitic medications, conventional medicine has achieved considerable strides. The management and treatment of parasitic infections have also benefited from the use of traditional medical systems, which are based on old knowledge and natural therapies. These two approaches could be combined with tremendous success (Yuan et al., 2016; Jayawardene et al., 2021).

### 8.2. Integrated Medicine System

Millions of people are still affected by parasitic infections, which continue to pose serious health issues on a global scale. An all-encompassing strategy for the therapy of parasite disorders is provided by integrative medicine, which blends the fundamental ideas and therapeutic modalities of several medical systems. This article examines the therapeutic advancements made possible by the fusion of homeopathy and allopathy, two well-known medical systems, in the management of parasite infections. Both allopathy and homeopathy are separate medical systems with unique methods of therapy. Based on the idea that "like cures like," homeopathy uses incredibly diluted medicines to encourage the body's natural healing processes. Conventional medicine, or allopathy, relies on using medications and other treatments to specifically target ailments (Ung et al., 2021).

Homeopathy and allopathy work together in an integrated medical system to provide comprehensive care. To improve treatment outcomes, homeopathic medicines can be taken in addition to prescription medications. By incorporating the best elements of both systems, this integration recognizes the advantages of each system and seeks to improve patient care. There have been substantial improvements in the treatment of parasitic infections as a result of the fusion of homeopathy and allopathy. The symptoms of parasitic diseases can be relieved and the immune system can be strengthened with the use of homeopathic treatments (Bellavite, 2015). These natural treatments are chosen based on the principle of customized treatment, taking into account each patient's distinct symptoms and constitution. Allopathic medications are essential for immediately attacking and getting rid of parasites from the body. Antiparasitic medications created through allopathic research and developments have been successful in treating a variety of parasites. For instance, drugs like artemisinin-based combination treatments (ACTs) have considerably decreased the mortality rates related to the parasite disease malaria (Yuan et al., 2016; Campbell and Soman-Faulkner, 2023).

Homeopathy and allopathy can be used to create individualized treatment plans that address the unique requirements of each patient. Homeopathic remedies can be used to strengthen the body's innate defenses, lessen the negative effects of prescription medications, and enhance general health. On the other hand, allopathic medicines specifically target the parasites to ensure efficient treatment and elimination. Homeopathy and allopathy have worked together to conduct research and advance the treatment of parasite disorders (Bellavite, 2015). The effectiveness and safety of mixing homeopathic remedies with traditional antiparasitic medications have been investigated in integrated clinical trials and investigations. These investigations seek to recognize synergistic effects and choose the most potent therapy combinations for particular parasite infections (Kleijnen et al., 1991).

Collaboration has also produced procedures and guidelines for combining homeopathy with allopathy in the treatment of parasitic infections. These recommendations make sure that the integration is supported by data and complies with both medical systems' guiding principles. They give medical professionals a framework for offering interdisciplinary care while preserving patient security and enhancing therapeutic results. Incorporating both allopathy and homeopathy into the management of parasitic infections gives a patient-centered strategy that takes into accounts each person's particular requirements and preferences (Mathie, 2003; Ghosh et al., 2014). By addressing both the patient's general well-being and the parasite illness, this integrated strategy offers holistic care. Healthcare professionals can give comprehensive treatment regimens that boost the body's innate healing processes while specifically targeting and getting rid of parasites by utilizing the strengths of both medical systems. Significant therapeutic improvements have resulted from the combination of homeopathy and allopathy in the treatment of parasitic infections. The personalized approach of homeopathy and the focused care of allopathy are combined in this integrated medical strategy (Jasemi et al., 2017; Chaughule and Barve, 2023).

### 8.3. Targeted Drug Delivery and Nanotherapeutics

Global health continues to be severely hampered by parasitic infections, demanding the creation of novel therapeutic strategies. Nanotherapeutics and targeted drug delivery have shown promise in the fight against parasitic illnesses. To tackle parasite infections, this article examines the therapeutic advancements made possible by the use of tailored drug delivery systems and nanotherapeutics (Singh et al., 2017). Targeted drug delivery systems are made to deliver drugs directly to the infection site, improving treatment effectiveness and reducing side effects. These systems have various benefits when it comes to parasite illnesses. They can increase drug concentration at the target site, boost drug stability, and increase medication bioavailability (Wen et al., 2015).

Antiparasitic medications have shown potential when delivered via nano-sized carriers such as liposomes, nanoparticles, and micelles to infected tissues or cells. These vehicles can enclose and safeguard the medication, allowing for a regulated release and extended circulation in the body. Additionally, the carriers' modified surfaces may enable particular interactions with parasite surfaces or infected cells, facilitating tailored medication administration (Sun et al., 2019). For instance, ligands that particularly bind to receptors on the surface of *Plasmodium* parasites can be added to liposomes or nanoparticles to treat malaria. This permits the targeted delivery of antimalarial medications to the parasites themselves, enhancing treatment effectiveness while lowering systemic toxicity (Anamika et al., 2020; Memvanga and Nkanga, 2021).

The term "nanotherapeutics" describes the use of nanoparticles as therapeutic agents to treat disease. Nanoparticles have special qualities that are appropriate for battling parasitic diseases, such as their small size, vast surface area, and customizable surface features. Nanotherapeutics has several benefits in the parasitology sector. They can enhance the solubility, stability, and bioavailability of drugs, enabling better medication delivery to parasites. Additionally, certain characteristics of nanoparticles can be modified to help them target and absorb parasites (Rudramurthy et al., 2016). Some nanoparticles naturally destroy parasites or prevent their proliferation by having antiparasitic properties. For instance, broad-spectrum antiparasitic activities of silver nanoparticles against a variety of parasites, such as protozoa and helminths, have been demonstrated. To increase treatment effectiveness, other nanoparticles, such as polymer-based nanocarriers, can be loaded with antiparasitic medications and released just at the infection site (Yin et al., 2020).

Additionally, nanotherapeutics can get past biological obstacles that prevent conventional drug delivery techniques from working. For instance, the blood-brain barrier may prevent medications from reaching parasites that infect the central nervous system. This barrier can be overcome by nanoparticles, allowing for the successful treatment of many difficult parasite infections (Teleanu et al., 2018). Although targeted medication delivery and nanotherapeutics show enormous potential, there are still a number of obstacles to overcome. Nanotherapeutics is susceptible to developing drug resistance, a problem that is particularly problematic in parasite diseases. Therefore, to combat resistance mechanisms, research must concentrate on creating novel drug delivery technologies and combination therapies (Patel et al., 2021). Additionally, a detailed investigation of nanotherapeutics' safety profile is required. Complex interactions between nanoparticles and biological systems have the potential to trigger toxicity or immunological reactions. Therefore, to ensure their safety and effectiveness, thorough preclinical and clinical investigations are required (Desai, 2012).

Future research in this area will focus on creating multifunctional nanosystems that can administer numerous medications or combination therapy. Nanotechnology advancements can also make it easier to create stimuli-responsive drug delivery systems, permitting regulated medication release that is triggered by particular circumstances at the infection site (Patra et al., 2018). Nanotherapeutics and targeted drug delivery systems are promising therapeutic developments for the treatment of parasitic infections. These methods improve treatment efficacy, increase drug distribution to the desired spot, and reduce side effects (Sethi et al., 2022).

## Conclusion

In conclusion, parasites and parasitism pose significant challenges to human health and ecosystem sustainability. However, through continuous research and collaborative efforts, modern therapeutic strategies have emerged to tackle these challenges effectively. The development of new drugs, advancements in diagnostic techniques, and the integration of multidisciplinary approaches provide hope for the prevention, control, and potential eradication of parasitic diseases. By addressing these challenges, we can strive towards a healthier and more sustainable future for individuals and ecosystems alike.

Finally, it should be noted that the medical sector has seen the cohabitation and development of numerous systems, including conventional or traditional medicine, integrated medicine (more particularly, homeopathy and allopathy), and targeted drug delivery with nanotherapeutics. These systems each provide distinctive viewpoints, methods, and healthcare strategies. Traditional or conventional medicine is still commonly practiced today, especially in areas where it has a rich historical background and is based on centuries-old cultural customs and empirical knowledge. It places a strong emphasis on natural cures, holistic treatment, and patient care that is tailored to each individual. Utilizing homeopathy and allopathy, integrated medicine aims to maximize each system's advantages. Allopathy relies on evidence-based medicine, diagnostic tools, and pharmacological interventions, whereas homeopathy focuses on treating patients with greatly diluted chemicals that encourage the body's self-healing capabilities. This integrative method offers patients a wider variety of therapeutic alternatives and promotes a more thorough comprehension of both health and sickness.

Nanotherapeutics and targeted drug delivery are revolutionary developments in contemporary medicine. Scientists can create medication delivery systems that specifically target sick cells or tissues using nanotechnology, increasing the effectiveness of treatment while reducing unwanted effects. With potential applications in the treatment of cancer, chronic illnesses, and regenerative medicine, this strategy holds considerable promise for the future of medicine. It is crucial to understand the benefits and drawbacks of each system and to promote cooperation between them in the context of a healthcare system that is continually changing. Traditional medicine, integrated medicine, targeted medication delivery, and nanotherapeutics can all be combined to provide more efficient, individualized healthcare solutions that ultimately improve patient outcomes and well-being. To guarantee that people throughout the world receive the greatest treatment possible as research and technological development proceed, it is essential to maintain an open-minded and evidence-based approach.

## References

Adam, R. D. (2001). Biology of *Giardia lamblia. Clinical Microbiology Reviews,* 14(3), 447-475.

Al-Janabi, A. A. (2014). Dermatophytosis: Causes, clinical features, signs and treatment. *Journal of Symptoms Signs*, 3(3), 200-203.

Anamika, J., Nikhar, V., Laxmikant, G., Priya, S., Sonal, V. & Vyas, S. P. (2020). Nanobiotechnological modules as molecular target tracker for the treatment and prevention of malaria: Options and opportunity. *Drug Delivery and Translational Research*, 10(4), 1095–1110.

Andrews, K. T., Fisher, G. & Skinner-Adams, T. S. (2014). Drug repurposing and human parasitic protozoan diseases. *International Journal for Parasitology: Drugs and Drug Resistance,* 4(2), 95-111.

Antinori, S. (2014). *Histoplasma capsulatum*: More widespread than previously thought. *The American Journal of Tropical Medicine and Hygiene*, 90(6), 982.

Arlian, L. G. (2007). Arthropod allergens and human health. *Annual Review of Entomology*, 47(1), 395-433.

Arroyo, R., Gonzalez-Robles, A., Martinez-Palomo, A. & Alderete, J. F. (1993). Signalling of *Trichomonas vaginalis* for amoeboid transformation and adhesion synthesis follows cytoadherence. *Molecular Microbiology*, 7, 299–309.

Arsenopoulos, K. V., Fthenakis, G. C., Katsarou, E. I. & Papadopoulos, E. (2021). Haemonchosis: A challenging parasitic infection of sheep and goats. *Animals*, 11(2), 363.

Babita, Panwar, P. & Upadhyay, S. K. (2019). A review on ecosegregation and parasitocoenosis of helminthes: Perspective to health and sustainability. *Bulletin of Pure and Applied Sciences– Zoology,* 38A(1), 40–51.

Babita, Upadhyay, S. K., Tuli, H. S., Dhama, K., Chandran, D., Mohapatra, R. K. & Singh, M. (2022). Morphotaxometry and ultratopography of *Lytocestus haryanii* n.sp. (Caryophyllidea: Lytocestidae) from the intestine of freshwater catfish *Clarias batrachus* Linnaeus 1758 (Siluriformes: Clariidae) of river Yamuna, Yamuna Nagar, Haryana, India. *Journal of Experimental Biology and Agricultural Sciences*, 13(3), 554–566.

Bahadur, A. (2022). Nematodes diseases of fruits and vegetables crops in India. *Intech Open*, 98850. https://doi.org/10.5772/intechopen.

Bahk, Y. Y., Shin, E. H., Cho, S. H., Ju, J. W., Chai, J. Y. & Kim, T. S. (2018). Prevention and control strategies for parasitic infections in the Korea Centers for Disease Control and Prevention. *Korean Journal of Parasitology*, 56(5), 401-408.

Baron, S. (1996). *Medical Microbiology* 4th edition. Medical Branch, University of Texas, Galveston (TX).

Bartnicki-Garcia, S. (1968). Cell wall chemistry, morphogenesis, and taxonomy of fungi. *Annual Reviews in Microbiology*, 22(1), 87-108.

Barwick, R. S., Levy, D. A., Braun, G. F., Beach, M. J. & Calderon, R. L. (2000). Surveillance for water-borne disease outbreaks—United States, 1997–1998. *Morbidity and Mortality Weekly Report Series, Centers for Disease Control and Prevention Surveillance Summaries,* 49(SS-4), 1–36.

Bellavite, P. (2015). Homeopathy and integrative medicine: Keeping an open mind. *Journal of Medicine and the Person*, 13(1), 1–6.

Bernard, G. C., Egnin, M. & Bonsi, C. (2017). The impact of plant-parasitic nematodes on agriculture and methods of control. *Intech Open*, 68958. https://doi.org/10.5772/intechopen.

Bhandari, J., Thada, P. K. & Nagalli, S. (2021). *Rhinocerebral mucormycosis*. In: StatPearls Publishing, Treasure Island (FL), https://www.ncbi.nlm.nih.gov/books/NBK559288.

Bhat, A. H., Chaubey, A. K. & Upadhyay, S. K. (2016). Morphotaxometric and molecular validation of entomopathogenic nematode, *Steinernema abbasi* (Rhabditida: Steinernematidae) with mucronate processes in adults of second generations off subhumid region, Uttar Pradesh, India. *World Journal of Pharmacy and Pharmaceutical Sciences,* 5(3), 1558-1579.

Bitam, I., Dittmar, K., Parola, P., Whiting, M. F. & Raoult, D. (2010). Fleas and flea-borne diseases. *International Journal of Infectious Diseases*, 14(8), e667-e676.

Bodey, G. P. & Vartivarian, S. (1989). Aspergillosis. *The European Journal of Clinical Microbiology and Infectious Diseases,* 8, 413-437.

Bogitsh, B. J., Carter, C. E. & Oeltmann, T. N. (2019). *Human parasitology*. Academic Press.

Bonilla, D. L., Durden, L. A., Eremeeva, M. E. & Dasch, G. A. (2013). The Biology and Taxonomy of Head and Body Lice- Implications for Louse-Borne Disease Prevention. *PLoS Pathogens*, 9(11), e1003724.

Brodsky, R. E., Spencer, H. C. & Jr Schultz, M. G. (1974). Giardiasis in American travelers to the Soviet Union. *Journal of Infectious Diseases,* 130, 319–323.

Brown, M. T. (1972). Trichomoniasis. *Practitioner,* 209, 639–644.

Calderone, R. A. & Clancy, C. J. (2011) *Candida and candidiasis*. American Society for Microbiology Press.

Campbell, S. & Soman-Faulkner, K. (2023). *Antiparasitic drugs*. In: StatPearls Publishing, Treasure Island (FL), http://www.ncbi.nlm.nih.gov/books/NBK544251/.

Casadevall, A. & Perfect, J.R. (1998). *Cryptococcus neoformans* Volume 595. American Society for Microbiology, Washington, DC.

Catterall, R. D. (1972). Trichomonal infections of the genital tract. *Medical Clinics of North America,* 56, 1203–1209.

CDC (2023a). *Leishmaniasis*. Centers for Disease Control and Prevention, https://www.cdc.gov/parasites/leishmaniasis/index.html. Accessed on 29th May, 2023.

CDC (2023b). *Giardia*. Centers for Disease Control and Prevention, https://www.cdc.gov/parasites/giardia. Accessed on 29th May, 2023.

Chai, J. Y. (2013). Praziquantel treatment in trematode and cestode infections: an update. *Infection and Chemotherapy,* 45(1), 32-43.

Chai, J. Y., Jung, B. K. & Hong, S. J. (2021). Albendazole and mebendazole as anti-parasitic and anti-cancer agents: An update. *The Korean Journal of Parasitology*, 59(3), 189–225.

Chakraborty, S., Gurusamy, M., Zawieja, D. C. & Muthuchamy, M. (2013). Lymphatic filariasis: Perspectives on lymphatic remodeling and contractile dysfunction in filarial disease pathogenesis. *Microcirculation,* 20(5), 349-364.

Chaughule, R. S. & Barve, R. S. (2023). Role of herbal medicines in the treatment of infectious diseases. *Vegetos*, https://doi.org/10.1007/s42535-022-00549-2.

Chauhan, P., Istkhar, & Chaudhary, A. (2023). Entomopathogenic nematodes and their mutualistic bacteria: Enemy of the enemies. In: *Parasitology: Risks and Challenges for Health and Sustainability* (Upadhyay, S.K., ed.). Nova Science Publishers, Inc., USA. pp.115-159.

Cheepsattayakorn, A. & Cheepsattayakorn, R. (2014). Parasitic pneumonia and lung involvement. *BioMed Research International,* 2014, 874021.

Chomicz, L., Conn, D. B., Szaflik, J. P. & Szostakowska, B. (2016). Newly emerging parasitic threats for human health: National and international trends. *BioMed Research International,* 2016, 4283270.

Chou, A. & Austin, R. L. (2023). *Entamoeba histolytica.* In: StatPearls Publishing, Treasure Island (FL), https://www.ncbi.nlm.nih.gov/books/NBK557718/.

Cibulskis, R. E., Alonso, P., Aponte, J., Aregawi, M., Barrette, A., Bergeron, L., Fergus, C. A., Knox, T., Lynch, M., Patouillards, E., Schwarte, S., Stewart, S. & Williams, R. (2016). Malaria: Global progress 2000–2015 and future challenges. *Infectious Diseases of Poverty,* 5, 61. https://doi.org/10.1186/s40249-016-0151-8.

Clapp, J. P., van der Stoel, C. D. & van der Putten, W. H. (2000). Rapid identification of cyst (*Heterodera* spp., *Globodera* spp.) and root-knot (*Meloidogyne* spp.) nematodes on the basis of ITS2 sequence variation detected by PCR-single-strand conformational polymorphism (PCR-SSCP) in cultures and field samples. *Molecular Ecology*, 9(9), 1223–1232.

Clendennen, T. E., Long, G. W. & Baird, K. J. (1995). QBC and Giemsa stained thick blood films: Diagnostic performance of laboratory technologists. *Transactions of the Royal Society of Tropical Medicine and Hygiene,* 89, 183–184.

Conterno, L. O., Turchi, M. D., Corrêa, I. & Monteiro de Barros Almeida, R. A. 92020). Anthelmintic drugs for treating ascariasis. *Cochrane Database Systematic Reviews*, 4(4), CD010599.

Cox, F. E. G., Wakelin, D., Gillespie, S. & Despommier, D. (2007). Parasitology. Volume 6. Topley and Wilson's Microbiology And Microbial Infections. Edward Arnold (Publishers) Ltd., London.

Cross, J. H. (1996a). Filarial nematodes. In: *Medical Microbiology* 4$^{th}$ edition (ed., Baron S.). Medical Branch, University of Texas, Galveston (TX), https://www.ncbi.nlm.nih.gov/books/NBK7844/.

Cross, J. H. (1996b). Enteric nematodes of humans. In: *Medical Microbiology* 4$^{th}$ edition (ed., Baron S.). Medical Branch, University of Texas, Galveston (TX), https://www.ncbi.nlm.nih.gov/books/NBK8261/.

Crump, A. (2017). Ivermectin: Enigmatic multifaceted 'wonder' drug continues to surprise and exceed expectations. *Journal of Antibiotics,* 70, 495–505.

Crutcher, J. M. & Hoffman, S. L. (1996). Malaria. In: *Medical Microbiology* 4th edition (ed., Baron S.). Medical Branch, University of Texas, Galveston (TX), https://www.ncbi.nlm.nih.gov/books/NBK8584/.

Cudmore, S. L., Delgaty, K. L., Hayward-McClelland, S. F., Petrin, D. P. & Garber, G. E. (2004). Treatment of infections caused by metronidazole-resistant *Trichomonas vaginalis*. *Clinical Microbiology Reviews,* 17, 783-793.

Desai, N. (2012). Challenges in development of nanoparticle-based therapeutics. *The American Association of Pharmaceutical Scientists Journal*, 14(2), 282–295.

Dhiman, U., Parihar, R. D., Rana, S., Upadhyay, S. K. & Kumar, V. (2021). Comparative *in silico* analysis of randomly selected heat shock proteins in *Caenorhabditis elegans* and *Photorhabdus temperate. Biointerface Research in Applied Chemistry,* 11(4), 11418-11430.

Dunne, J. A., Lafferty, K. D., Dobson, A. P., Hechinger, R. F., Kuris, A. M., Martinez, N. D., McLaughlin, J. P, Mouritsen, K. N., Poulin, R., Reise, K., Stouffer, D. B., Thieltges, D. W., Williams, R. J. & Zander, C. D. (2013). Parasites affect food web structure primarily through increased diversity and complexity. *PLoS Biology*, 11(6): e1001579.

Ellwanger, J. H. & Cavallero, S. (2023). Soil-transmitted helminth infections from a One Health perspective. *Frontiers in Medicine*, 10, 1167812.

Erickson, S. M., Xi, Z., Mayhew, G. F., Ramirez, J. L., Aliota, M. T., Christensen, B. M. & Dimopoulos, G. (2009). Mosquito infection responses to developing filarial worms. *PLoS Neglected Tropical Diseases,* 3(10): e529.

Eucker, J., Sezer, O., Graf, B. & Possinger, K. (2001). Mucormycoses. *Mycoses*, 44, 253-260.

Farris, V. K. & Honigberg, B. M. (1970). Behaviour and pathogenicity of *Trichomonas vaginalis* Donné in chick liver cells. *Journal of Parasitology*, 56, 849–882.

Flay, K. J., Hill, F. I. & Muguiro, D. H. (2022). A review: *Haemonchus contortus* infection in pasture-based sheep production systems, with a focus on the pathogenesis of anaemia and changes in haematological parameters. *Animals,* 12(10), 1238.

Frank, S., Bradley, L.K. & Moore. K.A. (2022). Integrated pest management. In: *North Carolina Extension Gardener Handbook*, 2nd edition (eds., Moore, K.A. & Bradley, L.K.). NC State Extension, Raleigh, NC, http://content.ces.ncsu.edu/8-integrated-pest-management-ipm.

Fraser, D., Bilenko, N., Deckelbaum, R. J., Dagan, R., El-On, J. & Naggan, L. (2000). *Giardia lamblia* carriage in Israeli Bedouin infants: Risk factors and consequences. *Clinical Infectious Diseases,* 30, 419–424.

Fuller, L. C. (2013). Epidemiology of scabies. *Current Opinion* in *Infectious Diseases,* 26(2), 123-126.

Gandra, S., Ram, S. & Levit, S. M. (2021). The black fungus in India: The emerging syndemic of COVID-19–associated Mucormycosis. *Annals of Internal Medicine*, 174, 1301-1302.

Garber, G. E. (2005). The laboratory diagnosis of *Trichomonas vaginalis*. *The Canadian Journal of Infectious Diseases and Medical Microbiology,* 16(1), 35-38.

Garber, G. E., Proctor, E. M. & Bowie, W. R. (1986). Immunogenic proteins of *Trichomonas vaginalis* as demonstrated by the immunoblot technique. *Infection and Immunity,* 51, 250-253.

George, O. P. (2018). Taxonomy and biology of Steinernematidae and Heterorhabditidae. *Entomopathogenic Nematodes in Biological Control*, 21–62.

Ghodeif, A.O. & Jain, H. (2023). *Hookworm.* In: StatPearls Publishing, Treasure Island (FL), https://www.ncbi.nlm.nih.gov/books/NBK546648/.

Ghosh, S., Saha, S., Koley, M., Kundu, M., Mondal, R. & Patra, S. (2014). Access to and utilization of the health services among the patients in a government homeopathic hospital in West Bengal, India: A cross-sectional study. *Journal of Evidence-Based Complementary & Alternative Medicine*, 19(4), 247–252.

Giari, L., Fano, E. A., Castaldelli, G., Grabner, D. & Sures, B. (2020). The ecological importance of amphipod–parasite associations for aquatic ecosystems. *Water, 12*, 2429.

Guo, S., Liu, H., Tang, X. & Yang, H. (2019). Clinical characteristics and prognoses of pulmonary mucormycosis in four children. *Pediatric Investigation,* 3, 223-227.

Gyasi, M. E., Okonkwo, O. N. & Tripathy, K. (2023). *Onchocerciasis*. In: StatPearls Publishing, Treasure Island (FL), https://www.ncbi.nlm.nih.gov/books/NBK559027/.

Haberland, A., Munoz, S. & Wallukat, G. (2013). Chronic Chagas disease: from basics to laboratory medicine. *Clinical Chemistry and Laboratory Medicine,* 51, 271-294.

Hall, A., Hewitt, G., Tuffrey, V. & de Silva, N. (2008). A review and meta-analysis of the impact of intestinal worms on child growth and nutrition. *Maternal and Child Nutrition,* 4(1) S118-S236.

Hanevik, K., Dizdar, V., Langeland, N. & Hausken, T. (2009). Development of functional gastrointestinal disorders after *Giardia lamblia* infection. *BMC Gastroenterology,* 9(1), 27.

Haque, R., Huston, C.D., Hughes, M., Houpt, E. & Petri, W. A. (2003). Amebiasis. *New England Journal of Medicine*, 348(16), 1565–1573.

Haque, R., Kress, K., Wood, S., Jackson, T. F. G. H., Lyerly, D., Wilkins, T. & Petri, W. A. (1993). Diagnosis of pathogenic *Entamoeba histolytica* infection using a stool ELISA based on monoclonal antibodies to the galactose specific adhesin. *Journal of Infectious Diseases*, 167(1), 247–249.

Hedegaard Clausen, J., Madsen, H., Murrell, K. D., Van, P. T., Thu, H. N., Do, D. T., Nguyen Thi, L. A., Nguyen Manh, H. & Dalsgaard, A. (2012). Prevention and control of fish-borne zoonotic trematodes in fish nurseries, Vietnam. *Emerging Infectious Diseases*, 18(9), 1438-1445.

Hemingway, J., Shretta, R., Wells, T. N., Bell, D., Djimdé, A. A., Achee, N. & Qi, G. (2016). Tools and strategies for malaria control and elimination: What do we need to achieve a grand convergence in malaria? *PLoS Biology*, 14(3), e1002380.

Heyneman, D. (1996). Cestodes. In: *Medical Microbiology* 4th edition (ed., Baron S.). Medical Branch, University of Texas, Galveston (TX), https://www.ncbi.nlm.nih.gov/books/NBK8399/.

Honigberg, B. M. & Brugerolle, G. (1990). *Structure.* In: Trichomonads parasitic in humans (Honigberg, B.M., ed.). Springer-Verlag, New York. pp. 5–35.

Honigberg, B. M. & King, V. M. (1964). Structure of *Trichomonas vaginalis* Donne. *Journal of Parasitology*, 50, 345–364.

Hooshyar, H., Rostamkhani, P., Arbabi, M. & Delavari, M. (2019). *Giardia lamblia* infection: Review of current diagnostic strategies. *Gastroenterology and Hepatology From Bed to Bench,* 12(1), 3-12.

Horiki, N., Furukawa, K., Kitade, T., Sakuno, T., Katsurahara, M., Harada, T., Tano, S., Yamada, R., Hamada, Y., Inoue, H., Tanaka, K., Gabazza, E. C., Ishii, N., Fukuda, K., Omata, F., Fujita, Y., Tachibana, H. & Takei, Y. (2015). Endoscopic findings and lesion distribution in amebic colitis. *Journal of Infection and Chemotherapy*, 21(6), 444–448.

Horwitz, P. & Wilcox, B. A. (2005). Parasites, ecosystems and sustainability: An ecological and complex systems perspective. *International Journal for Parasitology*, 35(7), 725–732.

IARC (1994). Infection with liver flukes (*Opisthorchis viverrini, Opisthorchis felineus* and *Clonorchis sinensis*). IARC Monographs on the evaluation of carcinogenic risks to humans. International Agency for Research on Cancer, 61. https://www.ncbi.nlm.nih.gov/books/NBK487790/.

Incani, R. N., Mughini-Gras, L., Homan, T., Sequera, I., Sequera, L., Serrano, R., Sequera, C., Salas, L., Salazar, M. 7 Santos, P. (2022). Risk of acquiring *Ascaris lumbricoides* infection in an endemically infected rural community in Venezuela. *Epidemiology and Infection,* 150, e151.

Incháustegui, A. (1918). De la leishmaniosis americana y de la úlcera de los chicleros en México. Tesis, Universidad Nacional de México.

Istkhar, Chaubey, A. K. & Upadhyay, S. K. (2016). Molecular phylogeny of three variable size juvenile isolates of *Steinernema abbasi* (Rhabditida: Steinernematidae) from the western part of Uttar Pradesh, India by the application of conserved genes sequence analyses. *International Journal of Global Science Research,* 3(5), 302–312.

Jaiswal, N., Upadhyay, S. K., Malhotra, A. & Malhotra, S. K. (2013). Multifactorial etiology of infections by larvae of *Eustrongylides tubifex* (Nematoda: Dioctophymidae) in silver whiting of the central west coast of India at Goa. *Asian Journal of Biological Sciences*, 6(1), 21–39.

Jaiswal, N., Upadhyay, S. K., Malhotra, A. & Malhotra, S. K. (2014a). Ecological morphotaxometry of trematodes of garfish (Teleostomi: Belonidae) from Gangetic riverine ecosystem in India. III. Principal Component Analysis for hydrobiological correlates to dynamics of infections by *Cephalogonimus yamunii* (Upadhyay, Jaiswal, Malhotra and Malhotra, 2012). *Journal of Parasitic Diseases,* 38(2), 153–162.

Jaiswal, N., Upadhyay, S. K., Malhotra, A., Blend, C. K., Dronen, N. O. & Malhotra, S. K. (2014b). A new species of *Neolebouria* Gibson, 1976 (Opecoelidae: Plagioporinae) from the whitecheek monocle bream, *Scolopsis vosmeri* (Perciformes: Nemipteridae), from the Panjim coast at Goa, with a checklist of parasites previously reported from this fish. *Zootaxa*, 3802(1), 098-108.

Jasemi, M., Valizadeh, L., Zamanzadeh, V. & Keogh, B. (2017). A concept analysis of holistic care by hybrid model. *Indian Journal of Palliative Care*, 23(1), 71–80.

Jayawardene, K. L. T. D., Palombo, E. A. & Boag, P. R. (2021). Natural products are a promising source for anthelmintic drug discovery. *Biomolecules*, 11(10), 1457.

Kali, A. (2015). Schistosome infections: An Indian perspective. *Journal of Clinical and Diagnostic Research,* 9(2), DE01-DE04.

Kantor, M., Abrantes, A., Estevez, A., Schiller, A., Torrent, J., Gascon, J., Hernandez, R. & Ochner, C. (2018). *Entamoeba histolytica*: Updates in clinical manifestation, pathogenesis, and vaccine development. *Canadian Journal of Gastroenterology and Hepatology,* 2, 2018.

Kaydos-Daniels, S. C., Miller, W. C., Hoffman, I., Banda, T., Dzinyemba, W., Martinson, F., Cohen, M. S. & Hobbs, M. M. (2003). Validation of a urine-based PCR-enzyme-linked immunosorbent assay for use in clinical research settings to detect *Trichomonas vaginalis* in men. *Journal of Clinical Microbiology*, 41(1), 318–323.

Kissinger, P. (2015). *Trichomonas vaginalis*: A review of epidemiologic, clinical and treatment issues. *BMC Infectious Diseases,* 15, 307. https://doi.org/10.1186/s12879-015-1055-0.

Kleijnen, J., Knipschild, P. & Riet, G. (1991). Clinical trials of homoeopathy. *British Medical Journal*, 302(6772), 316–323.

Kowalska, A., Kowalski, P. & Torres, M. (2011). Chagas Disease-American trypanosomiasis. *Polish Annals of Medicine,* 18, 156-167.

Krieger, J. N., Holmes, K. K., Spence, M. R., Rein, M. F., McCormack, W. M. & Tam, M. R. (1985). Geographic variation among isolates of *Trichomonas vaginalis*: Demonstration of antigenic heterogeneity by using monoclonal antibodies and the indirect immunofluorescence technique. *Journal of Infectious Diseases*, 152, 979-984.

Kumar, R., Thakur, A., Ahmad Hajam, Y., Datta, R., Sharma, A., Sharma, A. K. & Sonika (2022). *Parasitology.* In: Medical Microbiology (Sharma, A. K., Gupta, G. & Yadav, M., eds.). De Gruyter, Berlin, Boston. pp. 93-148.

Kumar, S., Jaiswal, N., Malhotra, A., Upadhyay, S. K., Capoor, V. N. & Malhotra, S. K. (2011). Application of numerical taxonomy for morphological and taxometric substantiation of cystidicolid nematodes, *Ascarophis alatae* n.sp. from Indian eels. *Proceedings of the Zoological Society of India*, 1, S45-S50.

Lafferty, K. D., Allesina, S., Arim, M., Briggs, C. J., De Leo, G., Dobson, A. P., Dunne, J. A., Johnson, P. T., Kuris, A. M., Marcogliese, D. J., Martinez, N. D., Memmott, J., Marquet, P. A., McLaughlin, J. P., Mordecai, E. A., Pascual, M., Poulin, R. & Thieltges, D. W. (2008). Parasites in food webs: The ultimate missing links. *Ecology Letters*, 11(6), 533-546.

Laga, M., Nzila, N. & Goeman, J. (1991). The interrelationship of sexually transmitted diseases and HIV infection: Implications for the control of both epidemics in Africa. *AIDS,* 5(1), S55–S63.

Lesh, E. J. & Brady, M. F. (2023). *Tapeworm.* In: StatPearls Publishing, Treasure Island (FL), https://www.ncbi.nlm.nih.gov/books/NBK537154/.

Limkittikul, K., Brett, J., LAzou, M., Epidemi, S. V., Hubert, J. & Li, Z. (2018). Human health problems and accidents associated with occurrence and control of storage arthropods and rodents. *Recent Advances in Stored Product Protection*, 19-43.

Liu, Q., Jin, X., Cheng, J., Zhou, H., Zhang, Y. & Dai, Y. (2023). Advances in the application of molecular diagnostic techniques for the detection of infectious disease pathogens (Review). *Molecular Medicine Reports*, 27(5), 104. https://doi.org/ 10.3892/mmr.2023.12991.

Lloyd, A. E., Honey, B. L., John, B. M. & Condren, M. (2014). Treatment options and considerations for intestinal helminthic infections. *Journal of Pharmacy Technology,* 30(4), 130-139.

Lopez-Romero, G., Quintero, J., Astiazarán-García, H. & Velazquez, C. (2015). Host defences against *Giardia lamblia*. *Parasite Immunology*, 37(8), 394-406.

MacMillan, J. R. (1991). Biological factors impinging upon control of external protozoan fish parasites. *Annual Review of Fish Diseases*, pp. 119-131.

Madsen, H. & Stauffer, R. Jr. (2022). Zoonotic trematode infections; Their biology, intermediate hosts and control. *Intech Open,* 102434. https://doi.org/ 10.5772/ intechopen.

Malhotra, A., Jaiswal, N., Upadhyay, S. K., Kumar, S. & Malhotra, S. K. (2009). Parasite stress response in zoonoses of *Cephalogonimus* sp. *Indian Journal of Helminthology*, 27, 73–80.

Mascarini-Serra, L. (2011). Prevention of soil-transmitted helminth infection. *Journal of Global Infectious Diseases,* 3(2), 175-182.

Mathie, R. T. (2003). The research evidence base for homeopathy: A fresh assessment of the literature. *Homeopathy*, 92(2), 84–91.

Mbong Ngwese, M., Prince Manouana, G., Nguema Moure, P. A., Ramharter, M., Esen, M. & Adégnika, A. A. (2020). Diagnostic techniques of soil-transmitted helminths: Impact on control measures. *Tropical Medicine and Infectious Disease,* 5(2), 93.

McCoy, O. R. (1935). The physiology of the helminth parasites. *Physiological Reviews,* 15(2), 221-240.

Memvanga, P. B. & Nkanga, C. I. (2021). Liposomes for malaria management: The evolution from 1980 to 2020. *Malaria Journal*, https://doi.org/10.1186/s12936-021-03858-0.

Miglianico, M., Eldering, M., Slater, H., Ferguson, N., Ambrose, P., Lees, R. S., Koolen, K. M. J., Pruzinova, K., Jancarova, M. & Volf, P. (2018). Repurposing isoxazoline veterinary drugs for control of vector-borne human diseases. *Proceedings of the National Academy of Sciences,* 115, E6920–E6926.

Mintz, E. D., Hudson-Wragg, M., Mshar, P., Cartter, M. L. & Hadler, J. L. (1993). Foodborne giardiasis in a corporate office setting. *Journal of Infectious Diseases,* 167, 250–253.

Morchón, R., Carretón, E., González-Miguel, J. & Mellado-Hernández, I. (2012). Heartworm disease (*Dirofilaria immitis*) and their vectors in Europe - New distribution trends. *Frontiers in Physiology,* 3, 196.

Moriyasu, T., Nakamura, R., Deloer, S., Senba, M., Kubo, M., Inoue, M., Culleton, R. & Hamano, S. (2018). *Schistosoma mansoni* infection suppresses the growth of *Plasmodium yoelii* parasites in the liver and reduces gametocyte infectivity to mosquitoes. *PLoS Neglected Tropical Diseases*, 12(1), e0006197.

Nguyen, K. & Hunt, D. (2007). *Entomopathogenic nematodes: Systematics, phylogeny and bacterial symbionts.* Brill. 816p. https://doi.org/10.1163/ej.9789004152939.i–816.

Odugbemi, T. O., Akinsulire, O. R., Aibinu, I. E. & Fabeku, P. O. (2006). Medicinal plants useful for malaria therapy in Okeigbo, Ondo State, Southwest Nigeria. *African Journal of Traditional, Complementary and Alternative Medicines*, 4(2), 191–198.

Olano, J. P., Weller, P. F., Guerrant, R. L. & Walker, D. H. (2011). *Principles of parasitism: Host–parasite interactions*. In: Tropical Infectious Diseases: Principles, Pathogens and Practice (Guerrant, R., Walker, D. H. & Weller, P. F. eds.), Saunders Elsevier, Philadelphia, pp. 1–7.

Olas, B. (2022). Bee products as interesting natural agents for the prevention and treatment of common cardiovascular diseases. *Nutrients*, 14(11), 2267. https://doi.org/10.3390/nu14112267.

PAHO (2003). *Zoonoses and communicable diseases common to man and animals 3rd Edition: Parasitoses Volume III*. Pan American Health Organization, Washington, D.C. 398p.

Paliwal, B., Dan, S., Modak, C. & Upadhyay, S. K. (2023). Zoonoses and foodborne diseases associated with parasites and vectors. In: *Parasitology: Risks and Challenges for Health and Sustainability* (Upadhyay, S. K., ed.). Nova Science Publishers, Inc., USA. pp. 231-268.

Panwar, P., Upadhyay, S. K., Singh, M., Yadav, M. & Sharma, A. K. (2022). Essence of amino acids as key biochemical variant for chemotaxonomic substantiation of cucullanid nematodes, *Dichelyne* (*Cucullanellus*) in catfish, *Rita rita*. *Journal of Xidian University*, 16(11), 264–274.

Patel, V., Chavda, V. & Shah, J. (2021). Nanotherapeutics in neuropathologies: Obstacles, Challenges and recent advancements in CNS targeted drug delivery systems. *Current Neuropharmacology*, 19(5), 693–710.

Patra, J. K., Das, G., Fraceto, L. F., Campos, E. V. R., Rodriguez-Torres, M. P., Acosta-Torres, L. S., Diaz-Torres, L. A., Grillo, R., Swamy, M. K., Sharma, S., Habtemariam, S. & Shin, H. S. (2018). Nano based drug delivery systems: Recent developments and future prospects. *Journal of Nanobiotechnology*, 16(1), 71. https://doi.org/10.1186/s12951-018-0392-8.

Peterson, K. M., Singh, U. & Petri Jr., W. A. (2011). *Enteric amebiasis*. In: Tropical Infectious Diseases: Principles, Pathogens and Practice (Guerrant, R., Walker, D. H. & Weller, P. F. eds.), Saunders Elsevier, Philadelphia, 614p.

Petrin, D., Delgaty, K., Bhatt, R. & Garber, G. (1998). Clinical and microbiological aspects of *Trichomonas vaginalis*. *Clinical Microbiology Reviews*, 11(2), 300-317.

Pires, D., Vicente, C. S. L., Menéndez, E., Faria, J. M. S., Rusinque, L., Camacho, M. J. & Inácio, M. L. (2022). The fight against plant-parasitic nematodes: Current status of bacterial and fungal biocontrol agents. *Pathogens*, 11(10), 1178.

Prakash, H., Ghosh, A. K., Rudramurthy, S. M., Singh, P., Xess, I. & Savio, J. (2019). A prospective multicenter study on mucormycosis in India: Epidemiology, diagnosis, and treatment. *Medical Mycology*, 57, 395-402.

Preston, D. & Johnson, P. (2010) Ecological consequences of parasitism. *Nature Education Knowledge,* 3(10), 47.

Pritchard, D. I. & Wilson, R. A. (1997). *Helminth infections*. In: Pulmonary Defences (Stockley, R.A. ed.). John Wiley and Sons Ltd.

Pritchard, D. I. (1993). Immunity to helminths: Is too much IgE parasite - rather than host-protective? *Parasite Immunology*, 15, 5-9.

Pritchard, D. I. (1997). The pro-allergic influences of helminth parasites: Understanding the dual role of eosinophils. *Memórias do Instituto Oswaldo Cruz,* 92(II), S15-S18.

Pritchard, D. I., Quinnell, R. J. & Walsh, E. A. (1995). Immunity in humans to *Necator americanus*: IgE, parasite weight and fecundity. *Parasite Immunology*, 17, 71-75.

Pulavarty, A., Egan, A., Karpinska, A., Horgan, K. & Kakouli-Duarte, T. (2021). Plant parasitic nematodes: a review on their behaviour, host interaction, management approaches and their occurrence in two sites in the Republic of Ireland. *Plants,* 10(11), 2352.

Raj, P., Vella, E. J. & Bickerton, R. C. (1998). Successful treatment of rhinocerebral mucormycosis by a combination of aggressive surgical debridement and the use of systemic liposomal amphotericin B and local therapy with nebulized amphotericin–a case report. *Journal of Laryngology and Otology,* 112, 367-370.

Rani, K. & Upadhyay, S. K. (2019). An introduction of monogenean parasites of fishes: Taxonomy and parasitocoenosis. In: *Parasitology Taxonomy and Bioecology* (Upadhyay, S.K., ed.). Write and Print Publications, New Delhi. pp. 84–99.

Riley, D. E., Roberts, M. C., Takayama, T. & Krieger, J. N. (1992). Development of a polymerase chain reaction-based diagnosis of *Trichomonas vaginalis*. *Journal of Clinical Microbiology*, 30, 465-472.

Roche, B. & Guégan, J. F. (2011). Ecosystem dynamics, biological diversity and emerging infectious diseases. *Comptes Rendus Biologies,* 334(5-6), 385-392.

Rodriguez, L., White, J. M., Richards, N. Q., You, A. X. & Couser, N. L. (2021). An adult *Loa loa* worm in the upper eyelid: An atypical presentation of loiasis in the United States. *Case Reports in Ophthalmological Medicine,* 2021, 6630875.

Ross, L. S. & Fidock, D. A. (2019). Elucidating mechanisms of drug-resistant *Plasmodium falciparum. Cell Host Microbe,* 26, 35–47.

Rudramurthy, G. R., Swamy, M. K., Sinniah, U. R. & Ghasemzadeh, A. (2016). Nanoparticles: Alternatives against drug-resistant pathogenic microbes. *Molecules*, 21(7), 836. https://doi.org/10.3390/molecules21070836.

Salit, I., Khairnar, K., Gough, K. & Pillai, D. (2009). A possible cluster of sexually transmitted. *Clinical Infectious Diseases,* 49(3), 346–353.

Sangweme, D. T., Midzi, N., Zinyowera-Mutapuri, S., Mduluza, T., Diener-West, M. & Kumar, N. (2010). Impact of schistosome infection on *Plasmodium falciparum* Malariometric indices and immune correlates in school age children in Burma Valley, Zimbabwe. *PLoS Neglected Tropical Diseases*, 4(11), e882.

Sato, S. (2021). *Plasmodium*-a brief introduction to the parasites causing human malaria and their basic biology. *Journal of Physiology and Anthropology,* 40(1), 3-12.

Schumann, J. A. & Plasner, S. (2023). *Trichomoniasis*. StatPearls Publishing, Teasure Island (FL), https://www.ncbi.nlm.nih.gov/books/NBK534826/.

Serban, G. (2019). Future prospects in the treatment of parasitic diseases: 2-Amino-1,3,4-Thiadiazoles in leishmaniasis. *Molecules*, *24*(8), 1557. https://doi.org/10.3390/molecules24081557.

Sethi, B., Kumar, V., Mahato, K., Coulter, D.W. & Mahato, R. I. (2022). Recent advances in drug delivery and targeting to the brain. *Journal of Controlled Release*, 350, 668–687.

She, R. C., Rawlins, M. L., Mohl, R., Perkins, S. L., Hill, H. R. & Litwin, C. M. (2007). Comparison of immunofluorescence antibody testing and two enzyme immunoassays in the serologic diagnosis of malaria. *The Journal of Travel Medicine,* 14, 105–111.

Sim, S., Aw, P. P. K., Wilm, A., Teoh, G., Hue, K. D. T. & Nguyen, N. M. (2015). Tracking dengue virus intra-host genetic diversity during human-to-mosquito transmission. *PLoS Neglected Tropical Diseases,* 9, e0004052.

Simpson, I., Woolley, I. J. & Gardiner, B. J. (2015). Caught in the act. A case of fulminant amoebic colitis. *JMM Case Reports,* 2(4), 1-3.

Singh, L., Kruger, H. G., Maguire, G. E. M., Govender, T. & Parboosing, R. (2017). The role of nanotechnology in the treatment of viral infections. *Therapeutic Advances in Infectious Disease*, 4(4), 105–131.

Singh, M., Kumar, V., Raj, M., Roy, S., Bhawana, Jarora, V. & Sharma, A. K. (2022). Reforming roadmap for vector control strategies for malaria elimination and eradication from transmission in context to the current evidence. *International Journal of Mosquito Research*, 9(3), 36-40.

Singh, M., Upadhyay, S. K., Gupta, S., Thakur, V. & Sharma, A. K. (2022). Effective management of *Aedes aegypti* Linn. (Diptera: Culicidae) population through conventional to genetic control and nanotechnology approaches: A short review. *International Journal of Mosquito Research*, 9(2), 95-99.

Smith, H. V. & Mank, T. G. (2011). *Diagnosis of human Giardiasis*. In: Giardia a model organism (Lujan, H.D. & Svard, S., eds.). Springer-Verlag, New York. pp. 353–374.

Steere, A. C. (2001). Lyme disease. *New England Journal of Medicine, 345*, 115–125.

Stejskal, V., Hubert, J. & Li, Z. (2018). Human health problems and accidents associated with occurrence and control of storage arthropods and rodents. *Recent Advances in Stored Product Protection*, 19-43.

Stock, S. P., Griffin, C. T. & Burnell, A. M. (2002). Morphological characterisation of three isolates of *Heterorhabditis* Poinar, 1976 from the `Irish group' (Nematoda: Rhabditida: Heterorhabditidae) and additional evidence supporting their recognition as a distinct species, *H. downesi* n. sp. *Systematic Parasitology*, *51*(2), 95–106.

Su, X. & Miller, L. H. (2015). The discovery of artemisinin and Nobel Prize in Physiology or Medicine. *Science China. Life Sciences*, 58(11), 1175–1179.

Subramanian, S. & Muthulakshmi, M. (2016). Entomopathogenic nematodes. *Ecofriendly Pest Management for Food Security*, pp. 367–410.

Sun, Y., Chen, D., Pan, Y., Qu, W., Hao, H., Wang, X., Liu, Z. & Xie, S. (2019). Nanoparticles for antiparasitic drug delivery. *Drug Delivery*, 26(1), 1206–1221.

Sures, B., Nachev, M., Selbach, C. & Marcogliese, D. J. (2017). Parasite responses to pollution: what we know and where we go in 'Environmental Parasitology'. *Parasites Vectors* 10, 65.

Sutherst, R. W. (2007). Arthropods as disease vectors in a changing environment. In: *Ciba Foundation Symposium 175-Environmental Change and Human Health: Environmental Change and Human Health: Ciba Foundation Symposium.* Chichester, UK: John Wiley & Sons, Ltd. 175, 124-145.

Talwani, R., Gilliam, B. L. & Howell, C. (2011). Infectious diseases and the liver. *Clinics in Liver Disease,* 15(1), 111-130.

Tangpukdee, N., Duangdee, C., Wilairatana, P. & Krudsood, S. (2009). Malaria diagnosis: A brief review. *Korean Journal of Parasitology,* 47(2), 93-102.

Taylor, J. W. & Barker, B. M. (2019). The endozoan, small-mammal reservoir hypothesis and the life cycle of Coccidioides species. *Medical Mycology*, 57(1), S16-S20.

Teleanu, D. M., Chircov, C., Grumezescu, A. M., Volceanov, A. & Teleanu, R. I. (2018). Blood-brain delivery methods using nanotechnology. *Pharmaceutics*, 10(4), 269. https://doi.org/10.3390/pharmaceutics10040269.

Torres-Guerrero, E., Quintanilla-Cedillo, M. R., Ruiz-Esmenjaud, J. & Arenas, R. (2017). *Leishmaniasis: A review.* 6, 750. https://doi.org/10.12688/f1000research.11120.1.

Ung, L., Stothard, J. R., Phalkey, R., Azman, A. S., Chodosh, J., Hanage, W. P. & Standley, C.J. (2021). Towards global control of parasitic diseases in the COVID-19 era: One Health and the future of multisectoral global health governance. *Advances in Parasitology*, 114, 1–26.

Upadhyay, S. K. (2018a). Morphotaxonomy, histopathology and population dynamics of natural enoplid infections in wild rat, *Rattus rattus* of eastern Uttar Pradesh, India. *AASCIT Journal of Bioscience,* 4(3), 22–27.

Upadhyay, S. K. (2020c). Autogenicity and precocious development of *Sturdynema multiembryonata* in *Xenentodon cancila* (Osteichthyes: Belonidae) from the Gangetic ecosystem. *Bulletin of Pure and Applied Sciences –Zoology*, 39A(1), 36–45.

Upadhyay, S.K & Singh, R. (2018). Polyfactorial etiology on demography of parasitic allocreodoidean trematodes in the Gangetic ecosystem. *AASCIT American Journal of Biomedical Science* and *Engineering,* 4(2), 17–23.

Upadhyay, S.K. & Nanware, S.S. (2020). Parasitoses and histological consequences of *Trichuris trichiura* (Nematoda: Enoplida) in rodents, *Rattus rattus* (Mammalia: Rodentia). *Asian Journal of Biological and Life Sciences,* 9(1), 74–78.

Upadhyay, S. K. (2012). *Transmission dynamics and environmental influence on foodborne parasitic helminthes of the Gangetic plains and central west coast of India.* Unpublished D.Phil. Thesis, University of Allahabad, India. 400p.

Upadhyay, S. K. (2017a). Morphotaxometry and molecular heterogeneity of *Sturdynema multiembryonata* gen. et sp.n. (Spiruroidea: Gnathostomatinae) of freshwater garfish, *Xenentodon cancilla* from the Gangetic riverine ecosystem in northern India with a revised key to genera of Gnathostomatinae. *Species,* 18(58), 1–13.

Upadhyay, S. K. (2017b). Environmental impact on helminth parasites of freshwater garfish from river Yamuna at Allahabad, Uttar Pradesh, India. *Proceeding of the Zoological Society of India,* 16(2), 63–75.

Upadhyay, S. K. (2018b). Molecular barcode analysis and phylogeny of parasitic helminthes: A laboratory manual. *Research Journal of Recent Sciences,* 7(3), 22–27.

Upadhyay, S. K. (2020a). *Parasitology: Taxonomy and Bioecology.* Write and Print Publication, New Delhi. 209p.

Upadhyay, S. K. (2020b). Biodiversity of parasites and parasitoses: Perspective to health and sustainability. In: *Biodiversity and Development Challenges of 21st Century* (Prakash, S., Ranjan, R. & Pandey, R. K. eds). Swaranjali Publication Pvt. Ltd., Ghaziabad, U.P. pp. 162–192.

Upadhyay, S. K. (2023a). *Emerging infectious zoonotic diseases: Causes and therapeutic approaches*. Rajsons Publications Pvt. Ltd., New Delhi. 126p.

Upadhyay, S. K. (2023b). *Parasitology: Risks and Challenges for Health and Sustainability*. Nova Science Publishers, Inc., New York. 274p.

Upadhyay, S. K., Babita & Singh, R. (2019c). The diversity and bioecology of cestodes in freshwater snakehead fish *Channa* sp. (Bloch) with a checklist of tapeworms previously reported from this fish in India. In: *Parasitology Taxonomy and Bioecology* (Upadhyay, S.K., ed.). Write and Print Publications, New Delhi. pp. 17–37.

Upadhyay, S. K., Babita, Panwar, P., Kumar, S. & Nanware, S. S. (2019a). Parasite–host interactions: A negative symbiotic association between organisms' perspective to health and sustainability. In: *Parasitology Taxonomy and Bioecology* (Upadhyay, S. K., ed.). Write and Print Publications, New Delhi. pp. 164–183.

Upadhyay, S. K., Babita, Panwar, P., Singh, M. & Singh, R. (2019b). Linking of DNA sequences and molecular heterogeneity with phylogeny for morphotaxonomic validation of parasites: A modern reliable technique in taxonomy. In: *Parasitology*

*Taxonomy and Bioecology* (Upadhyay, S.K., ed.). Write and Print Publications, New Delhi. pp. 134–154.

Upadhyay, S. K., Babita, Singh, M., Yadav, M., Kumar, V., Singh, R., Pandey, Y. P., Nanware, S. S. & Sharma, A. K. (2023a). A new species of *Allocreadium* Looss, 1900 (Allocreadoidea: Allocreadiidae) in *Wallago attu* Bloch and Schneider, 1801 (Siluriformes: Siluridae) from Yamuna River at Yamuna Nagar, Haryana. *Asian Journal of Biological and Life Sciences,* 12(1), 112-124.

Upadhyay, S. K., Jaiswal, N., Malhotra, A. & Malhotra, S. K. (2009). An aspidoderid round worm *Pseudaspidodera cordinae* n.sp. from rodents at Allahabad. *Indian Journal of Helminthology*, 27, 89-94.

Upadhyay, S. K., Jaiswal, N., Malhotra, A. & Malhotra, S. K. (2013a). Ecological morphotaxometry of trematodes of garfish (Teleostomi: Belonidae) from Gangetic riverine ecosystem in India. I. Morphology and taxometric assessment of *Cephalogonimus yamunii* n.sp. *Journal of Parasitic Diseases,* 37(2), 218–224.

Upadhyay, S. K., Jaiswal, N., Malhotra, A. & Malhotra, S. K. (2013b). Ecological morphotaxometry of trematodes of garfish (Teleostomi: Belonidae) from Gangetic riverine ecosystem in India. II. Correlation of seasonality and host biology with distribution pattern of *Cephalogonimus yamunii* n.sp. *Journal of Parasitic Diseases*, 37(2), 211–217.

Upadhyay, S. K., Pandey, Y. P., Singh, M., Dan, S., Upadhyay, K., Babita, Panwar, P., Singh, R., Kumar, S., Singh, D. P., Rani, K., Yadav, D. & Sharma, A. K. (2023c). Helminthoinformatics: In silico approaches in gene sequence analysis for taxonomic validation of parasitic helminths. In: *Parasitology: Risks and Challenges for Health and Sustainability* (Upadhyay, S. K., ed.). Nova Science Publishers, Inc., USA. pp. 77-113.

Upadhyay, S. K., Singh R., Babita, Panwar, P., Singh, D. P., Rani, K. & Yadav, D. (2020). Population ecology of parasitic helminthes *Oncodiscus* Yamaguti, 1934 (Cestoda: Bothriocephalidae) in Greater lizardfish *Saurida tumbil* Bloch (Aulopiformes: Synodontidae) from the coast of Visakhapatnam, Bay of Bengal. *Bulletin of Pure and Applied Sciences –Zoology*, 39A(2), 379–386.

Upadhyay, S. K., Singh, M., Singh, R., Sharma, A. K., Upadhyay, K. & Malhotra, S. K. (2021). Zoonoses and other communicable diseases: An emerging threat to human life, causes and therapy. In: *Proceedings of International Virtual Seminar on Recent Trends in Life Sciences and Biotechnology: Strategies to Combat COVID–19, Zoonoses and Other Communicable Diseases* (Upadhyay, S. K., Singh, M. & Sharma, A. K., eds). Rakesh Book Service, New Delhi. pp. 57–107.

Upadhyay, S. K., Upadhyay, K., Panwar, P., Babita, Singh, M., Yadav, M., Aggarwal, D., Pandey, Y. P., Kumar, S., Rana, N., Deshmukh, V. S., Nanware, S. S., Bhure, D. B., Dixit, Y. B. & Singh, R. (2023d). Emerging zoonotic diseases: Elementary concept, types, sources of infection and spreading, causes, control measures and therapeutic approaches. In: *Emerging infectious zoonotic diseases: Causes and therapeutic approaches* (ed., Upadhyay, S. K., ed.). Rajsons Publications Pvt. Ltd., New Delhi. pp. 1-43.

Upadhyay, S. K., Upadhyay, K., Singh, M., Yadav, M., Kumar, V., Babita, Panwar, P., Dan, S. & Malhotra, S. K. (2023b). Parasites and parasitism: an update on host-parasite-environment interactions to uncover the mystery of hidden and neglected infra-communities. In: *Parasitology: Risks and Challenges for Health and Sustainability* (Upadhyay, S. K., ed.). Nova Science Publishers, Inc., USA. pp. 1-33.

Upadhyay, S. K., Yadav, D. & Pathak, R. K. (2015). The impact of water quality on the population distribution pattern of cephalogonimid trematodes *Cephalogonimus yamunii* in freshwater fish *Heteropneustes fossilis* at Allahabad, Uttar Pradesh. *Journal of the Kalash Science,* 3(2), 11–17.

Warhurst, D. C. & Williams, J. E. (1996). Laboratory diagnosis of malaria. *Journal of Clinical Pathology*, 49, 533–538.

Warton, A. & Honigberg B. M. (1979). Structure of trichomonads as revealed by scanning electron microscopy. *Journal of Protozoology,* 26, 56–62.

Wen, H., Jung, H. & Li, X. (2015). Drug delivery approaches in addressing clinical pharmacology-related issues: opportunities and challenges. *The AAPS Journal*, 17(6), 1327–1340.

Wharton, R. H. & Norris, K. R. (2010). Control of parasitic arthropods. *Veterinary Parasitology*, 6(1-3), 135-164.

WHO (2009). Special programme for research and training in tropical diseases: Dengue-Guidelines for diagnosis, treatment, prevention, and control. *World Health Organization,* New ed. Geneva.

WHO (2023a), *Malaria*. World Health Organization, https://www.who.int/health-topics/malaria. Accessed on 28th May, 2023.

WHO (2023b). *Leishmaniasis*. World Health Organization, https://www.who.int/news-room/fact-sheets/detail/leishmaniasis. Accessed on 29th May, 2023.

Wilkinson, K., Grant, W. P., Green, L. E., Hunter, S., Jeger, M. J., Lowe, P., Medley, G. F., Mills, P., Phillipson, J., Poppy, G. M. & Waage, J. (2011). Infectious diseases of animals and plants: An interdisciplinary approach. *Philosophical Transactions of the Royal Society B: Biological Sciences,* 366(1573), 1933-1942.

Wisdom, A. R. & Dunlop, E. M. C. (1965). Trichomoniasis: Study of the disease and its treatment in women and men. *British Journal of Venereal Diseases,* 41, 90–96.

Yaeger, R. G. (1996). Protozoa: Structure, classification, growth, and development. In: *Medical Microbiology* 4th edition (ed., Baron S.). Medical Branch, University of Texas, Galveston (TX), https://www.ncbi.nlm.nih.gov/books/NBK8325/.

Yamaguti, S. (1958). *Systema helminthum vol. I. The trematode of vertebrates.* Inter Science Publications, NY. 979p.

Yamaguti, S. (1959). *Systema helminthum vol. II. The Cestodes of Vetebrates*. Inter Science Publications, NY. 860p.

Yamaguti, S. (1962). *Systema Helminthum vol. III. The Nematodes of Vertebrates*. Inter Science Publications, NY. 1261p.

Yan, L., Pape, T., Elgar, M. A., Gao, Y. & Zhang, D. (2019). Evolutionary history of stomach bot flies in the light of mitogenomics. *Systematic Entomology*, 44(4), 797-809.

Yin, I. X., Zhang, J., Zhao, I. S., Mei, M. L., Li, Q. & Chu, C. H. (2020). The antibacterial mechanism of silver nanoparticles and its application in dentistry. *International Journal of Nanomedicine*, 15, 2555–2562.

Yuan, H., Ma, Q., Ye, L. & Piao, G. (2016). The traditional medicine and modern medicine from natural products. *Molecules*, 21(5), 559. https://doi.org/10.3390/molecules 21050559.

Zeni, V., Baliota, G. V., Benelli, G., Canale, A. & Athanassiou, C. G. (2021). Diatomaceous earth for arthropod pest control: Back to the future. *Molecules*, 26(24), 7487.

# Chapter 2

# Parasites and Parasitic Diseases in Human: Risks, Challenges and Therapeutic Strategies

**Preeti Baxi**[1]
**Nishant Srivastava**[2,*]
**and Manoj Singh**[3]
[1]Phytosanitary Laboratory, Department of Plant Molecular Biology and Biotechnology, Indira Gandhi Agriculture University, Raipur, India
[2]Avishka Council of Industrial and Allied Biosciences (ACIAB), Greater Noida, India
[3]Department of Bio-Sciences and Technology, M.M.E.C., Maharishi Markandeshwar (Deemed to be University), Mullana-Ambala (Haryana), India

## Abstract

Parasitism is a fundamental association between two species: The parasite and the host. Parasitic illnesses cause noteworthy problems in the developing world. Zoonotic parasites are vital due to their human and animal health. The emergence and re-emergence of various zoonotic parasites have been described across the globe. Contaminated water and food pointedly increase the transmission of parasites. Climate changes associated with global warming, poverty, food trade, and scarcity of safe drinking water are the factors influencing the occurrence of these parasites. Therefore, there is a crucial need for surveillance and control.

**Keywords:** parasites, parasitism, helminths, zoonoses, modern therapy

In: Therapeutic Advances in Human Health and Diseases
Editors: Sushil Kumar Upadhyay, Manoj Singh and Anil Kumar Sharma
ISBN: 979-8-89113-304-4

## 1. Introduction

Parasites and parasitism are fundamental concepts in biology and describe a relationship between two organisms where one benefits at the cost of the other. A parasite is an organism that lives and feeds on or within another organism; known as the host, without providing any significant benefits in return (Poulin, 2007). Parasitism is a widespread ecological phenomenon found in various ecosystems and involves a wide range of organisms, including viruses, bacteria, fungi, protozoa, helminths (worms), and arthropods (Rollinson and Hay, 2011). Parasites have evolved numerous adaptations to exploit and survive within their hosts. They may derive nutrition from the host's tissues, blood, or other bodily fluids, often causing harm or disease in the process. Parasitic organisms have developed specialized structures or organs to facilitate attachment, feeding, and reproduction within their hosts (Poulin et al., 2015).

Parasites can infect humans, animals, and even plants, and their impact on their hosts can range from mild inconvenience to severe illness and death. The effects of parasitism can include nutrient depletion, tissue damage, immune system modulation, and interference with host reproductive capabilities (Herms, 1926; Suzuki, et al., 2019). Parasitism has shaped the course of evolution and has significant ecological and evolutionary implications. Parasites can exert selection pressures on host populations, driving the evolution of various adaptations in response to the parasitic threat. This includes the development of resistance mechanisms by hosts and counter-adaptations by parasites (Ebert, 2000; Ezenwa et al., 2016; Britt, 2018).

In human health, parasitic infections remain a global challenge, particularly in developing regions with limited access to clean water, sanitation, and healthcare. Parasitic diseases, such as malaria, schistosomiasis, leishmaniasis, and intestinal worm infections, affect millions of people worldwide and have substantial socio-economic impacts (Engels et al., 2006). Understanding parasites and parasitism is crucial for effective disease control, wildlife conservation, and ecological studies. Researchers investigate parasite life cycles, host-parasite interactions, transmission dynamics, and the development of novel therapeutic strategies to combat parasitic infections. In summary, parasites and parasitism represent a complex relationship between organisms, where one organism benefits at the expense of another. The study of parasites and their interactions with hosts is essential for understanding the intricacies of ecosystems, human health, and the ongoing battle against parasitic diseases.

## 2. Parasitism

The physiological association between two organisms in which the parasite which associate has vanished its individuality by losing its physiological independence and counts on the host, the other associate for its requirements like nutritional and sometimes for additional metabolic needs. In such type of association, the host has not gotten any benefit and habitually it gets actively injured by the parasite (Watson 1965; Olano et al., 2011; El-Tonsy, 2012). Humans can also get infected with these parasites, which trigger diseases. Medical parasitology comprises the study of different parasitic groups of animals: parasitic bacteria, parasitic protozoa, parasitic fungi, parasitic helminths (worms), and those arthropods that cause disease directly or act as vectors of many pathogens (Dubey, 1996). In general, the parasites are classified into categories: Protozoa, helminths, and arthropods (Figure 1) (Dhaiwal and Juyal, 2013).

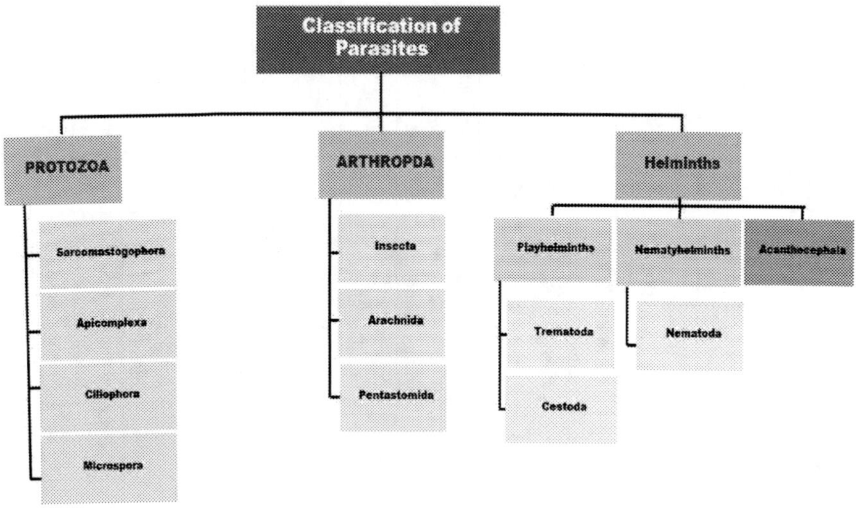


**Figure 1.** Classification of parasites.

## 3. Types of Parasites

According to the nature of the relationship/interaction between host-parasite, environmental factors, and type of life cycle, the parasites are grouped biologically into the following types (Table 1):

**Table 1.** Different parasites, host, their transmission, and diseases caused by the parasites

| Group | Parasite | Host | Disease | Transmission | References |
|---|---|---|---|---|---|
| Protozoa | *Entamoeba histolytica* | Man | Pulmonary infection, Amoebiasis | Ingestion of food/ water contaminated with cyst, sexual contact, vector | Isabella and Rohit, 2018; Kantor et al., 2018 |
| | *Toxoplasma gondii* | Definitive host: Cats, felines Intermediate host: Man, other mammals (sheep, goat, pig, cattle) | Toxoplasmosis | Ingestion of sporulated oocyst from soil, food, water, ingestion of tissue cyst, blood transfusion. | Dubey, 1996; Isabella and Rohit, 2018 |
| | *Leishmania donovani* | Vertebrate host: Man, dog, rodents; Insect vector: Sandfly | Leishmaniasis | Bite of an infected sandfly, blood transfusion | Isabella and Rohit, 2018 |
| | *Balantidium coli* | Natural host: Pig Accidental host: Man | Balantidiasis | Ingestion of food/water contaminated with cysts | Isabella and Rohit, 2018 |
| | *Plasmodium falciparum* | Definitive host: Female Anopheles mosquito Accidental host: Man | Malaria | Bite of female Anopheles mosquito, blood transfusion. | Isabella and Rohit, 2018; Zekar and Sharman, 2022 |
| Helminthes | *Echinococcus multilocularis* | Definitive host: Foxes, wolves, dogs, cats Intermediate host: Small wild rodent's Accidental intermediate host: Man | Alveolar echinococcosis | Ingestion of food contaminated with eggs Mechanical vectors for eggs: flies | Peregrine et al., 2012; Isabella and Rohit, 2018 |
| | *Schistosoma haematobium* | Definitive host: Man, Intermediate host: Freshwater snails | Bilharzia | Penetration of skin by infective cercariae present in contaminated water | Isabella and Rohit, 2018 https://www.cdc. |

| Group | Parasite | Host | Disease | Transmission | References |
|---|---|---|---|---|---|
| | | | | | gov/parasites/schistosomiasis/gen |
| | *Ancylostoma* sp. | Man | Ancylostomiasis | Penetration of skin by third stage (filariform) larva | Isabella and Rohit, 2018 |
| | *Ascaris lumbricoides* | Man | Ascariasis | Ingestion of embryonated eggs from contaminated soil, water, food | Isabella and Rohit, 2018; de Lima Corvino et al., 2022 |
| | *Ascaris suum* | Pigs. Human infection is rare | | Ingestion of egg with an L2 larva | Isabella and Rohit, 2018 |
| | *Paragonimus westermani* | pigs, dogs, and a variety of feline species | Paragonimiasis (possible areas: Lung parenchyma, pleura, thoracic cavity) | by eating infected crab or crawfish that is either, raw, partially cooked, pickled, or salted | Dalia and Ahmad, 2020 |
| | *Dracunculus medinensis* | Humans: principal definitive host, and Cyclops: intermediate host. | Dracunculiasis (guinea-worm disease) | drinking unsafe, stagnant water contaminated by copepods (water fleas) that contain *Dracunculus* medinensis larvae | Dalia and Ahmad, 2020; Rawala and Jan 2022 |

### 3.1. Endoparasites

These parasites live inside the host body. A large number of endoparasites are intestinal such as nematodes like Ascarids (roundworm), hookworms, threadworms, whipworms, cestodes like tapeworms, and trematodes like flukes are also intestinal endoparasites. Some endoparasites live in the liver like larvae of Echinococcus spp. and liver flukes (Watson, 1965; El-Tonsy, 2012).

### 3.2. Ectoparasites

Taxonomically these parasites belong to a diverse group of organisms that survive by attaching them outside the host's body. Examples are fleas, lice, mosquitoes, mites, ticks, bugs, etc. Usually, ectoparasites attach to the skin of the host to feed but do not continue on the host for their whole life. Some ectoparasitic arthropods and nematodes can cause visible skin lesions. Such kinds of infections are often itchy, causing annoyance and discomfort. Plague of head and body lice i.e., pediculosis and scabies are found in all human races to some extent. The rate of mortality is low in the case of ectoparasitic infection while cumulative morbidity is considerable (Watson, 1965; El-Tonsy, 2012).

### 3.3. Permanent and Temporary Parasites

Permanent parasites spend the major span of their lives inside the body of the host like a tapeworm. In some cases, they are attached to the surface of the host's body. On the other hand, temporary parasites make time-to-time contact with the host body such as mosquitoes (Watson, 1965; El-Tonsy, 2012).

### 3.4. Facultative and Obligate Parasites

The facultative parasite is capable of living their life both way free living in the environment and parasitic, according to circumstances, for example, tapeworms, *Rhabditis hominis*. Contrary obligatory parasites are totally dependent on the host and cannot continue their life away from the host, for example, hookworms (Watson, 1965; El-Tonsy, 2012).

### 3.5. Monoxenous, Heteroxenous and Auto heteroxenous Parasites

Monoxenous parasites, like hookworms, *Coccidoa*, *Amoeba*, live in only a single host during the course of their normal life cycle. Heterogenous parasite, such as tapeworms, require two or more types of hosts, viz a definite host and one or other intermediate hosts, in each life cycle. Auto-heterogenous parasites e.g., Trichina worms, *Trichinella spiralis*, are the type in which one generation's definite host will become the next generation's intermediate host (Watson, 1965).

### 3.6. Accidental Parasites

These parasites affect an unusual host, they can maintain their life for some time but not permanently. For example, a dog tapeworm, *Dipylidium caninum*, can start itself for a while in man (Watson 1965).

## 4. Host-Parasite Relationship

The relationship between the host and the parasite and the struggle for supremacy is term as host-parasite relationship. There are different types of hosts, as given in Figure 2 (Isabella and Rohit, 2018). The term infection and disease are two different phenomena. A person can get infected but that may not turn into a disease. If the supremacy is in the host, cause of increased host resistance, the person remains healthy. In such cases, the parasite either leaves or adopts a benign relationship with the host body. But if the host body loses the competition, a disease may develop. In the living world, the association between two organisms is primarily in the form of symbiosis, which means "life together" viz, two organisms living in a relationship with each other (Solomon et al., 2014). Thus, three different types of symbiotic relationships have developed namely:

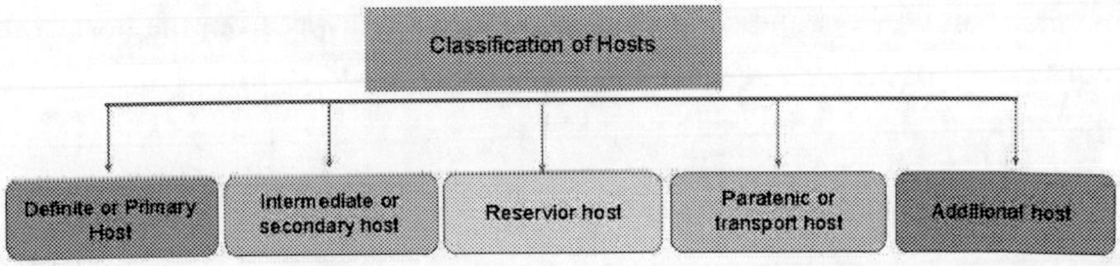


**Figure 2.** Classification of hosts.

### 4.1. Parasitism

One of the organisms, the parasite, either troubles or survives at the cost of the host. Parasites may induce mechanical injury, such as skin or tissue digging, causing an immune response (Watson, 1965; El-Tonsy, 2012).

### 4.2. Mutualism

An association in which both organisms benefit from each other is called mutualism. In general, mutualism is obligatory, as in many cases physiological dependence has grown to such a grade that one organism cannot continue its life without the other one e.g., blood-sucking leeches, filarial nematodes, etc. (Watson, 1965; El-Tonsy, 2012).

### 4.3. Commensalism

Relationship in which one partner (parasite) benefits, but the host is neither benefited nor harmed e.g., *Entamoeba polecki*, *Endolimax nana,* etc. (Watson, 1965; El-Tonsy, 2012).

## 5. Risks and Challenges

Parasites influence host nature and fitness, and can also regulate the population size of the host, sometimes with deep effects on food webs, competition, trophic interaction, biodiversity, etc. Parasites are being progressively recognized as significant pathogens with important global, environmental, economic, and human health impacts. Worldwide, more than three billion people are infected with one or other parasites with changing morbidity and mortality. (Daniel and Jonhson, 2010; Preston and Johnson, 2010; Elsheikha, 2014). The increasing number of parasites and the emergence of diseases in wildlife and humans, make it a relevant time to further study and improve our understanding of the role of parasitism in public health, ecosystem, biodiversity, etc. To understand in a better way this book focuses on the different types of parasites, the role of climate change in the population and behavior of the parasites, the diagnosis, detection and therapeutic aspects, and recent trends in parasitology.

## 6. National and International Trends on Newly Emerging Parasitic Threats

Parasites spoil healthy life and growth in hundreds of millions of entities throughout the world. Various human populations are at serious risk of sickness and even demise from these pathogens. Evidence indicates that changes in natural and anthropogenic environments affect the emergence and spread of parasitic diseases. Climate change, population, agriculture intensification, human intrusion into wildlife, alterations, and degradation in microbial and other ecosystems stimulate the spread, occurrence, and epidemiological dynamics of parasitic infections (Patz, 2000; Jonsson, 2012; Nahid, 2020).

### 6.1. Vector-Borne Diseases

Parasitic diseases transmitted by vectors such as mosquitoes, ticks, and flies continue to pose significant threats globally. Diseases like malaria, dengue fever, Lyme disease, and Chagas disease have seen increases in certain regions due to factors such as climate change, urbanization, and human travel (Pollitt et al., 2011; Poulin et al., 2015).

### 6.2. Neglected Tropical Diseases

Neglected Tropical Diseases (NTDs) including several parasitic infections, affect millions of people in low-income countries. These diseases, such as schistosomiasis, soil-transmitted helminthiasis, and lymphatic filariasis, often occur in impoverished areas with limited access to clean water, sanitation, and healthcare (Engels et al., 2006).

### 6.3. Drug Resistance

The emergence of drug-resistant parasites is a growing concern. Some parasites, such as Plasmodium falciparum (the parasite that causes malaria), have developed resistance to commonly used antimalarial drugs. This trend underscores the need for ongoing research and the development of new treatment strategies. (Marfurt et al., 2010; Picot et al., 2022).

### 6.4. Zoonotic Parasitic Infections

Parasites that can be transmitted between animals and humans, known as zoonotic parasites, are a significant concern. Zoonotic diseases can be triggered by bacteria, viruses, parasites, and fungi. Examples include *Toxoplasma gondii*, which can be contracted from cats, and *Cryptosporidium*, which can be transmitted through contaminated water sources (Moratal, 2020).

### 6.5. Foodborne Parasitic Infections

Parasites transmitted through contaminated food or water can cause significant health issues. For instance, parasites like *Cyclospora cayetanensis* and *Trichinella spiralis* can be contracted by consuming contaminated produce or undercooked meat, respectively (Bintsis, 2017).

### 6.6. Increased Travel and Globalization

Global travel and migration contribute to the spread of parasitic infections. People may acquire parasites during their travels and bring them back to their home countries, leading to the emergence of previously uncommon parasitic threats in new regions (Buss, 2002).

### 6.7. One Health Approach

The One Health concept recognizes the interconnection between human, animal, and environmental health. It highlights the importance of collaborative efforts among human and veterinary medicine, ecology, and other disciplines to address emerging parasitic threats more effectively (Blake et al., 2017).

## 7. Modern Therapeutic Stratégies in Parasitologie

Parasitology incorporates the study of parasites and the diseases they root. Over time, various therapeutic strategies have been developed to combat parasitic infections. Here are some modern therapeutic strategies in parasitology:

### 7.1. Chemotherapy

Chemotherapy involves the use of drugs to kill or inhibit the growth of parasites. Antiparasitic drugs target specific aspects of the parasite's life cycle, metabolism, or molecular pathways. For example, antimalarial drugs like chloroquine and artemisinin derivatives are used to treat malaria, while anti-helminthic drugs like albendazole and mebendazole are effective against intestinal worm infections (Van den Bossche, 1978; Horn and Duraisingh, 2013).

### 7.2. Combination Therapy

Combining multiple antiparasitic drugs with different mechanisms of action has become a common strategy to enhance efficacy, prevent drug resistance, and improve treatment outcomes. For instance, combination therapy is widely used in the treatment of malaria to counter resistance and achieve better parasite clearance (Nosten and Brasseur, 2002).

### 7.3. Vaccination

The development of vaccines against parasitic infections is a promising approach. Vaccines can stimulate the immune system to recognize and mount a response against specific parasites, preventing infection or reducing disease severity. Vaccines have been developed for certain parasitic diseases such as malaria and leishmaniasis (Sharma et al., 2015).

### 7.4. Targeted Therapies

Advancements in understanding parasite biology and genomics have led to the identification of specific parasite proteins or enzymes that are essential for survival or virulence. Targeted therapies aim to inhibit or disrupt these vital parasite components selectively. For example, protease inhibitors have been developed for the treatment of diseases caused by the protozoan parasite Trypanosoma cruzi, such as Chagas disease, Chloroquine inhibits heme detoxification and nucleic acid biosynthesis (McKerrow et al., 2008; Campbell and Soman, 2022).

### 7.5. Host-Directed Therapies

Host-directed therapies focus on modulating the host's immune response to control or eliminate parasites. These strategies aim to enhance the immune system's ability to recognize and eliminate parasites effectively. Immunomodulatory drugs and adjuvants are being investigated for their potential to enhance host immunity against parasitic infections (Singh et al., 2019).

### 7.6. Drug Repurposing

Existing drugs approved for other indications are being explored for their potential activity against parasitic infections. This approach, known as drug repurposing, offers the advantage of leveraging known safety profiles and established manufacturing processes. Examples include the use of the antiparasitic drug ivermectin for onchocerciasis and lymphatic filariasis

(Andrews et al., 2014). It's important to note that the choice of therapeutic strategy depends on the specific parasite, the nature of the infection, drug availability, local resistance patterns, and other factors. Ongoing research and collaborations between scientists, clinicians, and public health experts continue to drive the development of new and improved therapeutic approaches in parasitology.

## Conclusion

Directly or indirectly Parasites like protozoa, helminths, and arthropods interact mostly with bacteria in different possible ways. This interaction could be either advantageous or, occasionally, harmful to either or both classes of pathogens. In contrast, if the host is human, the parasite-bacteria interaction is frequently detrimental but can, occasionally, be beneficial. Clarification of the degree and significance of this communication as well as the basic mechanisms can be decoded into improved understanding of parasite biology and also better management of clinical cases. Furthermore, detection of the molecular basis could expose novel drug target therapy for both types of pathogens. Lastly, assessment of the nature of the parasite–host relationship may strengthen the prevention of an array of communicable diseases.

## References

Andrews, K. T., Fisher, G. & Skinner-Adams, T. S. (2014). Drug repurposing and human parasitic protozoan diseases. *International Journal for Parasitology: Drugs and Drug Resistance*, 4(2), 95–111.

Baron, S. (1996). Introduction to parasitology. *In: Medical Microbiology*. 4th edition. University of Texas Medical Branch at Galveston, Galveston (TX). https://www.ncbi.nlm.nih.gov/books/NBK8262/.

Bintsis, T. (2017). Foodborne pathogens. *AIMS Microbiology*, 3(3), 529.

Blake, D. P. & Betson, M. (2017). One health: Parasites and beyond. *Parasitology*, 144(1), 1–6.

Buss, P. M. (2002). Globalization and disease: In an unequal world, unequal health. *Cadernos de Saúde Públication*, 18, 1783–1788.

Campbell, S. & Soman-Faulkner, K. (2023). *Antiparasitic drugs*. StatPearls Publishing, Treasure Island (FL). https://www.ncbi.nlm.nih.gov/books/NBK544251/.

de Lima Corvino, D. F. & Horrall S. (2022). *Ascariasis*. StatPearls Publishing, Treasure Island (FL). https://www.ncbi.nlm.nih.gov/books/NBK430796/.

Dhaliwal, B. B. S. & Juyal, P. D. (2013). *Parasitic zoonoses*. Springer India. https://doi.org/10.1007/978-81-322-1551-6_1.

Dubey, J.P. (1996). *Toxoplasma gondii. In: Medical microbiology*. 4th edition. https://www.ncbi.nlm.nih.gov/books/NBK7752/.

Ebert, D., Lipsitch, M. & Mangin, K. L. (2000). The effect of parasites on host population density and extinction: Experimental epidemiology with *Daphnia* and six microparasites. *American Naturalist,* 156, 459–477.

Elsheikha, H. M. (2014). The future of parasitology: challenges and opportunities. *Frontiers in Veterinary Science*, 1, 25. https://doi.org/10.3389/fvets.2014.00025.

El-Tonsy, M. M. (2012). *Introduction to medical parasitology*. Encyclopedia of Life Support System (EOLSS-UNESCO). 53p.

Engels, D. & Savioli, L. (2006). Reconsidering the underestimated burden caused by neglected tropical diseases. *Trends in Parasitology*, 22(8), 363–366.

Ezenwa, V. O., Archie, E. A., Craft, M. E., Hawley, D. M., Martin, L. B., Moore, J. & White, L. (2016). Host behaviour–parasite feedback: an essential link between animal behaviour and disease ecology. *Proceedings of the Royal Society B: Biological Sciences*, 283(1828), 20153078.

Hay, S. I. & Rollinson, D. (2011). This first volume of 2011 brings with it five diverse and strong chapters. Preface. *Advances in Parasitology*, 74, xxi–xxii.

Herms, W. B. (1926). The Effects of Parasitism on the Host and on the Parasite. *Journal of Economic Entomology*, 19(2), 316–325.

Horn, D. & Duraisingh, M. T. (2014). Antiparasitic chemotherapy: from genomes to mechanisms. *Annual Review of Pharmacology and Toxicology,* 54, 71–94.

Jonsson, M., Buckley, H. L., Case, B. S., Wratten, S. D., Hale, R. J. & Didham, R. K. (2012). Agricultural intensification drives landscape-context effects on host–parasitoid interactions in agroecosystems. *Journal of Applied Ecology*, 49(3), 706–714.

Kantor, M., Abrantes, A., Estevez, A., Schiller, A., Torrent, J., Gascon, J., Hernandez, R. & Ochner, C. (2018). *Entamoeba histolytica*: Updates in clinical manifestation, pathogenesis, and vaccine development. *Canadian Journal of Gastroenterology and Hepatology*, 4601420. https://doi.org/10.1155/2018/4601420.

Koskella, B. (2018). Resistance gained, resistance lost: an explanation for host–parasite coexistence. *PLoS Biology*, 16(9), e3000013.

Marfurt, J., Smith, T.A., Hastings, I. M., Müller, I., Sie, A., Oa, O., Baisor, M., Reeder, J. C., Beck, H. P. & Genton, B. (2010). *Plasmodium falciparum* resistance to anti-malarial drugs in Papua New Guinea: Evaluation of a community-based approach for the molecular monitoring of resistance. *Malaria Journal,* 9, 8. https://doi.org/10.1186/1475-2875-9-8.

McKerrow, J. H., Rosenthal, P. J., Swenerton, R. & Doyle, P. (2008). Development of protease inhibitors for protozoan infections. *Current Opinion in Infectious Diseases*, 21(6), 668–672.

Moratal, S., Dea-Ayuela, M. A., Cardells, J., Marco-Hirs, N. M., Puigcercós, S., Lizana, V. & López-Ramon, J. (2020). Potential risk of three zoonotic protozoa (*Cryptosporidium* spp., *Giardia duodenalis*, and *Toxoplasma gondii*) transmission from fish consumption. *Foods*, 9(12), 1913.

Nahid, M. I., Fossøy, F., Stokke, B. G., Begum, S., Røskaft, E. & Ranke, P. S. (2020). How does human disturbance affect brood parasitism and nest predation in hosts inhabiting a highly fragmented landscape? *Global Ecology and Conservation,* 24, e01295. https://doi.org/10.1016/j.gecco.2020.e01295.

Nosten, F. & Brasseur, P. (2002). Combination therapy for malaria: the way forward? *Drugs*, 62, 1315–1329.

Olano, J. P., Weller, P. F., Guerrant, R. L. & Walker, D. H. (2011). Principles of parasitism: host–parasite interactions. *Tropical Infectious Diseases: Principles, Pathogens and Practice,* pp. 1–7. https://doi.org/10.1016/B978-0-7020-3935-5.00001-X.

Patz, J. A., Graczyk, T. K., Geller, N. & Vittor, A. Y. (2000). Effects of environmental change on emerging parasitic diseases. *International Journal for Parasitology*, 30(12-13), 1395–1405.

Peregrine, A. S., Jenkins, E. J., Barnes, B., Johnson, S., Polley, L., Barker, I. K., De Wolf, B. & Gottstein, B. (2012). Alveolar hydatid disease (*Echinococcus multilocularis*) in the liver of a Canadian dog in British Columbia, a newly endemic region. *Canadian Veterinary Journal,* 53(8), 870–874.

Picot, S., Beugnet, F., Leboucher, G. & Bienvenu, A. L. (2022). Drug resistant parasites and fungi from a one-health perspective: A global concern that needs transdisciplinary stewardship programs. *One Health,* 14, 100368. https://doi.org/10.1016/j.onehlt.2021.100368.

Pollitt, L. C., MacGregor, P., Matthews, K. & Reece, S. E. (2011). Malaria and trypanosome transmission: Different parasites, same rules? *Trends in Parasitology*, 27(5), 197–203.

Poulin, R. & Randhawa, H. S. (2015). Evolution of parasitism along convergent lines: from ecology to genomics. *Parasitology*, 142(S1), S6–S15.

Poulin, R. (2011). Evolutionary ecology of parasites. *In: Evolutionary ecology of parasites*. Princeton University Press.

Preston, D. & Johnson, P. (2010). Ecological consequences of parasitism. *Nature Education Knowledge*, 3(10), 47.

Princess, I. & Vadala, R. (2018). Pleuropulmonary parasitic infections of present times- A brief review. *Journal of Microbiology and Infectious Diseases,* 8(4), 165–180.

Rawla, P. & Jan, A. (2022). Dracunculiasis. StatPearls Publishing, Treasure Island (FL). https://www.ncbi.nlm.nih.gov/books/NBK538231/.

Sharma, N., Singh, V. & Shyma, K. P. (2015). Role of parasitic vaccines in integrated control of parasitic diseases in livestock. *Veterinary World*, 8(5), 590–598.

Singh, B., Varikuti, S., Halsey, G., Volpedo, G., Hamza, O. M. & Satoskar, A. R. (2019). Host-directed therapies for parasitic diseases. *Future Medicinal Chemistry*, 11(16), 1999–2018.

Solomon, N. U., James, M., Alphonsus, O. N. & Nkiruka, R. U. (2015). A review of host-parasite relationships. *Annual Research and Review in Biology*, 5(5), 372–384.

Suzuki, S. U. & Sasaki, A. (2019). Ecological and evolutionary stabilities of biotrophism, necrotrophism, and saprotrophism. *American Naturalist*, 194(1), 90–103.

Van den Bossche, H. (1978). Chemotherapy of parasitic infections. *Nature*, 273, 626–630.

Watson, J. M. (1965). An introduction to parasitology. *In: Medical Microbiology.* University of Texas Medical Branch, Galveston (TX). pp.1–14.

Zekar, L. & Sharman, T. (2022). *Plasmodium falciparum* Malaria. StatPearls Publishing, Treasure Island (FL). https://www.ncbi.nlm.nih.gov/books/NBK555962/.

## Chapter 3

# The Role of Nanobiotechnology in Drug Discovery: Recent Developments, Molecular Diagnostics and Future Prospects

**Mayank Raj**[1]
**Manoj Singh**[1,2,*]
**Tamanna Devi**[1]
**Vikas Kumar**[1,3]
**Sushil Kumar Upadhyay**[1]
**and Mukesh Yadav**[1]
[1]Department of Bio-Sciences and Technology, MMEC,
Maharishi Markandeshwar (Deemed to be University), Mullana-Ambala, Haryana, India
[2]Laboratory of Biomedical Nanomaterials, National University of Science and Technology "MISiS," Moscow, Russia
[3]Department of Microbiology, International Medical School, UIB, Almaty, Kazakhstan

### Abstract

Nanobiotechnology has already established its worth in a range of life science and biotechnology fields. Nanomedicine and nano-delivery systems are part of a young but fast-emerging science in which tiny materials are used as diagnostic tools or to deliver therapeutic drugs to specifically targeted locations in a controlled manner. It plays a critical role in several biological applications such as molecular imaging, biomarkers, biosensors, gene therapy, and medication delivery. It also leads to advancements in this sector. Future potential is truly related to

---

* Corresponding Author's Email: lookformanoj@gmail.com.

In: Therapeutic Advances in Human Health and Diseases
Editors: Sushil Kumar Upadhyay, Manoj Singh and Anil Kumar Sharma
ISBN: 979-8-89113-304-4

new modifications to such applications. Despite significant impediments, this technology offers enormous optimism for the future. The current review provides an up-to-date summary of recent advances in the field of nanomedicine and nano-based drug delivery systems by conducting a thorough examination of the discovery and application of nanomaterials in improving the efficacy of both new and old drugs, as well as selective diagnosis via disease marker molecules. Nanomedicine possibilities and limitations in drug transport from synthetic/natural sources to clinical applications are also highlighted.

**Keywords:** nanomaterials, nanomedicine, drug delivery, nanobiotechnology, natural products

## Introduction

Nanotechnology is the study of structures and devices in the 1-100 nanometer range, and it relates to the development of novel science and technology at the atomic, molecular, and macromolecular levels with controlled manipulation (Liu et al., 2009). This nano field could offer a slew of new study opportunities for biologists. Nanomaterials-based nanotechnology can interact with complex biological organs while consuming only a small amount of biomolecules. Nanoparticles have been used to power the field of biomedicine, which includes nanobiotechnology, drug delivery, biosensors, and tissue engineering (Mirza and Siddiqui, 2014; Yadav et al., 2016). The development and design of multifunctional nanoparticles provide interdisciplinary researchers with new opportunities to target, diagnose, and cure diseases such as cancer. As a result, they can move more easily in the human body than larger materials (Rudramurthy et al., 2016). Nanomedicine has gained popularity in recent years because nanostructures can be used as delivery agents by encapsulating or attaching therapeutic pharmaceuticals and delivering them to target tissues more accurately with a controlled release (Lam et al., 2017). Nanomedicine is a new area that applies nanoscience knowledge and technology to medical biology and illness prevention and treatment.

Despite the benefits, pharmaceutical corporations are cautious about investing more in natural product-based drug development and drug delivery systems, preferring to explore existing chemical compound libraries to discover novel medications (Beutler, 2009). Natural substances are currently being tested for the treatment of many serious illnesses, including cancer, diabetes, cardiovascular, inflammatory, and microbial diseases. This is mostly due to the special benefits that natural medicines provide, such as reduced toxicity and side effects, low cost, and strong therapeutic potential. However, concerns about the biocompatibility and toxicity of natural chemicals make employing them as medication more difficult. As a result of these issues, numerous natural substances are failing to progress through the clinical trial stages (Watkins et al., 2015). As a result, nanotechnology has had a significant impact on modern drug formulations, controlled drug release, and successful delivery. While using nanomaterials for drug delivery, the physicochemical characteristics of the drug are taken into consideration when choosing the nanoparticle. The combination of nanoscience and bioactive natural substances is highly appealing and has grown significantly in recent years. When it comes to the delivery of natural remedies for the treatment of cancer and many other diseases, it offers some benefits (Wang and Feng, 2015; Yadav et al., 2016).

The biophysical and biochemical characteristics of the targeted medications chosen for therapy are the primary factors considered when choosing the best nano-drug delivery technology. When considering the use of nanomedicine, issues like the toxicity demonstrated by nanoparticles must be disregarded. In order to reduce toxicity issues, nanoparticles have primarily been used recently in conjunction with natural products. The green chemistry technique of developing drug-loaded nanoparticles is widely promoted since it reduces the hazardous elements in the biosynthetic process. Thus, utilizing green nanoparticles for medicine delivery can reduce pharmaceutical adverse effects (Ouattara et al., 1997). Thus, nanotechnology has numerous advantages in the treatment of chronic human diseases through site-specific and target-oriented drug delivery. However, a lack of knowledge regarding nanostructure toxicity is a key concern, necessitating additional studies for better efficacy with higher safety, allowing for safer practical deployment of these medications. As a result, properly constructing these nanoparticles may be beneficial in addressing the issues related to their use. Given the foregoing, the purpose of this review is to present various nano-based drug delivery systems, significant applications of natural compound-based nanomedicine, bioavailability, targeting sites, and controlled release of nano-drugs, as well as other challenges associated with nanomaterials in medicine (Jahangirian et al., 2017).

Cancer nanomedicine is a rapidly developing discipline that uses nanoparticles to diagnose and cure cancer (Rhodes and Green, 2018). The nanoparticles are capable of better transporting ordinarily insoluble medications to local and distant tumor locations, lowering the systemic side effects associated with conventional therapeutic therapy. These nano drugs are invariably biocompatible, non-immunogenic, non-toxic, and biodegradable, lowering the possibility of unexpected loss of function or side consequences seen in standard therapy (Wang et al., 2021). Nanoparticles' versatility in terms of size, shape, selective binding capacity, high permeability and retention impact, surface modification, and so on put them in an excellent position in cancer therapy, particularly in ovarian, breast, and non-small cell lung malignancies. Modern designs and methodologies including the interaction between nano drugs and receptors on immune cells (such as antigen-presenting cells) are being used in cancer therapy for long-term anti-tumor effects (Sun et al., 2014).

## 1. Nanoparticles Used in Drug Delivery System

There are several biopolymer materials used in drug delivery systems. These materials and their qualities will be described further below.

### 1.1. Inorganic Nanoparticles

Silver, gold, iron oxide, and silica nanoparticles are examples of inorganic nanoparticles. Despite having some potential uses, there are not as many studies on them as there are on the other types of nanoparticles covered in this area. However, only a small number of nanoparticles have been approved for use in medicine, and the majority of them are still undergoing clinical trials (Choi et al., 2013). Silver and gold metal nanoparticles exhibit unique features like SPR (Surface Plasmon Resonance), whereas liposomes, dendrimers, and micelles do not possess them. They demonstrated a number of benefits, including strong biocompatibility and adaptability in terms of surface functionalization. Studies on their drug delivery-related activity have not been able to determine whether the particulate or ionized form is related to their toxicity, and despite the fact that two mechanisms, namely par cellular transport and transcytosis, have been proposed, there is insufficient information about their in vivo transport and uptake mechanism. Drugs can be conjugated to the surfaces of gold nanoparticles (AuNPs) via ionic or covalent bonding and physical absorption, and they can be delivered and controlled via biological stimuli or light activation (Kong et al., 2017).

### 1.2. Metallic Nanoparticles

The use of metallic nanoparticles in several medical applications, such as bioimaging, biosensors, target/sustained drug delivery, hyperthermia, and light ablation therapy, has grown in recent years (McNamara and Tofail, 2017). Furthermore, by modifying and functionalizing these nanoparticles with specific functional groups, they can bind to antibodies, medicines, and other ligands, making these systems more attractive in biomedical applications. Although gold, silver, iron, and copper are the most researched metallic nanoparticles, a growing interest has been shown in other types of metallic nanoparticles, including zinc oxide, titanium oxide, platinum, selenium, gadolinium, palladium, and cerium dioxide among others (Kudr et al., 2017).

### 1.3. Quantum Dots

Quantum dots (QDs) are a distinct type of fluorescent marker with unique optical qualities such as high brightness and long-term colloidal and optical stability; they are excellent for optical imaging, drug delivery and optical tracking, fluorescence assays, and other therapeutic applications. The unique optical property of QDs allows one to explore real-time dynamic events in living cells, such as interactions between intracellular proteins, intracellular signal transmission pathways, and cell development (Niemeyer, 2001). The QDs have received a lot of attention in the field of nanomedicine because, unlike typical organic dyes, the QDs emit in the near-infrared region (650 nm), Because of the low absorption by tissues and the reduction in light scattering, this is a particularly desirable quality in the field of biomedical imaging (Volkov, 2015). Furthermore, QDs of varying sizes and/or compositions can be excited by the same light source, resulting in distinct emission colors throughout a wide spectrum range (Xu et al., 2016). In this regard, QDs are ideal for multiplex imaging. QDs have been intensively explored in the realm of medicine as targeted drug delivery, sensors, and bioimaging. The literature now contains a considerable number of researched studies on the use of QDs as contrast agents for in vivo imaging (Shi et al., 2015).

## 1.4. Cellulose

Cellulose and its derivatives are widely used in drug delivery systems, primarily to modify the solubility and gelatin of medicines, allowing for modulation of the drug's release profile (Sun et al., 2019). Hansen et al. (2015) studied four cellulose derivatives for use in drug release into the nasal mucosa: methylcellulose, hydroxyl propyl methylcellulose, sodium carboxyl methylcellulose, and cationic hydroxyl ethyl cellulose. The interaction of these cellulose derivatives with another excipient was also investigated. Acyclovir was the drug model used in this technique. The polymers' viability as excipients for nasal release applications was also investigated in terms of ciliary beat frequency (CBF) and infusion through the tissue system of the nose cavity. An increase in thermally induced viscosity was seen when the cellulose derivatives were combined with polymer graft copolymer. Acyclovir penetration into the nasal mucosa was also boosted when coupled with cationic hydroxyl ethyl cellulose. According to CBF, none of the cellulose derivatives had a detrimental effect on nasal mucosa tissues and cells.

## 1.5. Xanthan Gum

Xanthan gum (XG) is a polysaccharide with a high molecular weight generated by *Xanthomonas campestris*. It's a polyanionic polysaccharide with excellent bioadhesive characteristics. Xanthan gum is commonly utilized as a medicinal excipient since it is non-toxic and non-irritating (Goswami and Naik, 2014). To treat sialorrhea, (Laffleur and Michalek, 2017) created a carrier made of xanthan gum that has been thiolated with l-cysteine to release tannin in the buccal mucosa. When compared to native xanthan gum, thiolation of xanthan gum increased buccal mucosa adherence. Tannic acid astringes and dries up the oral mucosa, but xanthan gum thiolate has higher saliva absorption. This system might be effective in lowering sialorrhea patients' salivary flow in this manner. Angiogenesis is a crucial component of soft tissue regeneration.

## 1.6. Chitosan

Chitosan can be used to function at the constrictive epithelial junctions since it has muco-adhesive qualities. As a result, continuing drug-release systems for many types of epithelia, including buccal, intestinal, nasal, ocular, and pulmonary epithelia, are frequently made of chitosan-based nanoparticles (Portero et al., 2002). To potentially administer medications into the oral cavity, Pistone et al. (Pistone et al., 2017) created nanoparticles of chitosan, alginate, and pectin. Based on the nanoparticles' solubility in saliva and their potential for cytotoxicity in oral cell lines, the formulations' biocompatibility was calculated. For at least 2 hrs, alginate nanoparticles remained the most stable in the artificial saliva, while pectin and particularly chitosan nanoparticles were unstable. Alginate and pectin nanoparticles have shown cytotoxicity in all of the test settings, although chitosan nanoparticles were the most cytocompetitive (concentration and time). The observed cytotoxicity might be brought on by the presence of $Zn^{++}$ (a cross-linking agent). Each formulation has advantages and disadvantages for oral cavity release, needing additional modification.

## 1.7. Alginate

Alginate is another biopolymer substance that has been utilized for medication delivery. When compared to cationic and neutral polymers, this anionic mucoadhesive biopolymer, which has final carboxyl groups, exhibits better mucoadhesive strength (Sosnik, 2014). For an antibacterial effect, Costa et al. (2015) created chitosan-coated alginate nanoparticles to improve daptomycin absorption into the ocular epithelium. Utilizing models made from ocular epithelial cell culture, in vitro permeability was evaluated. The pathogens involved in bacterial endophthalmitis were susceptible to the antibacterial action of nanoencapsulated daptomycin. Additionally, the ocular permeability investigations showed that daptomycin nanoparticles encapsulated in chitosan/alginate nanoparticles were able to cross the HCE and ARPE-19 cells after 4 hours of treatment. These findings suggested that drug retention in the ocular epithelium has increased with the use of this technology.

## 2. Natural Product-Based Nanotechnology and Drug Delivery

According to a World Health Organization (WHO) report, traditional medicine in poor nations provides for the fundamental medical needs of 80% of the population or more (Robinson and Zhang, 2011). The scientific community is currently concentrating on research on bioactive substances, their chemical makeup, and the pharmacological potential of various plant species in order to create novel active components that have fewer negative side effects than current ones (David et al., 2015). Plants have long been recognized as a significant source of natural substances with important therapeutic uses, and they continue to provide a wealth of resources for the development of novel, highly effective medications. However, because they come from living things whose metabolite composition shifts under stress, the finding of active chemicals from natural sources is linked to a number of problems. In order to produce synthetic substances, the pharmaceutical industries have decided to pool their resources (Namdari et al., 2017). Numerous natural chemicals' makeup and activities have already been investigated and established. The bioactive molecules present in plants include, among others, alkaloids, flavonoids, tannins, terpenes, saponins, steroids, and phenolic compounds. However, these substances typically have low absorption capacities due to their inability to pass lipid membranes due to their large molecular sizes, which results in decreased bioavailability and efficacy (Yuan et al., 2016). These compounds also have high systemic clearance, which calls for frequent administration and/or high doses and reduces the therapeutic efficacy of the medicine (Patra et al., 2016). The scientific advancement of nanotechnology has the potential to change the creation of formulations based on natural products by bringing instruments capable of resolving the issues that have hitherto prevented the widespread use of these substances in nanomedicine. The use of nanotechnology techniques in the medical area has been the subject of substantial research in recent years (Duncan and Gaspar, 2011).

Figure 1 gives some illustrations of biological substances derived from higher plants and their applications in the field of nanomedicine. For the advancement and design of contemporary pharmaceuticals as well as the improvement of current ones, the pharmaceutical industries have consistently attempted to develop and apply new technologies (Grazu et al., 2012). In this way, the rapid advancement of nanotechnology has prompted the development of new formulations using a variety of strategies, including delivering the drug to the site of action (nano-pharmaceutics), imaging and diagnosing (nano-diagnostic), creating medical implants (nano-biomaterials), and treating diseases while simultaneously diagnosing and treating those nano-theranostics (Devasena, 2017).

These natural product-based materials are currently regarded as the primary components in the manufacture and processing of new nano-formulations due to their appealing properties, such as their availability, biocompatibility, renewable nature, and low toxicity (Khan et al., 2018). Biomaterials typically allow for chemical modification in addition to the aforementioned characteristics, ensuring that they have distinctive and desired qualities for their prospective applications in the field of nanomedicine (Aravamudhan et al., 2014). Several bacteria, including *Escherichia coli, Pseudomonas aeruginosa*, *Bacillus subtilis*, and *Klebsiella pneumonia,* have been used to produce gold, silver, cadmium sulfide, and titanium dioxide with a variety of morphological properties. Due to their higher potential than all other metal nanoparticles, these nanoparticles, particularly the silver ones, have received extensive in vitro research on their ability to fight bacteria, fungi, and cytotoxicity (Pajardi et al., 2016).

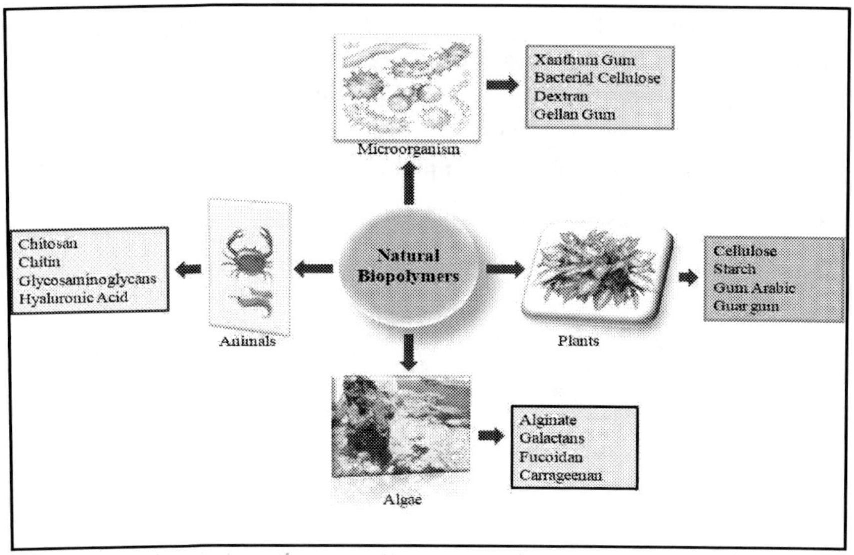


**Figure 1.** Different sources of natural biopolymers are used in nanomedicine applications. Natural biopolymers could be obtained from higher plants, animals, microorganisms, and algae.

## 3. Nano-Biotechnology in Molecular Diagnostic

In recent decades, interest in nanotechnology has exploded. Nanotechnology, to put it simply, is the use of the least amount of input to produce the greatest amount of output. The term "nano" refers to size. This technology is praised for being an excellent fusion of physics and chemistry. When this method is combined with biology, a new discipline known as nanobiotechnology is created, in which biochemical processes are altered to produce outcomes that are significantly better than those of straightforward biotechnological techniques. The successful exploitation of nano-biotechnology for diagnostic purposes has been achieved in the medical arena (Figure 2). It helps create diagnostic kits that are more accurate than the ones currently available. These tools are suited for probing biological issues at the level of cellular pores and receptors. Additionally, because of the small size of diagnostic materials, hazardous and unfavorable effects have been significantly diminished. With the help of this cutting-edge method, new diagnostic tool dimensions have been investigated. Numerous changes are currently in the planning stages (Theron et al., 2010).

It is now clear that direct analysis of DNA and protein could significantly outperform traditional molecular diagnostic techniques in terms of speed, accuracy, and sensitivity. Nanobiotechnology-based techniques can offer more accurate measurements since DNA, RNA, protein, and their functional scaffolds and compartments are assessed on the nanoscale scale.

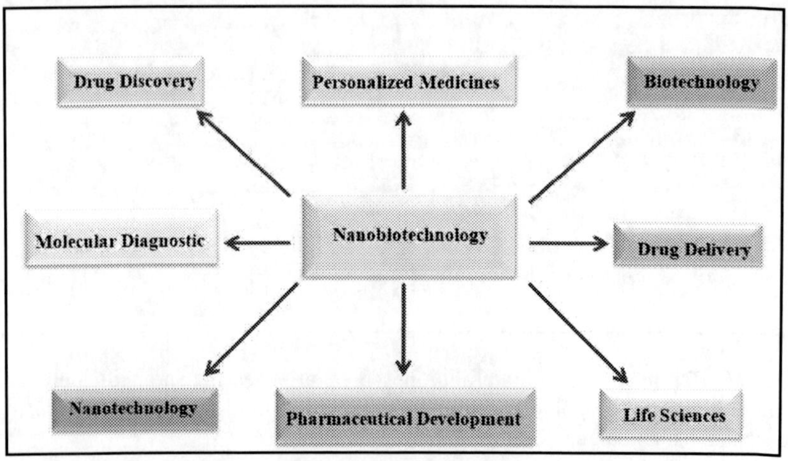


**Figure 2.** Nanobiotechnology for molecular diagnosis.

By enabling point-of-care diagnosis, integrating diagnostics with medicines, and extending the capabilities of current molecular diagnostics, nanobiotechnology is advancing the field of personalized medicine (Jain, 2007). Molecular imaging is a crucial diagnostic tool that can be used in conjunction with therapies and is a crucial foundational technology for individualized treatment. In-depth research is being done on nanoparticulate agents, such as superparamagnetic contrast agents and perfluorocarbon nanoparticles, as revolutionary molecular imaging tools that would enable noninvasive patient segmentation and characterization for the delivery of customized medicine (Caruthers et al., 2006).

## 4. Role of Nanotechnology in Cancer Diagnosis and Treatment

Across the world, researchers are working tirelessly to provide an effective alternative to chemotherapy and a better cancer cure. Whereas efforts to use nanotechnology to cure cancer and improve therapeutic efficacy are still in the early stages, nanoparticles have been widely used in biomedical applications (Setyawati et al., 2017). Because of their nano-size and extremely particular features (such as mass density, surface charge, and so on), nanoparticles have a comparatively large surface area, which permits functionalization with diverse ligands such as DNA, RNA, peptides, aptamers, antibodies, and so on. This will aid in the direct transport of the modified nanoparticle to its target spot (*in vivo*). This trait has a significant impact on the development of a broader repertoire of active theranostic substances to be integrated with nanoparticles, thereby improving the pharmacokinetic property (and thus the efficacy) of the nanoparticle for cancer treatment (Bakshi et al., 2019). The role of nanoparticles as immunogenic cargo in traditional radio- and chemotherapies, as well as advanced adjuvant therapy, is also being investigated (Das et al., 2019). The biocompatibility of nanoparticles encouraged the development of novel nanostructures, which are now being used in completely unexpected roles (as artificial antigen-presenting cells (aAPCs) or as in vivo repository of immunostimulatory molecules, for long-term antitumor activity (González-Ballesteros et al., 2019). APCs are a novel technology in cancer immunotherapy in which a nanoparticle-based system mimics the antigen-presenting cell by activating critical signal proteins against cancer, making nano-aAPCs one of the next-generation cancer nanomedicine (Song et al., 2019). Nanotechnology is important in the development of cancer therapies and the identification of cancer biomarkers. It also adds comprehensive procedures and worthy approaches against cancer through prognosis, individualized therapy, diagnosis, medication, and cancer prevention (Misra et al., 2010).

## 5. Mechanism of Action of Nanoparticles

In general, nanoparticles induce apoptosis in cancer cells by a variety of mechanisms, the best researched of which is reactive oxygen species (ROS)-mediated apoptosis. Other methods of action of nanoparticles in apoptosis induction in cancer cells include protein up- and down-regulation, immunological interventions, transcription inhibition, site-specific cytotoxicity, and so on (Ganbold et al., 2019). It is critical to note at this point that several of these events interact with one another, but the end result is apoptotic cell death (Figure 3).

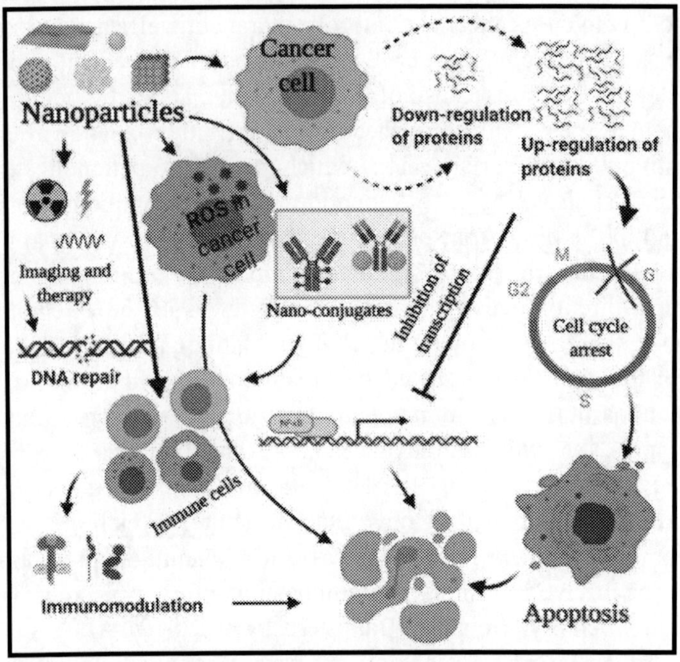


**Figure 3.** Mechanisms of cell death in cancer induced by nanoparticles.

### 5.1. Generation of ROS

ROS-induced apoptosis is one of the fundamental modes of action explored in the context of nanoparticle-induced cytotoxicity. In general, ROS acts as a double-edged sword, causing both anti-apoptotic and pro-apoptotic actions. ROS's pro-apoptotic effect includes cell cycle arrest, apoptosis, and necrosis, whereas its anti-apoptotic effect includes cell proliferation, invasion, and metastasis while blocking apoptosis (Kim et al., 2020). Proteins have the ability to cause ROS-mediated apoptosis. Most cancers lose fragile histidine triad (Fhit) proteins, but when they are recovered, they can induce apoptosis. Fhit interacts with ferrodoxin reductase to cause ROS production in Fhit-deficient cancer cells after peroxide therapy. ROS-induced apoptosis was observed in lung cancer cells after oxidative stress was generated. Fhit-negative cells were found to be resistant to ROS overproduction and, most likely, oxidative damage (Druck, 2019). Nanoparticles are more effective at inducing apoptosis because of their enhanced reactivity due to greater surface area, resulting in the excessive production of ROS. When oxidative stress develops in the cells, it releases inflammatory intermediates, which lead to DNA and protein damage, resulting in cytotoxicity (Raj et al., 2021). Silver nanoparticles encased in polysaccharides were shown to generate considerable levels of ROS, which resulted in cell death mostly via autophagy and the extension of apoptosis. Nanoparticles delivered to mitochondria through pyruvate generate ROS, which inhibits ATP generation. By suppression of ATP generation, silica carbon nanoparticles coated with lipid membranes were reported to reduce the growth of multidrug-resistant malignancies with no evidence of systemic damage (Wang et al., 2018).

## 6. Targeting the Cancerous Micro-Environment

In several proteins, the arginine-aspartic acid-glycine motif has been demonstrated to have great selectivity and affinity for the cell surface; thus, it is a good ligand for therapeutic NPs targeting cancer. A drug with a short half-life or that is particularly cytotoxicity in circulation can now be regulated in an inactive form as a pro-drug or nanoformulation. These medications target the tumor microenvironment using tumor-specific chemicals. When the tumor arrives at its target, the microenvironment facilitates its change to an active state. This tumor-activated nanoformulation treatment works by targeting stroma and tumor cells (Mansour et al., 2015). Metronomic therapy contains a given schedule that lacks extensive periods of relaxation and consists of a lower dose of chemotherapeutic medications (Hanahan et al., 2000). The innovative aspect of this notion is that it targets the tumor microenvironment, specifically endothelial cells, which are more responsive to low-dose medication administration than malignant cells. As a result, tumor angiogenesis is prevented, resulting in tumor growth suppression. Poly-base NPs become trapped in the fenestrated malignant vasculature after aggregating in the low-PH micro-environment offered by tumor tissue (Pietras and Hanahan, 2005).

## 7. Targeting Drug-Resistant Tumors

PEGylated liposomes modified with a fibronectin-mimetic peptide were discovered to target metastatic colon carcinoma cells that over-express integrin. When examining multiple types of drug resistance in cancer cells, NPs have been developed to promote endocytosis when targeting multidrug-resistant tumors, or to bypass or inhibit efflux pumps on the membrane (Garg et al., 2009). TPGS 1000 (D-α-Tocopheryl polyethylene glycol 1000 succinate) has become one of the prominent surfactants that promote the cytotoxicity of colchicines, doxorubicin, paclitaxel, and vinblastine in G-185 cells as compared to parental cells (Constantinides and Wasan, 2007). The Pluronic block copolymer (P85) is another potential and noteworthy example of a P-gb (P-glycoprotein) altering chemical (P85). In P85 treatment, membrane fluidization disrupts metabolic processes and inhibits the P-gb ATPase drug efflux pathway (Dintaman and Silverman, 2010). The NP (nanoparticle) system consists of a lipid shell and a doxorubicin-conjugated polylactic-co-glycolic acid (PLGA) core comprised of cholesterol, PEG (Polyethylene glycol) distearoylphos-phatidylethanolamine, and phosphatidylcholine. These NPs are loaded with combretastatin, a natural phenolic chemical that causes vascular disruption in cancer cells. NPs containing folic acid ligands that can connect to folate receptors were observed to accumulate in malignant cells and be over-expressed on the surface of drug-resistant cancer cells. Attempts to co-govern medications with ultrasound, photodynamic therapy, and thermo-sensitive therapy may improve the NP transport system for the comprehensive and synergistic roles of cancer nano-chemotherapy (Alexis et al., 2010).

## 8. Personalized Therapy for Cancer

The 3-targeted Para-magnetic NPs have been utilized to analyze angiogenesis in great detail, as well as non-intrusively study emerging melanoma tumors. Early detection has the potential to improve treatment efficacy, particularly in the case of melanomas (Choi et al., 2005). To target malignant tumors with increased specificity and affinity, NPs can be combined with bio-targeting ligands such as small molecules, peptides, and monoclonal antibodies. These improvements, in terms of each person's molecular profile, provide prospects for the creation of personalized oncology, in which tumor therapy, diagnostics, and detection are, personalized (Wang et al., 2007). Iron oxide NPs, when directed at tumors, tissue, cells, or organs and guided by an external magnetic field, can bind to nucleotides, proteins, antibodies, and medicines. Magnetic iron oxide nanoparticles (NPs) are currently being used to target cellular receptors such as the urokinase plasminogen activator receptor. This nano-construct permits the immersion of drug-delivering NPs in the endothelial cell layer of the tumor, tissues, or malignant cells with the goal of boosting the efficacy of drug transport via receptor-mediated endocytosis and the killing of cancer stromal fibroblasts. These iron oxide NPs may find substantial applications in cancer treatment and imaging due to their spatial imaging capacity and enhanced biocompatibility (Harisinghani et al., 2010). Breast cancer cells expressing HER2 receptors (Human epidermal growth factor receptor 2) can be connected using the HER2 antibody (Herceptin) trastuzumab, which has been coupled with iron oxide nanoparticles. When magnetically linked to the tumor, it can display improved anticancer activity with cytotoxicity compounds like doxorubicin (Tsivgoulis et al., 2014).

## 9. Cancer Treatment through Thermal Ablation

Metallic NPs have demonstrated the ability to be used in targeted hyperthermia therapy, particularly carbon nanotubes, gold silica nanoshells, iron oxide nanoparticles, and solid gold NPs (Cherukuri et al., 2010). Iron oxide nanoparticles (NPs) have been used to treat deep tissue malignancies as both therapeutic and diagnostic nanoscale agents. A greater quantity of gold NPs could be achieved by labeling gold NPs with antibodies against specific tumor cells. After the integration of NPs, the application of radio-frequency fields to cells resulted in restricted heat and tumor cell death (Mody et al.,

2010). Magnetic nanoparticles (NPs) use magnetically induced heat to provide an encouraging method for the minimally invasive excision of tiny breast tumors (Samanta et al., 2008). This technology has the advantage of allowing for the precise and selective adjustment of the degree of energy deposition, as well as adequate temperature control at the target region (Jain, 2005). It also satisfies the increased need for breast-conserving therapies. The anti-human epidermal growth factor receptor 2 antibodies can be used to transport medicines to tumors that express human epidermal growth factor receptor 2 and can trigger an anticancer response (Hilger et al., 2005). CYT-6091, a PEGylated colloidal GNP (gold nanoparticle) with tumor necrosis factor bound to its surface, has been demonstrated to augment thermal therapy and is being studied as an adjuvant (Pearce, 2011). Additionally, superparamagnetic NPs have the potential to cure malignancies by inducing hyperthermia. When these NPs are exposed to an alternating magnetic field of sufficient frequency and strength, magnetic energy is converted into thermal energy. The heat generated is subsequently transferred to the cells that revolve around the NPs. As the protein denatures and the limited temperature rises above 40°C, tumor cells die by apoptosis (Giustini et al., 2008).

## 10. Nanotechnology in the Treatment of Genetic Disorders

### 10.1. Alzheimer's Disease

Alzheimer's disease (AD), the most common form of dementia, is a neurodegenerative ailment with initial signs of decreased memory and diminishing cognitive abilities that proceed to motor system dysfunction (Sanchez-Lopez et al., 2018). A large body of data suggests a favorable link between the concentration of a peptide's soluble aggregates and the degree of dementia in Alzheimer's disease patients (Liao et al., 2012). They combine to produce insoluble fibrils, which then aggregate to form distinctive plaques. As a result, the majority of current research is focused on preventing their aggregation. Nanomaterials are used for this purpose because of their extremely small size and ability to cross the BBB. Grape resveratrol (a neuroprotective, anti-inflammatory chemical) (Cartiera et al., 2010) and OX26 mAB-conjugated solid lipid nanoparticles (SLNs) have the ability to suppress aggregation. The hydrophobic lipid core of SLNs helps the medication to disperse, enhancing its bioavailability (Goel et al., 2008). Furthermore, they are swiftly opsonized and cleared from the bloodstream, providing evidence that these SLN do not accumulate in the bloodstream unnecessarily, reducing the related dangers (Kaur et al., 2008). Similarly, a monoclonal antibody directed against fibrillary human amyloid 42 was coupled with iron oxide nanoparticles, which successfully targeted aggregates in mouse arterioles. Amyloid conjugates can also be destroyed by curcumin and water-soluble PLGA-NPs conjugated with Tet-1 peptide (Neves et al., 2013). Curcumin is an ideal candidate for AD treatment due to its anti-mutagenic, anti-inflammatory, antioxidant, anti-cholesterol, anti-tau hyperphosphorylation, and anti-amyloid characteristics. B6 peptide was coupled with curcumin-loaded PLGA-NPs (Bi et al., 2016) which reduced curcumin diameter and increased its cellular absorption. They also improved learning and memory in mice by preventing tau hyperphosphorylation and deposition. Memantine, a neuron-death-preventive medication, was similarly placed into PEG-coated PLGA-NPs, which reduced amyloid plaques and the typical inflammation of AD (Kumar and Singh, 2015). Negatively charged gold nanoparticles (AuNPs) have also been shown to be effective against amyloids since they impede fibrillization and separate fibrils in their bare state (DeTure and Dickson, 2019). This discovery identifies them as potential carriers of anti-AD medications. Protein-capped cadmium sulfate (PC-CdS) and iron oxide nanoparticles have anti-tau aggregation effects while maintaining neuroblastoma cell viability. Moreover, PC-CdS NPs can disaggregate Tau cells (Helmschrodt et al., 2017).

## 10.2. Parkinson's Disease

The second most common neurodegenerative disease is Parkinson's disease (PD). Dopaminergic (DA) neurons of the substantial nigra pars compact die selectively, resulting in the formation of synLewy bodies (Esteves et al., 2015). Six mutations have been identified as the cause of familial Parkinson's disease: SNCA, DJ-1, parkin, PINK 1, ATP13A2, and LRKK2. Because syn has been linked to the onset of PD, scientists are now looking for new ways to interfere with its expression (Desplats et al., 2012). An N-isopropyl acrylamide derivative was immobilized on oleic acid with short hairpin RNA (shRNA) and loaded in magnetic iron oxide nanoparticles in a recent work. N-isopropyl acrylamide was also treated with nerve growth factor. ShRNA successfully interfered with syn production, making it a viable treatment for Parkinson's disease. NPs containing retinoic acid (a neuroprotective substance) have also been employed and proved to be therapeutic for DA neurons. They also stimulated the creation of mRNA and transcription factor proteins that allow DA neurons to survive, especially Nurr 1 and PitX. This qualifies them for use in the prevention of Parkinson's disease (Ozansoy and Basak, 2013). Curcumin and piperine, which have exceptional cognitive and antioxidant capabilities, were recently co-loaded on glyceryl monoleate NPs. These NPs were coated with a variety of surfactants, which improved the bioavailability of the loaded chemicals. According to in vivo data, they can inhibit syn and reduce oxidative stress, apoptosis, rotenone toxicity, and the neuronal degeneration process of DA (DeCoteau et al., 2016). RNA interference (RNAi) can be used to silence certain genes. A study combined syn-targeting RNAi and polyethylenimine NPs to treat incurable neurodegenerative illnesses such as Parkinson's disease (Barber et al., 2006). The syn level was reduced by about 50% in 5 days, with no side effects (such as the induction of toxicity) identified. PEG has also been used to treat Parkinson's disease. Lactoferrin-coated PLGA-laden NPs improved the distribution of loaded rotigotine. The results showed that the cells that came into touch with it did not lose viability. In reality, free rotigotine was poisonous. It was also shown that rotigotine was heterogeneously distributed to the striatum, which is a key afflicted region in Parkinson's disease (Chen et al., 2017).

### 10.3. Amyotrophic Lateral Sclerosis

Amyotrophic lateral sclerosis (ALS) is another neurodegenerative condition in which upper and lower motor neurons, the spinal cord, and the motor cortex region are affected. Mutant superoxide dismutase (SOD) levels are also elevated in ALS patients. Misfolded SOD 1 has been proposed as the cause of the disease's orderly course. As a result, most research is focused on lowering SOD levels (Debnath et al., 2017). Although antisense Oligonucleotides (ASOs) can effectively quiet the proteins, their inability to cross the BBB rendered them ineffective. To address this issue, ASOs were loaded onto calcium phosphate lipid-coated NPs. They successfully transported ASO into a neuron-like cell line when negatively charged (Bhatt et al., 2015). It has also been observed that oxidative stress and damage contribute to ALS. DNA, RNA, and other molecules are harmed by reactive oxygen species (ROS) and reactive nitrogen species (RNS). Cerium nanoparticles can participate in redox processes that neutralize ROS and RNS. As a result, they are appropriate for use in antioxidant therapy for a variety of neurodegenerative illnesses, including ALS (Sandhir et al., 2014).

## 10.4. Huntington's Disease

Anxiety, uncontrollable movements, and chorea define Huntington's disease (HD), as an autosomal-dominant neurodegenerative disorder (Tabrizi et al., 2018). Biological materials taken from patients with neurodegenerative disorders such as Huntington's disease have been found to have oxidative stress and mitochondrial abnormalities. Electron transport chains in HD brains are also defective (Lin and Beal, 2006). 3-nitroproponoic acid (3-NP) is a neurotoxin that produces ROS; thus, researchers are looking for novel medicines that can potentially limit 3-NP formation. Curcumin, in conjunction with SLN, has also been used to treat Huntington's disease. They can alleviate the effects of 3-NP in HD mice by reducing the quantity of intermediate complex II activity. Reduced swelling of the mitochondria, lipid peroxidation, and ROS generation are among the symptoms noted. Neuromotor coordination was improved as well (Tureli et al., 2017). SLNs were loaded with rosmarinic acid and administered to 3-NO-induced mice, yielding promising outcomes. CD NPs have also been utilized to carry siRNA, which can suppress or change mutant HTT expression. CDNPs significantly reduced the amount of mutant gene mRNA and demonstrated partial toxicity, although the overall toxicity profile was satisfactory (Vij et al., 2010). Trehalose-loaded zwitterions NPs reduce amyloid and polyglutamine aggregation in the brains of Alzheimer's disease mice. Its zwitterionic shell promotes cell absorption while avoiding cytotoxicity. By creating multivalent bonds, it inhibited aggregation. This approach requires trehalose in microgram quantities; however, when employed in molecular form, millimolar concentrations are required. Other anti-amyloidogenic compounds include trehalose and zwitterions (Gibson et al., 2003).

## 10.5. Cystic Fibrosis

A mutation in the cystic fibrosis transmembrane conductance (CFTR) gene causes the deadly genetic condition cystic fibrosis. It is distinguished by aberrant trafficking in endothelial cells of various tissues. This results in extremely thick and sticky mucus that clogs organs.

**Table 1.** Summary of the various nanosystems used for treating genetic disorders

| Genetic Disease | Nanosystems | Effects | References |
|---|---|---|---|
| Alzheimer's Disease | Solid lipid nanoparticles (SLNs)<br>PLGA NPs conjugated with Tet-1 peptide | inhibited Aβ aggregation improved cellular uptake | Cartiera et al., 2010 |
| Parkinson's Disease | Retinoic acid NPs | Increased bioavailability of loaded compounds, prevented apoptosis, oxidative stress, and toxicity | Chen et al., 2017 |
| Amyotrophic Lateral Sclerosis | Calcium phosphate lipid-coated NPs | able to pass through the BBB, neutralized RNS, and ROS reactions | Bhatt et al., 2015 |
| Huntington's Disease | Curcumin SLN<br>Trehalose-loaded zwitterion NPs | Reduced the activity of intermediate complex II<br>Inhibited amyloid and polyglutamine aggregation | Vij et al., 2010 |
| Cystic Fibrosis | Lipid NPs<br>PLGA NPs coated with PEG | Increased the amount of membrane-localized CFTR<br>Effectively delivered anti-inflammatory compounds | Sato et al., 2012 |

The lung is the most commonly obstructed organ. These results in the establishment of recurring bacterial infections, which gradually degrade the lung tissues, causing pulmonary illness to proceed to the point of death (Chen et al., 2006). Correction of the CFTR gene appears to be an appealing strategy for treating this condition. Chemically modified mRNA was loaded onto lipid nanoparticles. This resulted in an increase in the number of membrane-localized CFTR, restoring its primary function as a chloride channel. Furthermore, nasal administration of these NPs reactivated chloride transport to nasal airway epithelial cells. This has proven to be a successful CFTR treatment method that can be tweaked in the future. PEG-coated PLGA-NPs have been used to treat practically every genetic/ neurodegenerative condition, including cystic fibrosis. They efficiently provided anti-inflammatory chemicals and CFTR correctors in this circumstance (Papa et al., 2014). Another intriguing strategy for treating CFTR infections was to load biodegradable NPs with antibiotics like ciprofloxacin complex. This strategy was used to combat the infections that are common with the condition. *Pseudomonas aeruginosa* was the organism targeted by these antibiotic-loaded NPs. Following treatment, mucus was tested and studied. Colloidal stability was demonstrated, and the mucus became noticeably less turbid, indicating a decrease in harmful bacteria (Sato et al., 2012). Table 1 outlines the results of certain nanomaterials used to treat genetic diseases.

## 11. Future Prospectus

One of the most exciting fields of research nowadays is nanomedicine. Cancer seems to be the best example of a disease for which non-medical technology has helped with both diagnosis and treatment, as discussed in the several sections above. The use of nanomedicine and nano-drug delivery systems is undoubtedly the trend that will continue to be the future field of research and development for decades to come by delivering the precise dosage of medication to the affected cells, such as cancer/tumor cells, without disturbing the physiology of the normal cells (Iravani, 2014). Nanobiotechnology has a great deal of credibility, but its usage has been limited because of its toxicity and environmental issues. Despite this, researchers in the domains of drug delivery, drug discovery, gene therapy, molecular imaging, biomarkers, and biosensors are investigating the potential of nanobiotechnology. The field of targeted drug delivery and clinical diagnosis has a promising future thanks to nanobiotechnology. Because it is now simpler to identify unhealthy cells quickly in the field of diagnosis, it is now possible to stop defective cells from spreading throughout the body (Fakruddin et al., 2012). This is still a futuristic research that has not yet become a reality but which humanity may achieve in the very near future. But just as with their advantages, nanomedicine's potential drawbacks must also be thoroughly investigated, both for humans and the ecosystem as a whole. Therefore, a thorough examination of the potential acute or long-term harmful consequences of novel nanomaterials on people and the environment is required. The affordability of nanomedicine would be another area of research that requires more research input as it becomes more and more popular. This discipline is currently undergoing steady development, and several previously incurable diseases could likely one day be treated using the tools of nanobiotechnology (Desai, 2012).

## Conclusion

Nanobiotechnology is now in its early stages of development. Nano-biotechnology is having a significant impact on many scientific and technological disciplines as a result of its widespread use and ongoing inventive research. A number of novel opportunities in medicine, diagnosis, and the biomedical sciences are being presented by nano-biotechnology. With the advent of something new as a result of nano-biotechnology innovation in drug delivery systems, it now appears viable to treat some incurable diseases. Novel natural biomaterials have remained in demand because of their biodegradability, biocompatibility, availability, renewable nature, and low toxicity. It's safe to state that nano-biotechnology will play a fantastic and distinctive role in the future in the treatment of human diseases and the investigation of human physiology. A conclusion that can be drawn from recent research on nano-biotechnology is that this field will play an increasingly important role in our daily lives.

## References

Alexis, F., Pridgen, E. M., Langer, R. & Farokhzad, O. C. (2010). Nanoparticle technologies for cancer therapy. *Drug Delivery,* 55–86.

Aravamudhan, A., Ramos, D. M., Nada, A. A. & Kumbar, S. G. (2014). Natural polymers: polysaccharides and their derivatives for biomedical applications. In: *Natural and synthetic biomedical polymers*. New York: Elsevier, p. 67–89.

Bakshi, S., Zakharchenko, A., Minko, S., Kolpashchikov, D. & Katz, E. (2019). Towards nanomaterials for cancer theranostics: A system of DNA-modified magnetic nanoparticles for detection and suppression of rna marker in cancer cells. *Magneto chemistry*, 5, 24.

Barber, S. C., Mead, R. J. & Shaw, P. J. (2006). Oxidative stress in ALS: A mechanism of neurodegeneration and a therapeutic target. *Biochimica et Biophysica Acta,* 1762, 1051–1067.

Beutler, J. A. (2009). Natural products as a foundation for drug discovery. *Current Protocols in Pharmacology*, 46(1), 9–11.

Bhatt, R., Singh, D., Prakash, A. & Mishra, N. (2015). Development, characterization and nasal delivery of rosmarinic acid-loaded solid lipid nanoparticles for the effective management of Huntington's disease. *Drug Delivery*, 22, 931–939.

Bi, C., Wang, A., Chu, Y., Liu, S., Mu, H., Liu, W., Wu, Z., Sun, K. & Li, Y. (2016). Intranasal delivery of rotigotine to the brain with lactoferrin-modified PEG-PLGA nanoparticles for Parkinson's disease treatment. *The International Journal of Nanomedicine,* 11, 6547–6559.

Cartiera, M. S., Ferreira, E. C., Caputo, C., Egan, M. E., Caplan, M. J. & Saltzman, W. M. (2010). Partial correction of cystic fibrosis defects with PLGA nanoparticles encapsulating curcumin. *Molecular Pharmaceutics,* 7, 86–93.

Caruthers, S. D., winter, P. M., Wickline, S. A. & Lanza, G. M. (2006). Targeted magnetic resonance imaging contrast agents. *Methods in Molecular Medicine,* 124, 387–400.

Chen, J., Patil, S., Seal, S. & McGinnis, J. F. (2006). Rare earth nanoparticles prevent retinal degeneration induced by intracellular peroxides. *Nature Nanotechnology*, 1, 142–150.

Chen, L., Watson, C., Morsch, M., Cole, N. J., Chung, R. S., Saunders, D. N., Yerbury, J. J. & Vine, K. L. (2017). Improving the delivery of SOD1 antisense oligonucleotides to motor neurons using calcium phosphate-lipid nanoparticles. *Frontiers in Neuroscience,* 11, 476.

Cherukuri, P., Glazer, E. S. & Curley, S. A. (2010). Targeted hyperthermia using metal nanoparticles. *Advanced Drug Delivery Reviews,* 62, 339–345.

Choi, S. J., Lee, J. K., Jeong, J. & Choy, J. H. (2013). Toxicity evaluation of inorganic nanoparticles: considerations and challenges. *Molecular and Cellular Toxicology,* 9, 205–210.

Choi, Y., Thomas, T., Kotlyar, A., Islam, M. T. & Baker, J. R. (2005). Synthesis and functional evaluation of DNA-assembled polyamidoamine dendrimer clusters for cancer cell-specific targeting. *Chemistry and Biology*, 12, 35–43.

Constantinides, P. P. & Wasan, K. M. (2007). Lipid formulation strategies for enhancing intestinal transport and absorption of P-glycoprotein (P-gp) substrate drugs: In vitro/in vivo case studies. *Journal of Pharmaceuticals Science,* 96, 235–248.

Costa, J., Silva, N., Sarmento, B. & Pintado, M. (2015). Potential chitosan-coated alginate nanoparticles for ocular delivery of daptomycin. *The European Journal of Clinical Microbiology and Infectious Diseases,* 34, 1255–1262.

Das, M., Shen, L., Liu, Q., Goodwin, T. J. & Huang, L. (2019). Nanoparticle delivery of RIG-I agonist enables effective and safe adjuvant therapy in pancreatic cancer. *Molecular Therapy* 27, 507–517.

David, B., Wolfender, J. L. & Dias, D. A. (2015). The pharmaceutical industry and natural products: historical status and new trends. *Phytochemistry Reviews*, 14, 299–315.

Debnath, K., Pradhan, N., Singh, B. K., Jana, N. R. & Jana, N. R. (2017). Poly (trehalose) nanoparticles prevent amyloid aggregation and suppress polyglutamine aggregation in a Huntington's disease model mouse. *ACS Applied Materials and Interfaces*, 9, 24126–24139.

DeCoteau, W., Heckman, K. L., Estevez, A. Y., Reed, K. J., Costanzo, W., Sandford, D., Studlack, P., Clauss, J., Nichols, E. & Lipps, J. (2016). Cerium oxide nanoparticles with antioxidant properties ameliorate strength and prolong life in mouse model of amyotrophic lateral sclerosis. *Nanomedicine,* 12, 2311–2320.

Desai, N. (2012). Challenges in development of nanoparticle-based therapeutics. *The AAPS Journal,* 14(2), 282–300.

Desplats, P., Patel, P., Kosberg, K., Mante, M., Patrick, C., Rockenstein, E., Fujita, M., Hashimoto, M. & Masliah, E. (2012). Combined exposure to Maneb and Paraquat alters transcriptional regulation of neurogenesis-related genes in mice models of Parkinson's disease. *Molecular Neurodegeneration*, 7, 49.

DeTure, M. A. & Dickson, D. W. (2019). The neuropathological diagnosis of Alzheimer's disease. *Molecular Neurodegeneration,* 14, 32.

Devasena, T. (2017). Diagnostic and therapeutic nanomaterials. In: *Therapeutic and diagnostic nanomaterials.* New York: Springer, p. 1–13.

Dintaman, J. M. & Silverman, J. A. (2010). Inhibition of P-glycoprotein by D-tocopheryl polyethylene glycol 1000 succinate (TPGS). *Pharmaceutical Research,* 16, 1550–1556.

Druck, T., Cheung, D. G., Park, D., Trapasso, F., Pichiorri, F., Gaspari, M., Palumbo, T., Aqeilan, R. I., Gaudio, E. & Okumura, H. (2019). Fhit–Fdxr interaction in the mitochondria: Modulation of reactive oxygen species generation and apoptosis in cancer cells. *Cell Death Disease,* 10, 1–10.

Duncan, R. & Gaspar, R. (2011). Nanomedicine (s) under the microscope. *Molecular Pharmaceutics,* 8, 2101–2141.

Esteves, M., Cristovao, A. C., Saraiva, T., Rocha, S. M., Baltazar, G., Ferreira, L. & Bernardino, L. (2015). Retinoic acid-loaded polymeric nanoparticles induce neuroprotection in a mouse model for Parkinson's disease. *Frontiers Aging Neuroscience,* 7, 20.

Fakruddin, M. D., Afroz, H. & Hossain, Z. (2012). Prospects and applications of nanobiotechnology: A medical perspective. *Journal of Nanbiotechnology,* 10(31), 1–8.

Ganbold, T., Han, S., Hasi, A. & Baigude, H. (2019). Receptor-mediated delivery of therapeutic RNA by peptide functionalized curdlan nanoparticles. *International Journal of Biological Macromolecules,* 126, 633–640.

Garg, A., Tisdale, A. W., Haidari, E. & Kokkoli, E. (2009). Targeting colon cancer cells using PEGylated liposomes modified with a fibronectin-mimetic peptide. *International Journal of Pharmaceuticals* 366, 201–210.

Gibson, R. L., Burns, J. L. & Ramsey, B. W. (2003). Pathophysiology and management of pulmonary infections in cystic fibrosis. *The American Journal of Respiratory and Critical Care Medicine,* 168, 918–951.

Giustini, A. J., Petryk, A. A., Cassim, S. M., Tate, J. A., Baker, I. & Hoopes, P. J. (2010). Magnetic nanoparticle hyperthermia in cancer treatment. *Nano Life,* 1, 17–32.

Goel, A., Kunnumakkara, A. B. & Aggarwal, B. B. (2008). Curcumin as "Curecumin": From kitchen to clinic. *Biochemical Pharmacology,* 75, 787–809.

Gonzalez-Ballesteros, N., Diego-González, L., Lastra-Valdor, M., Rodríguez-Argüelles, M. C., Grimaldi, M., Cavazza, A., Bigi, F. & Simón-Vázquez, R. (2019). Immunostimulant and biocompatible gold and silver nanoparticles synthesized using the: *Ulva intestinalis* L. aqueous extract. *The Journal of Materials Chemistry,* 7, 4677–4691.

Goswami, S. & Naik, S. (2014). Natural gums and its pharmaceutical application. *Journal of Scientific and Innovative Research,* 3, 112–21.

Grazu, V., Moros, M. & Sánchez-Espinel, C. (2012). Nanocarriers as nanomedicines: design concepts and recent advances. In: *Frontiers of nanoscience.* Vol. 4, New York: Elsevier,. p. 337–440.

Hanahan, D., Bergers, G. & Bergsland, E. (2000). Less is more, regularly: Metronomic dosing of cytotoxic drugs can target tumor angiogenesis in mice. *The Journal of Clinical Investigation*, 105, 1045–1047.

Hansen, K., Kim, G., Desai, K. G., Patel, H., Olsen, K. F., Curtis-Fisk, J., Tocce, E., Jordan, S. & Schwendeman, S. P. (2015). Feasibility investigation of cellulose polymers for mucoadhesive nasal drug delivery applications. *Molecular Pharmaceutics*, 12, 2732–41.

Harisinghani, M. G., Saini, S., Weissleder, R., Hahn, P. F., Yantiss, R. K., Tempany, C., Wood, B. & Mueller, P. (2010). MR lymphangiography using ultrasmall super paramagnetic iron oxide in patients with primary abdominal and pelvic malignancies: Radiographic pathologic correlation. *American Journal of Roentgenology*, 172, 1347–1351.

Helmschrodt, C., Hobel, S., Schöniger, S., Bauer, A., Bonicelli, J., Gringmuth, M., Fietz, S. A., Aigner, A., Richter, A. & Richter, F. (2017). Polyethylenimine nanoparticle-mediated siRNA delivery to reduce Synuclein expression in a model of Parkinson's disease. *Molecular Therapy Nucleic Acids*, 9, 57–68.

Hilger, I., Hergt, R. & Kaiser, W. (2005). Use of Magnetic Nanoparticle Heating in the Treatment of Breast Cancer. *IEE Proceedings - Nanobiotechnology*, 152, 33–39.

Iravani, S. (2014). Bacteria in nanoparticle synthesis: current status and future prospects. *International Scholarly Research Notices*, 359316.

Jahangirian, H., Lemraski, E. G., Webster, T. J., Rafiee-Moghaddam, R. & Abdollahi Y. (2017). A review of drug delivery systems based on nanotechnology and green chemistry: Green nanomedicine. *International Journal of Nanomedicine*, 12, 2957.

Jain, K. (2005). Role of nanobiotechnology in developing personalized medicine for cancer. *Cancer Research and Treatment*, 4, 645–650.

Jain, K. K. (2007). Applications of nanobiotechnology in clinical diagnostics. *Clinical Chemistry*, 53(11), 2002–2009.

Kaur, I. P., Bhandari, R., Bhandari, S. & Kakkar, V. (2008). Potential of solid lipid nanoparticles in brain targeting. *The Journal of Controlled Release*, 127, 97–109.

Khan, H. A., Sakharkar, M. K., Nayak, A., Kishore, U. & Khan, A. (2018). 14-nanoparticles for biomedical applications: An overview. In: Narayan R, editor. *Nanobiomaterials.* Cambridge: Woodhead Publishing, p. 357–84.

Kim, U., Kim, C. Y., Lee, J. M., Oh, H., Ryu, B., Kim, J. & Park, J. H. (2020). Phloretin inhibits the human prostate cancer cells through the generation of reactive oxygen species. *Pathology and Oncology Research*, 26, 977–984.

Kong, F. Y., Zhang, J. W., Li, R. F., Wang, Z. X., Wang, W. J. & Wang, W. (2017). Unique roles of gold nanoparticles in drug delivery, targeting and imaging applications. *Molecules*, 22, 1445.

Kudr, J., Haddad, Y., Richtera, L., Heger, Z., Cernak, M., Adam, V. & Zitka, O. (2017). Magnetic nanoparticles: from design and synthesis to real world applications. *Nanomaterials,* 7, 243.

Kumar, A. & Singh, A. (2015). A review on Alzheimer's disease pathophysiology and its management: An update. *Pharmacological Reports*, 67, 195–203.

Laffleur, F. & Michalek, M. (2017). Modified xanthan gum for buccal delivery– a promising approach in treating sialorrhea. *The International Journal of Biological Macromolecules*, 102, 1250–6.

Lam, P. L., Wong, W. Y., Bian, Z., Chui, C. H. & Gambari, R. (2017). Recent advances in green nanoparticulate systems for drug delivery: efficient delivery and safety concern. *Nanomedicine*, 12, 357–85.

Liao, Y. H., Chang, Y. J., Yoshiike, Y., Chang, Y. C. & Chen, Y. R. (2012). Negatively charged gold nanoparticles inhibit Alzheimer's amyloid fibrillization, induce fibril dissociation, and mitigate neurotoxicity. *Small,* 8, 3631–3639.

Lin, M. T. & Beal, M. F. (2006). Mitochondrial dysfunction and oxidative stress in neurodegenerative diseases. *Nature,* 443, 787–795.

Liu, Y., Zhu, F., Dan, W., Fu, Y. & Liu, S. (2014). Construction of carbon nanotube based nanoarchitectures for selective impedimetric detection of cancer cells in whole blood. *Analyst,* 139, 5086–5092.

Mansour, A. M., Drevs, J., Esser, N., Hamada, F. M., Badary, O. A., Unger, C., Fichtner, I. & Kratz, F. (2015). A new approach for the treatment of malignant melanoma: Enhanced antitumor efficacy of an albumin-binding doxorubicin prodrug that is cleaved by matrix metalloproteinase. *Cancer Research,* 63, 4062–4066.

Martinho, N., Damge, C. & Reis, C. P. (2011). Recent advances in drug delivery systems. *Journal of Biomaterials and Nanobiotechnology*, 2, 510.

McNamara, K. & Tofail, S. A. (2017). Nanoparticles in biomedical applications. *Advances in Physics,* 2, 54–88.

Mirza, A. Z. & Siddiqui, F. A. (2014). Nanomedicine and drug delivery: A mini review. *International Nano Letters*, 4, 94.

Misra, R., Acharya, S. & Sahoo, S. K. (2010). Cancer nanotechnology: Application of nanotechnology in cancer therapy. *Drug Discovery Today*, 15, 842–850.

Mody, V. V., Siwale, R., Singh, A. & Mody, H. R. (2010). Introduction to metallic nanoparticles. *The Journal of Pharmacy and Bioallied Sciences,* 2, 282–289.

Namdari, M., Eatemadi, A., Soleimaninejad, M. & Hammed, A. T. (2017). A brief review on the application of nanoparticle enclosed herbal medicine for the treatment of infective endocarditis. *Journal of Biomedical and Pharmacology*, 87, 321–331.

Neves, A. R., Lucio, M., Martins, S., Lima, J. L. C. & Reis, S. (2013). Novel resveratrol nanodelivery systems based on lipid nanoparticles to enhance its oral bioavailability. *International Journal of Nanomedicine*, 8, 177–187.

Niemeyer, C. M. (2001). Semi-synthetic nucleic acid-protein conjugates: Applications in life sciences and nanobiotechnology. *Journal of Biotechnology,* 82(1), 47-66.

Ouattara, B., Simard, R. E., Holley, R. A., Piette, G. J. P. & Begin, A. (1997). Antibacterial activity of selected fatty acids and essential oils against six meat spoilage organisms. *International Journal of Food Microbiology,* 37, 155–62.

Ozansoy, M. & Basak, A. N. (2013). The central theme of Parkinson's disease: Synuclein. *Molecular Neurobiology*, 47, 460–465.

Pajardi, G., Rapisarda, V., Somalvico, F., Scotti, A., Russo, G. L., Ciancio, F., Sgro, A., Nebuloni, M., Allevi, R. & Torre, M. L. (2016). Skin substitutes based on allogenic fibroblasts or keratinocytes for chronic wounds not responding to conventional therapy: a retrospective observational study. *International Wound Journal,* 13, 44–52.

Papa, S., Ferrari, R., De Paola, M., Rossi, F., Mariani, A., Caron, I., Sammali, E., Peviani, M., DellOro, V. & Colombo, C. (2014). Polymeric nanoparticle system to target activated microglia/macrophages in spinal cord injury. *Journal of Controlled Release*, 174, 15–26.

Patra, J. K., Das, G. & Baek, K. H. (2016). Towards a greener environment: Synthesis and applications of green nanoparticles. *Pakistan Journal of Agricultural Sciences*, 53, 59–79.

Pearce, J. (2011). Mathematical models of laser-induced tissue thermal damage. *International Journal of Hyperthermia,* 27, 741–750.

Pietras, K. & Hanahan, D. (2005). A multitargeted, metronomic, and maximum-tolerated dose “chemo-switch” regimen is antiangiogenic, producing objective responses and survival benefit in a mouse model of cancer. *Journal of Clinical Oncology*, 23, 939–952.

Pistone, S., Goycoolea, F. M., Young, A., Smistad, G. & Hiorth, M. (2017). Formulation of polysaccharide-based nanoparticles for local administration into the oral cavity. *The European Journal of Pharmaceutical Sciences,* 96, 381–389.

Portero, A., Remunan-Lopez, C., Criado, M. & Alonso, M. (2002). Reacetylated chitosan microspheres for controlled delivery of anti-microbial agents to the gastric mucosa. *Journal of Microencapsulation,* 19, 797–809.

Raj, S., Khurana, S., Choudhari, R., Kesari, K. K., Kamal, M. A., Garg, N., Ruokolainen, J., Das, B. C. & Kumar, D. (2021). Specific targeting cancer cells with nanoparticles and drug delivery in cancer therapy. *Seminars in Cancer Biology*, 69, 166–177.

Rhodes, K. R. & Green, J. J. (2018). Nanoscale artificial antigen presenting cells for cancer immunotherapy. *Molecular Immunology,* 98, 13–18.

Robinson, M. & Zhang, X. (2011). The world medicines situation. Traditional medicines: Global situation, issues and challenges. *Geneva: World Health Organization*, p. 1–12.

Rudramurthy, G. R., Swamy, M. K., Sinniah, U. R. & Ghasemzadeh, A. (2016). Nanoparticles: Alternatives against drug-resistant pathogenic microbes. *Molecules*, 21, 836.

Samanta, B., Yan, H., Fischer, N. O., Shi, J., Jerry, D. J. & Rotello, V. M. (2008). Protein-passivated $Fe_3O_4$ nanoparticles: Low toxicity and rapid heating for thermal therapy. *Journal of Materials Chemistry*, 18, 1204–1208.

Sanchez-Lopez, E., Ettcheto, M., Egea, M. A., Espina, M., Cano, A., Calpena, A. C., Camins, A., Carmona, N., Silva, A. M. & Souto, E. B. (2018). Memantine loaded PLGA PEGylated nanoparticles for Alzheimer’s disease: In vitro and in vivo characterization. *Journal of Nanobiotechnology,* 16, 32.

Sandhir, R., Yadav, A., Mehrotra, A., Sunkaria, A., Singh, A. & Sharma, S. (2014). Curcumin nanoparticles attenuate neurochemical and neurobehavioral deficits in experimental model of Huntington’s disease. *NeuroMolecular Medicine,* 16, 106–118.

Sato, S., Hiruma, Y., Nagata, H. & Takenaka, T. (2012). Excess Potassium and Microstructure Control for Producing Dense KNbO3 Ceramics. *Transactions of the Materials Research Society of Japan*, 37, 65–68.

Setyawati, M. I., Tay, C. Y., Bay, B. H. & Leong, D. T. (2017). Gold nanoparticles induced endothelial leakiness depends on particle size and endothelial cell origin. *ACS Nano*, 11, 5020–5030.

Shi, Y., Pramanik, A., Tchounwou, C., Pedraza, F., Crouch, R. A., Chavva, S. R., Vangara, A., Sinha, S. S., Jones, S. & Sardar, D. (2015). Multifunctional biocompatible graphene oxide quantum dots decorated magnetic nanoplatform for efficient capture and two-photon imaging of rare tumor cells. *ACS Applied Materials and Interfaces,* 7, 10935–10943.

Song, S., Jin, X., Zhang, L., Zhao, C., Ding, Y., Ang, Q., Khaidav, O. & Shen, C. (2019). PEGegylated and CcD47-conjugated nanoellipsoidal artificial antigen-presenting cells minimize phagocytosis and augment anti-tumor T-cell responses. *International Journal of Nanomedicine,* 14, 2465–2483.

Sosnik, A. (2014). Alginate particles as platform for drug delivery by the oral route: state-of-the-art. *ISRN Pharmaceutics*, 926157.

Sun, B., Zhang, M., Shen, J., Fatehi, P. & Ni, Y. (2019). Applications of cellulose based materials in sustained drug delivery systems. *Current Medicinal Chemistry,* 24, 2485–2501.

Sun, T., Zhang, Y. S., Pang, B., Hyun, D. C., Yang, M. & Xia, Y. (2014). Engineered nanoparticles for drug delivery in cancer therapy. *Angewandte Chemie, 53,* 12320–12364.

Tabrizi, S., Cleeter, M., Xuereb, J., Taanman, J. W., Cooper, J. & Schapira, A. (2018). Biochemical abnormalities and excite toxicity in Huntington's disease brain. *Annals of Neurology,* 45, 25–32.

Theron, J., Cloete, T. E. & Kwaadsteniet M. D. (2010). Molecular techniques for determining microbial diversity and community structure in natural environments. *Critical Reviews in Microbiology,* 36, 318–339.

Tsivgoulis, G., Katsanos, A. H. & Alexandrov, A. V. (2014). Reperfusion therapies of acute ischemic stroke: Potentials and failures. *Frontiers in Neurology*, 5, 215.

Tureli, N. G., Torge, A., Juntke, J., Schwarz, B. C., Schneider-Daum, N., Tureli, A. E., Lehr, C. M. & Schneider, M. (2017). Ciprofloxacin-loaded PLGA nanoparticles against cystic fibrosis *P. aeruginosa* lung infections. *European Journal of Pharmaceutics and Biopharmaceutics*, 117, 363–371.

Vij, N., Min, T., Marasigan, R., Belcher, C. N., Mazur, S., Ding, H., Yong, K. T. & Roy, I. (2010). Development of PEGylated PLGA nanoparticle for controlled and sustained drug delivery in cystic fibrosis. *Journal of Nanobiotechnology,* 8, 22.

Volkov, Y. (2015). Quantum dots in nanomedicine: recent trends, advances and unresolved issues. *Biochemical and Biophysical Research Communications,* 468, 419–27.

Wang, H., Gao, Z., Liu, X., Agarwal, P., Zhao, S., Conroy, D. W., Ji, G., Yu, J., Jaroniec, C. P. & Liu, Z. (2018). Targeted production of reactive oxygen species in mitochondria to overcome cancer drug resistance. *Nature Communications,* 9, 1–16.

Wang, J., Li, Y. & Nie, G. (2021). Multifunctional biomolecules nanostructures for cancer therapy. *Nature Reviews Materials*, 6, 766–783.

Wang, M. D., Shin, D. M., Simons, J. W. & Nie, S. (2007). Nanotechnology for targeted cancer therapy- Expert review. *Anticancer Therapy*, 7, 833–837.

Wang, N. & Feng, Y. (2015). Elaborating the role of natural products-induced autophagy in cancer treatment: achievements and artifacts in the state of the art. *BioMed Research International,* 934207.

Watkins, R., Wu, L., Zhang, C., Davis, R. M. & Xu, B. (2015). Natural product-based nanomedicine: recent advances and issues. *International Journal of Nanomedicine*, 10, 6055.

Xu, G., Zeng, S., Zhang, B., Swihart, M. T., Yong, K. T. & Prasad, P. N. (2016). New generation cadmium-free quantum dots for biophotonics and nanomedicine. *Chemical Reviews,* 116, 12234–12237.

Yadav, D., Upadhyay, S. K., Anwar, M. F. & Unnithan, J. S. (2016). A review on the patents of various metal nanoparticles: preparations and formulations. *World Journal of Pharmacy and Pharmaceutical Sciences*, 5(2), 1309–1317.

Yuan, H., Ma, Q., Ye, L. & Piao, G. (2016). The traditional medicine and modern medicine from natural products. *Molecules*, 21, 559.

## Chapter 4

# Nanotechnology-Based Biosensors to Detect Coronavirus

**Tamanna Devi**[1]
**Mayank Raj**[1]
**Manoj Singh**[1,2,*]
**Sushil Kumar Upadhyay**[1]
**Nirmala Sehrawat**[1]
**Vikas Kumar**[1, 3]
**Prabhakar Mishra**[4]
**and Nishant Srivastava**[5]
[1]Department of Bio-Sciences and Technology, MMEC,
Maharishi Markandeshwar (Deemed to be University), Mullana-Ambala, Haryana, India
[2]Laboratory of Biomedical Nanomaterials, National University of Science and Technology "MISiS," Moscow, Russia
[3]Department of Microbiology, International Medical School, UIB, Almaty, Kazakhstan
[4]Department of Biotechnology, School of Applied Sciences,
REVA University, Bengaluru, Karnataka, India
[5]Avishka Council of Industrial and Allied Biosciences, Greater Noida, India

## Abstract

By creating diagnostics and therapies, nanotechnology has the ability to create novel COVID-19 defense mechanisms. Due to the appearance of novel variations all over the world, the identification of the emerging

* Corresponding Author's Email: manoj.singh@mmumullana.org.

In: Therapeutic Advances in Human Health and Diseases
Editors: Sushil Kumar Upadhyay, Manoj Singh and Anil Kumar Sharma
ISBN: 979-8-89113-304-4

coronavirus (COVID-19) has captured the attention of the research community since December 2019. Coronavirus early diagnosis is difficult to regulate and difficult to avoid. By applying suppressing tactics, this epidemic can be ended, improving outcomes and saving more lives. As a result, the study demonstrated that COVID-19 must only be controlled by using public health strategies like testing, isolation, and social exclusion. It has taken a lot of effort to diagnose coronavirus. Different testing techniques have been created, selected, and modified for quick and precise detection. The detection of SARS-CoV-2 is necessary for advanced molecular identification because it is thought to be the primary cause of this epidemic. According to studies, a number of molecular assays are crucial for confirming coronavirus infection. Numerous serology-based techniques, such as point-of-care assays and high-throughput enzyme immunoassays that support the detection of COVID-19, are also utilized in the detection and identification of coronavirus. Both of these assays take a lot of time and are less reliable in terms of diagnosis. To stop the spread of SARS-CoV-2, we have concentrated on nanotechnology-based detection methods in this review, including nanoparticles and biosensors.

**Keywords:** COVID-19, SARS-CoV-2, nanotechnology, molecular diagnosis, biosensors

## Introduction

Nanomaterials have lately received a lot of awareness, due to the rising need to manage desired molecules existing in humans and their environment (Tansil et al., 2006). A nanomaterial is made up of nanoparticles (NPs) that seem to be at least 100 nm in one dimension or smaller than that. The term "nanotechnology" is used when referring to materials that are several hundred nanometers or sub-nanometers in size (Ozin et al., 2009). Due to its potential use in the fields of nanoelectronics, structural components, catalysis, magnetic data storage, biosensors, and biomaterials, Nanomaterials are currently undergoing rapid development (Cao et al., 2004).

A biosensor is defined as a device with a biological receptor unit or bioinspired receptor unit, having distinct specificities towards related analytes. These analytes are commonly biological in origin and include DNA or genetic material from bacteria, viruses, proteins originated by the immune system (antibodies and antigens), and living organisms that have been infected or polluted. Whenever a biological receptor component with uniqueness is present, such analytes may also include simple biomolecules like glucose or sugars. The effective signal recording of the bio-recognition event is one of the different difficulties in biosensor development (transduction). These transducers convert the electrochemical, electro-chemiluminescent, magnetic, gravimetric, or optical signals that result from analytes' interaction with the biological element. Nanomaterials are intriguing options for improving sensitivities and lowering detection limits to even single molecules since they have the potency to trap a good amount of bioreceptor components in smaller quantities and even operate as a transduction element. Among these nanomaterials, graphene, carbon nanotubes, gold nanoparticles, semiconductor quantum dots, polymer nanoparticles, and nanodiamonds have all been the subject of extensive research. Due to the extensive development of this study subject, this analysis focuses on nanoparticles that offer additional positive features that "only" an increased surface area in order to present a non-exhaustive summary of the benefits of nanomaterials (Michael et al., 2014).

The coronavirus is a polyadenylated, 30 kb enclosed RNA virus that is spherical or pleomorphic and is single-stranded, positive-sense (Dharmendra and Rishabha, 2020). It has always been difficult to diagnose viral antigens worldwide. When compared to DNA viruses, RNA viruses' rate of mutation is substantially higher, which leads to the accumulation of changes in their genomes and the generation of false-negative results. Due to the symptoms' resemblance to those of many other potential pathogens, such as para-influenza viruses and respiratory syncytial viruses, SARS-CoV-2 is difficult to diagnose.

The most crucial element in ensuring the demand for healthcare is testing. Coronavirus diagnostics have been developed after extensive investigation. There are numerous detection methods for the various coronavirus strains. RT-PCR is the most reliable and cost-effective method for identifying this etiological agent, although it has several significant drawbacks.

a. Patients may not accept the sample collection, particularly infants small children, and older patients,
b. Some RT-PCR assays exhibited greater sensitivity difficulties.
c. RT-PCR has a high operational cost. For the identification of COVID-19, a number of serological-based methods are being initiated.

For the purpose of keeping track of the SARS-CoV-2 infection, certain point-of-care (POC) tests have also been used. These assays, however, have some drawbacks, such as more cumbersome procedures, higher cost-effectiveness, and increased sensitivity, which make them less advantageous than recently developed nano-based detection approaches (Loeffelholz and Tang, 2021). There is a novel technology in which antibody arrays are bound with nanoparticles that have the potency to detect antigenic proteins in samples of nasal swabs as shown in Figure 1.

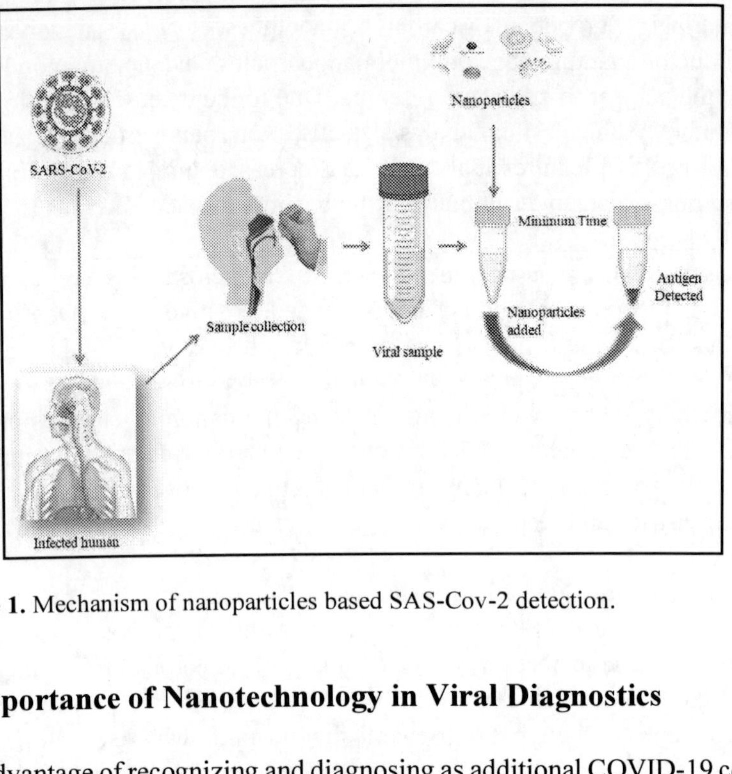


**Figure 1.** Mechanism of nanoparticles based SAS-Cov-2 detection.

## 1. Importance of Nanotechnology in Viral Diagnostics

The advantage of recognizing and diagnosing as additional COVID-19 control tools was regarded to be the rapid deployment of control actions to isolate and manage contamination. Due to the reaction of the vaccination and the simple fact that any virus multiplies quickly, it is crucial to develop robust, sensitive, and advanced detection methods in order to stop viral outbreaks. Nanotechnology shows potential in this situation. Nanotechnology has actually been crucial to rescuing COVID-19. The market for diagnostic processes, testing, PPE, coverings, air filters, disinfectants, and numerous additional products has already been addressed (Sivasankarapillai et al., 2020).

The Nanotechnology Products Database (NPD), utilized in several number of COVID-19 applications is a reliable source of information related to nanotechnology products. Nanomaterials may have a significant positive impact on the treatment of viral infectious diseases such as the human immunodeficiency virus (HIV), the Ebola virus, and the SARS-CoV, according to research (Iannazzo et al., 2018). Numerous viral infections can be successfully treated with the help of nanotechnology, as demonstrated in this case (Chakraborty et al., 2020). We will have access to a variety of nano-based diagnostic methods developed for the speedy identification and effective management of diseases like COVID-19 here. Virus detection is particularly challenging because of its small size and also due to the intracellular life cycle, which makes it difficult for smaller lab-scale optical microscopes to differentiate (Draz et al., 2018).

Similar to other viral infections, SARS-CoV-2 required rapid response tests with simplified operating and effective detection limits (Cheng et al., 2009). In the early stages of this diagnosis, when no characteristic initial appearances had been seen, it was difficult to examine COVID-19 purely on clinical signs (Huang et al., 2021). Although speedy diagnosis for significant clinical cases was not possible with whole-genome sequencing due to its lengthy sequencing time and high equipment requirements, it was incredibly accurate for the diagnosis of COVID-19 (Wu et al., 2020). Real-time reverse transcription polymerase chain reaction (rRT-PCR) was employed in public health and clinical research facilities during the COVID-19 outbreak to identify SARS-CoV-2 due to its high specificity and sensitivity (Corman et al., 2020). Apart from this, the RT-PCR methods rely substantially on high-end equipment, knowledgeable personnel, and a reliable power source.

The RT-PCR test needs a few hours to complete, starting with the clinical cases and ending with the dissemination of the results. Several areas, in particular, where the COVID-19 pandemic commonly occurred lacked the infrastructure required for dependable diagnostic facilities for RT-PCR, field studies, and laboratories (Chu et al., 2020). Given the enormous number of patients and the inherent shortcomings of the RT-PCR and other procedures, particularly in terms of accessibility and test cost, the need for new, inexpensive testing techniques that can aid in the early detection of the illness cannot be stressed. The development of SARS-CoV-2 detection tools and sensors based on nanoparticles has taken a lot of time and effort. It is crucial to design biosensing techniques that benefit from particular NP properties, such as their quantum effects, high surface-to-volume ratio, high adsorption capacity, side effects, and reactive capacity compared to their bulk form.

Additionally, because NPs are easily customizable in terms of shape and size, it is possible to alter or immobilize the exteriors with a wide range of biological species via covalent or non-covalent bonding, enhancing their biosensing characteristics in regards to low limits of detection (boosted up to a few orders of magnitudes), highly sensitive selectivity, and rapid response to the sample analytes. (Srivastva et al, 2021; Kokkinos, 2019). Capturing the extremely minute signals that take place between different biological species (bio-receptors and analytes), such as those between DNA and RNA, is one of the most challenging aspects of building biosensors. This issue can be resolved by using nanomaterials as labels to create a considerable signal boost that is prominent enough to be easily identifiable. Labeling is possible by attaching the appropriate DNA/bio-recognizing sensor to metal nanoparticles (Au NPs/Ag NPs) and quantum dots (Cd/Pb) (Sivasankarapillai et al., 2021). Quantum dots and polymeric nanoparticles are examples of organic nanoparticles used in diagnostics, while silica, gold, and silver nanoparticles are examples of inorganic nanoparticles.

## 2. Detection of COVID-19 by Different Kind of Nanoparticles

Detection of viral antigens is a challenging task as they acquire variation in their genomic sequences a lot of studies and research have been done to diagnose for coronavirus. However, all other methods are less preferred over the latest nanoparticle-based detection methods. Coronavirus can be detected by different nanoparticles as shown in Figure 2.

### 2.1. Gold Nanoparticles

The ability to accurately detect coronavirus in the genome of humans may be provided by nanoparticles (NPs). Molecular-based detections are not much preferred as compared to serological detections because they are more economical and take less time to perform. Point-of-care (POC) devices made of gold nanoparticles are very effective for detecting IgG, IgM, and IgA antibody reactions in human hosts against spike 1 and spike 2 coronavirus structural proteins, as well as the nucleocapsid N protein (Jiao et al., 2020). Gold nanoparticles show unique properties for coronavirus genome diagnosis, including reduced sample consumption, higher stability and cytocompatibility, relatively inexpensive testing, no need for expensive tools, and quick reaction time (Ranjan et al., 2021). In this latest method, gold nanoparticles (AuNP) and antibody arrays were used to identify antigenic proteins in nasopharyngeal swab samples. For this, a very sensitive lateral-flow chromatographic (AuNP-LF) test based on gold nanoparticles was created (Du et al., 2020).

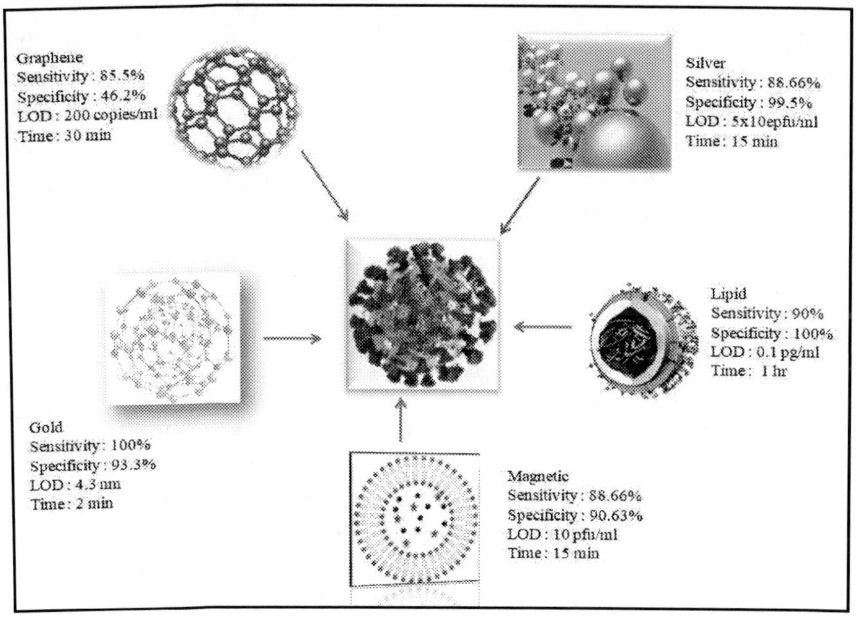


**Figure 2.** Different nanoparticles for the detection of SARS-CoV-2.

## 2.2. Silver Nanoparticles

When it comes to various bacterial, fungal, and viral species, silver (Ag) possesses a broad spectrum of antibacterial activity. Researchers assert that silver nanoparticles (AgNPs) are less likely to cause microbial resistance than other antibiotics, which is a common concern in modern society (McKaya et al., 2020) and in this context; silver nanoparticles are expected to be much more efficacious against SARS-CoV-2 for its suppression. By limiting the respiratory enzymes and reducing the electron transport systems, $Ag^{+}$ ions prevent the proliferation of viruses and impede DNA activity. Using a variety of AgNP sizes and concentrations, the promising antimicrobial effect of AgNPs against new coronaviruses was openly examined. The COVID-19-

infected patient's nasal swab was used to culture the veroE6 cell line to create virus propagation. 5-10 cells were used to fertilize 96-well plates. After that, the plates were dissolved in 10% FBS/DMEM and let to develop overnight. Then, supernatants were removed and added to the appropriate virus-diluted wells. For 96 hours, incubation took place at 37°C. A quadruplicated test was used to estimate MOI (Multiplication of infection) and the median tissue culture-infecting dose and the required amount of Ag nanoparticles was created. The Cell Titer-Glow assay for cell feasibleness was carried out, and GIoMax was used to measure luminescence intensities. The amount of viral copies in the culture supernatant was measured using RT-qPCR. Results indicate that AgNPs demonstrate cytotoxicity at the highest level from 20 parts per million veroE6 cells through the generation of reactive oxygen species (ROS) (Jeremiah et al., 2020).

## 2.3. Magnetic Nanoparticles

The use of nanoparticles to treat viral infections produced excellent and encouraging outcomes. Recently, it was found that metallic oxide NPs with a great detection level have antibacterial action (Abo-zeid and Williams, 2020). Reactive oxygen species (ROS) production has antimicrobial effects; it oxidizes many microorganism sites, which causes cell death owing to non-resistive activity (Abo-zeid et al., 2020). Additionally, investigations into the antibacterial activity of $Fe_3O_4$ nanoparticles against rotavirus, dengue virus, and H1N1 influenza viruses as well as other viruses have been described (Paunovic et al., 2020). Molecular docking investigations have identified the potential antiviral effect of iron oxide NPs on HCV and SARS-CoV-2 (Gutierrez et al., 2009). This demonstrates the effective engagement of the new coronavirus and HCV glycoproteins E1 and E2 with the receptor-binding region of $Fe_2O_3$ and $Fe_3O_4$. While $Fe_3O_4$ is associated with the S1-RBD antigen, $Fe_2O_3$ forms a stable complex with HCV E1 and E2. These interactions could affect the antiviral activity as well as conformational changes in the virus structure (Abo-zeid and Williams, 2020).

## 2.4. Graphene Nanoparticles

To create graphene-based nano-sheets, graphite, a sp2 hybridized allotropic form of carbon, is organized in a configuration resembling a honeycomb lattice (Raval et al., 2020). These nano-sheets are notable for their lightweight, distinctive physical, chemical, optical, thermal, and electrical properties, as well as their high surface-to-mass ratio, surface-enhanced Raman scattering, and large surface area. These characteristics make them beneficial for biosensing and imaging virus-based antigens in human hosts (Alphandery, 2020; Vermisoglou et al., 2020). When used as a diagnostic tool, graphene-based nanoparticles (GBNs) can detect human coronavirus (SARS-CoV-2). To improve the sensitivity and specificity of graphene nanoparticles, scientists can add functional groups to the surface of the particles. Reduced graphene, functionalized graphene, and graphene oxide are some of the graphene-based complexes that are created when graphene is combined with other substances and are beneficial for biomedical operations, drug administration, and a variety of therapeutic uses (Cordaro et al., 2020). For the synthesis of GBNs, mechanical and physicochemical exfoliation-based top-down methods are employed (Seo et al., 2020).

## 2.5. Lipid Nanoparticles

The challenges of nanotechnology and the development of treatments for SARS-CoV-2 are similar to those of other infections (Kostarelos, 2020). In order to produce vaccines against the coronaviruses that have previously been identified, similar methods include MERS and SARS (Nicogossian, 2012). Researchers might focus on particular intracellular and cellular processes that are implicated in the pathological processes of SARS-CoV-2. The greatest way to prevent viral rebounds while treating viral infections is with controlled nanocarrier drug release (Sago et al., 2018). As a result, techniques based on nanomedicine can enhance the development of therapeutics against SARS-CoV-2. Lipid nanoparticles carrying siRNA are used in nanobiotechnology to help fight diseases (Adams et al., 2018). There are numerous instances of lipid-based NPs that help with antiviral activities, such as mesoporous silica lipid nanoparticles that improve the systemic circulation time and biocompatibility through an *in vivo* procedure and suppress some viral activities (LaBauve et al., 2018). Additionally, protein-based pharmacological systemic immunotoxicity can be avoided by using nanocarriers, which can also advance immuno-oncology therapies (Zhang et al., 2020).

## 3. Developments in Nanotechnology-Based Corona Virus Detection

### 3.1. Colorimetric Assay

A "naked-eye" colorimetric SARS-CoV-2 diagnosis test that is simple, quick, and precise is currently urgently needed. Specialized antisense nucleotide sequences (ASOs) for the N phosphoprotein of SARS-CoV-2 were altered by thiol for its conjugation, and colorimetric assays take advantage of AuNPs' optical characteristics. After RNA isolation, detection was carried out in less than ten minutes. Thiol-modified ASOs covered the NPs (ASO) aggregate whenever the targeted RNA sequence from SARS-CoV-2 was detected as shown in Figure 3, and a modification in surface Plasmon resonance was noticed. When RNase is added, the RNA segment is separated from the RNA-DNA hybrid, which causes the aggregation of AuNPs to help produce a visually discernible precipitate. This approach yielded an LOD of 0.18 mg/L of RNA with a SARS-CoV-2 virus load when RS-CoV viral RNA is present (Moitra et al., 2020).

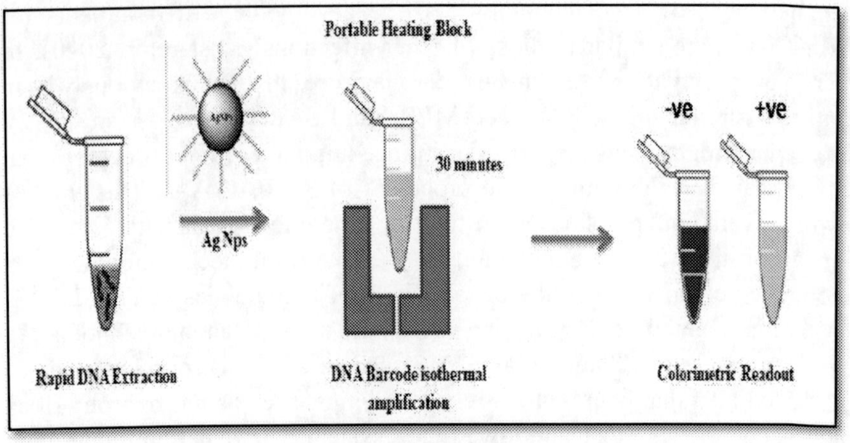


**Figure 3.** Colorimetric test for fast detection of SARS-CoV-2.

### 3.2. Micro Fluidic Devices

Another method for use as a proof-of-concept test is microfluidic devices. Using materials like poly-dimethylsulfoxide, paper, or glass, these palm-sized chips are imprinted with micrometer-sized channels and reaction chambers, offering benefits including reduced size and acquiring just a little sample volume and a quick detection time. These microfluidic chips' fundamental working idea is to mix and separate liquid samples utilizing capillary action as well as electro-kinetic characteristics (Foudeh et al., 2012). Various antibodies against three STIs can be found using microfluidic devices and an app attachment for smartphones. In Rwanda, the platform demonstrated sensitivity and specificity of 100% and 87%, respectively, when evaluated on 96 patients (Laksanasopin et al., 2015). Microfluidic devices can be used because of how simple and dependable they are and that's why they are used to detect viruses.

The nucleocapsid (N) protein, which is among the most common COVID-19 biomarkers, may now be detected using a microfluidic chip immunoassay that is based on platinum-decorated gold nanoparticles (Au-Pt NPs) (Figure 4). This method's sensitivity surpasses that of paper-based detection. Excellent stability and catalytic performance in challenging conditions are displayed by the synthesized Au-Pt NPs. Unaided identification of N protein in the small hectogram range (about 0.1 pg/mL) and throat swab sample detection in less than 40 minutes are made possible by the catalytic amplification of Au-Pt NPs. Because this microfluidic chip immunoassay is simple to use and read out without apparatus assistance, it is more suited for on-site diagnosis and future pathogen surveillance. Within 40 minutes, this microfluidic chip immunoassay could identify SARS-CoV-2 N protein at concentrations as low as 0.1 pg/mL. By switching detecting antibodies, the microfluidic chip immunoassay platform has the potential to be expanded for the diagnosis of additional viruses and biomarkers. It also displayed great sensitivity and ease of operation and readout without equipment. Future research could lead to the development of multiplex microfluidic systems for the simultaneous and multiple recognition of respiratory viruses including SARS-CoV-2, influenza, respiratory syncytial virus (RSV), parainfluenza virus, and adenovirus. The strong catalytic activity of Au-Pt NPs is responsible for the proposed microfluidic chip immunoassay's exceptional performance. The benefits of Au-Pt NPs include good stability, affordability, ease of manufacture, and simplicity in combining with the microfluidic chip immunoassay, which expands the range of potential applications (Feng et al., 2022).

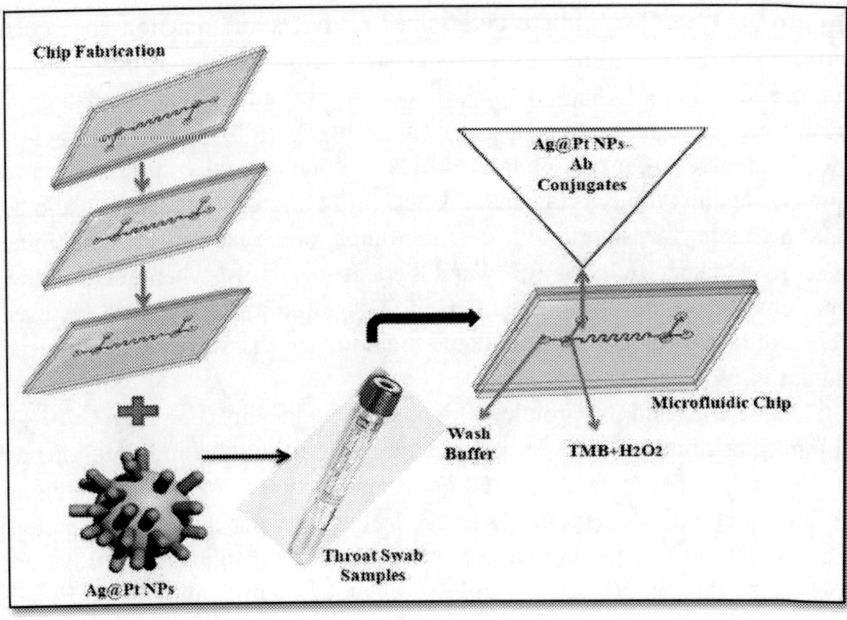


**Figure 4.** Platinum-decorated gold nanoparticle-based microfluidic chip.

## 3.3. Point-of-Care Testing

PoC testing is explained as testing carried out at a house or in a facility in which the patient or infected is receiving care utilizing a kit or strip as shown in Figure 5. The biosensor, which is utilized to conduct a biochemical assay to diagnose the pathogen, is a very crucial part of PoC testing (Vashist., 2017). The benefits of adopting PoC testing include: I minimum storage and testing space requirements; (ii) extensive analysis; (iii) analysis can be conducted in a lot of different places; and (iv) flexibility in fulfilling various medical demands. Despite sending samples to specialized labs, PoC testing allows for diagnosis. One such PoC approach being developed for the detection of COVID-19 is an LFA for SARS-CoV-2 (Xiang et al., 2020). The gadget is more dependable and sensitive when an LFA is coupled with nanoparticles. The membrane of lateral flow strips is typically constructed of nitrocellulose and is covered with two lines: the test line, which is an antibody coupled with a nanoparticle, and the control line, which is an antibody capture line.

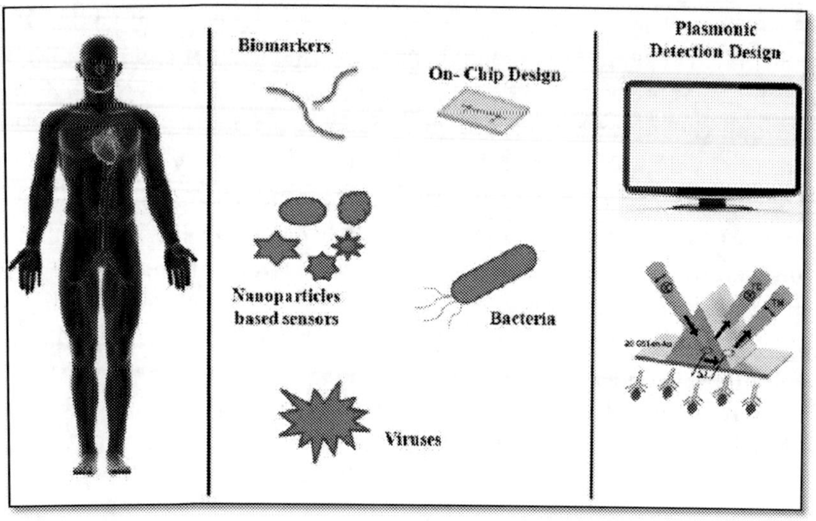


**Figure 5.** Point of care testing.

The sample is placed on the membrane, also referred to as the sample pad, and analytes move along the strip by capillary action until they reach the first line. Antigens in the analytes bond to the conjugate as they progress through the initial test line, and this complex passes through the membrane. A colored line appears when it combines with the detected antibodies at the second line. IgG and IgM (IgM) have corresponding clinical sensitivity, specificity, and precision values of 81, 100, and 86% and 57, 100, and 69% from an LFA. With a sensitivity of 82%, this test can identify IgM and IgG (Xiao et al., 2020).

## 3.4. Separation Based on Magnetic Nanoparticles

Magnetic nanoparticles (MNPs) have been employed in biomagnetic separation and immunoassays to bind particular target molecules shown in Figure 6 (Huang et al., 2019; Wang and Lin., 2020). Due to its high specificity and simplicity as well as the low cost of the necessary fundamental resources, biomagnetic separation is receiving a lot of attention from a variety of sectors (Safarik and Safarikova, 1999). To improve immunoassay sensitivity and the efficacy of biomagnetic separation, MNPs have undergone a number of alterations. The polymer coating is one such modification (Nagaoka et al., 2011). Due to their distinctive features, magnetic nanoparticles (MNPs) have drawn attention as potential materials for quick and highly sensitive diagnosis procedures (Xu et al., 2019). First, when an external magnet is present, MNPs behave as "nano-magnets". Whenever the magnetic field is eliminated, they migrate quickly in the direction of the external magnet (Ha et al., 2018). Second, it is widely known that MNPs can be magnetically stabilized when conjugated with a variety of biomaterials. These properties allow MNPs to magnetically pre-concentrate target materials from a very low concentration in two steps: (i) the target materials communicate with bioconjugated MNPs, and (ii) the target material-bioconjugated MNPs are obtained with a magnet from the outside and re-dispersed into a small amount of matrix for the pre-concentration of the samples to increase the detection sensitivity. Additionally, because the biological components that have no contact with MNPs are non-magnetic, MNPs provide low background noise (Gowri et al., 2021).

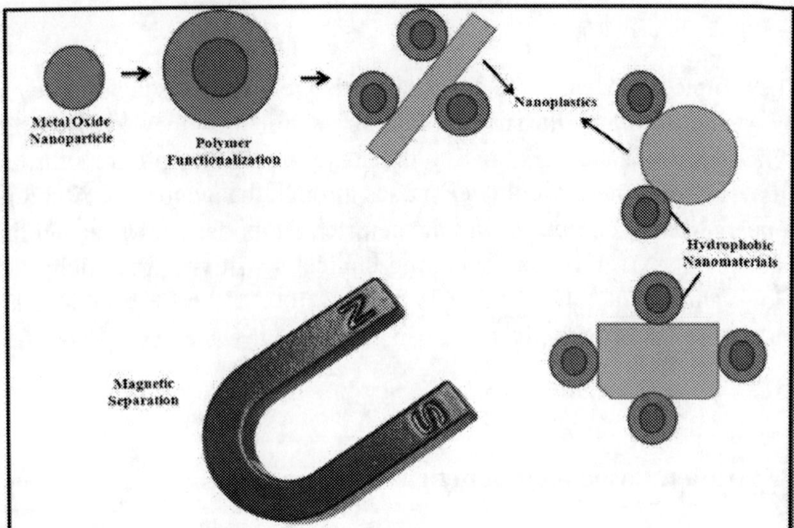


**Figure 6.** Separation based on the magnetic nanoparticle.

Additionally, MNPs have a large surface area, which enables quick interaction between bioconjugated MNPs and the target materials to enable quick detection times. In fact, MNPs have been successfully used to quickly and very sensitively detect a variety of specific analytes from bacteria (Sánchez-Cano et al., 2021) and viruses (Mun et al., 2010). It is also important to point out that the most recent research has used MNPs-based immunoassays with a CRISPR (clustered regularly interspaced short palindromic repeats)/Cas system, an appealing technique for precise detection of infectious bacteria and viruses. For instance, Kim et al., 2020 used MNPs to detect multidrug-resistant (MDR) bacteria using a CRISPR/Cas system in conjunction with a surface-enhanced Raman scattering (SERS) assay. Due to their superparamagnetic characteristics, which are suited to SERS and allow for the efficient separation and purification of targeted samples, MNPs attain great sensitivity in the experiment. To identify *Salmonella typhimurium* (*S. typhimurium*) in food samples, MNPs were also added to a CRISPR/Cas system (Cai et al., 2021). In this study, magnetic separation of the target bacteria is made possible by polyclonal antibody-conjugated MNPs, enabling quick and extremely sensitive detection.

## 4. Future Aspects and Challenges

The COVID-19 pandemic posed a terrifying risk to human societies everywhere, but it should also be viewed as an opportunity to reaffirm to our international community that adopting multi- and inter-disciplinary approaches, supporting diversity in the formation of problem-solving groups, and exchanging knowledge between nations would all be crucial to arriving at novel and important scientific solutions. Nanotechnology is anticipated to play a significant role in the struggle against COVID-19 by developing biosensors to detect the virus in its initial stages of infection, avoiding its spread using nanocomposites which may also be utilized to disinfect public health care equipment, and ultimately using vaccines to provide resistance against transmission. The development of diagnostic test kits can make use of the optical and magnetic properties of various NPs. However, more research is necessary for early and instant virus detection (Pandey et al., 2020). Additionally, it has been successfully demonstrated that adding NPs to preference-based biosensing systems enables the rapid, accurate, and reliable detection of COVID-19, MERS, and SARS. Nanomaterial-based biosensors have enabled the development of improved biosensor capabilities, such as high selectivity, sensitivity, and low thresholds for detection. Silicon and gold nanoparticles have been successfully used in the development of an immunosensor and a DNA sensor for MERS and COVID-19, respectively. One of the important features of nano biosensors is their potential for downsizing into inexpensive, integrated devices that function equivalent to handheld electrochemical readers. Despite these encouraging characteristics, only a tiny number of nano biosensor detection samples have been developed and successfully applied in actual clinical research up to this point. The ones that are sold are thin membrane segments that look like paper and are covered in gold nanoparticle-antigen combined in the conjugation pad and nitrocellulose membrane antigens (Antiochia, 2020). Moving forward, compared to the SARS-CoV-1 outbreak in 2003, artificial intelligence (AI) has had a higher impact on the identification of COVID-19 infections in medical images (chest X-rays and CT scans), contact tracing, and evidence-based policymaking. Artificial intelligence-enabled devices like AI robots, digital toilets, and smartphones could be very useful for tracing, diagnosing, and treating diseases. Since the smart toilet is a non-invasive device that may gather and analyze feces and urine, it might be crucial in assisting with the diagnosis of COVID-19. The robot can work in dangerous situations, relieving pressure on front-line medical staff. The AI robot can collect throat samples. The diagnostic and service robots will be employed in crowded public locations including customs, airports, ports, and train stations. Ideally, as AI technology develops, robotics will become more intelligent and effective (Jamshidi et al., 2020). Patients with COVID-19 who are asymptomatic and who have been distributed are more likely to transmit the disease to others who are nearby, making preventing and controlling an epidemic challenging and needing long-term surveillance and tracking. The virus detection in urine and stool specimens of certain validated patients, including asymptomatic cases, is further proof of the great demand for ultrasensitive diagnostic methods. A smartphone equipped with different opt mechanical add-ons that allow the accuracy of bright field, fluorescence, spectroscopy, or phase imaging is a suitable read-out platform. These instruments allow for precise diagnosis in remote locations. Due to the miniaturized sequencing instruments, it may now be used on-site outside of the lab. Combining several assays, such as CT imaging, lateral flow immunoassay, clinical symptoms, and viral RNA detection, can lead to a more accurate diagnosis. In actual therapeutic settings, however, it is necessary to strike a compromise between cost, time, precision, and specificity (Yuan et al., 2020). In the end, there is still much work to be done in order to develop quick nano biosensors that can detect diseases like coronaviruses that could spread quickly and jeopardize human life. But because of their outstanding potential for performing quick, accurate, in-person diagnostics and, most importantly, for tracking infectious diseases and preventing new pandemic outbreaks, NPs, like other occupations, are undeniably advantageous and inspire a lot of hope for future advancements.

## 5. Current Issues and Solutions

Similar to other forms of technology, nanotechnology is composed of numerous technical fields, such as physics, biology, chemistry, material science, self-assembly, and electronics. It also has some disadvantages related to the use of nanomaterials or nanoparticles in the creation of nanotechnology products. The toxicological and hazardous impacts that nanoparticles have on the environment and human health are fundamentally different from those that the same bulk materials have because of their exceptional physicochemical properties. Additionally, nanoparticles degrade very slowly, increasing the likelihood of their buildup in the administration area. Nanoparticles age in different ways in both the atmosphere and living things, which causes cytotoxicity and organ damage. Cellulose nanomaterials, clay, starch nanocrystals, halloysite nanotubes, nanocarbon (graphene nanoplatelets, graphene, graphite, etc.), and carbonaceous nanomaterials are examples of biodegradable and safer nanoparticles that can be used to solve this problem (carbon nanotube, nanospheres, etc.). The absence of high selectivity and specificity in nano-biosensors, which increases the inaccuracy in the identification process of samples as a result of virus proteins and mRNA alterations, is one of the main obstacles to diagnosing COVID-19. It appears from the reports that the specificity and selectivity of the sensors can be significantly increased by combining a number of diagnostic factors, such as nucleocapsid and spike proteins (N- and S-proteins), widening RNA-dependent RNA polymerase (RdRp) genes, reading frame 1a/b (ORF1a/b), etc. 109 The origin of the examined samples has an impact on any ambiguities that may result in the susceptibility and specificity of the nano-biosensors for detection of COVID-19. The susceptibility and specificity of COVID-19 detection can be increased by locating the source of contamination in the larynx, olfactory ducts, and mouth.

## Conclusion

The threat posed by COVID-19 plagues the entire world. Although scientists have been successful in discovering, analyzing, and finding numerous facts about the virus, COVID-19 treatment and detection remain difficult. The first step in treating COVID-19 patients is to make an accurate diagnosis. The traditional methods used for SARS-CoV2 detection still are ineffective as methods for mass screening. Therefore, it is necessary to develop and market diagnostic instruments that are more trustworthy, quick, precise, affordable, convenient, easy to use, and widely available. This review has emphasized certain cutting-edge nanotechnology methods based on fluorescent markers, electrochemical reactions, colorimetric detection, and magnetic field-induced identifications. The number of qualitative and quantitative tests conducted each day has expanded thanks to this cutting-edge equipment. However, developing nano-biosensors that are able to detect identical pollutants or analyzers at much lower concentrations while maintaining excellent specificity is still difficult. Therefore, the present nano-biosensor research should concentrate on developing sensors that are more accurate and have quicker response times, require fewer post-processing processes, are regenerable for reuse, have longer lives, and are more affordable. To use as diagnostic tools for unforeseen medical emergencies, the binding affinity and sensitivity of the nano-biosensors for such viruses of SARS COV-2 should be further enhanced.

## References

Abid, R., Shahzad, M. K., Sulaman, S. K., Faheem, M., Naeem, M., Khan, R., Khalil, A. A. K., Haider, A., Ahmad, B., Gul, R., Bukhari, N. & Jama, S. B. (2022). Therapeutic significance of nano- and biosensor technology in combating SARS-CoV-2: A review. *Applied Nanoscience*, 12, 3127–3140.

Abo-zeid, Y. & Williams, G. R. (2020). The potential anti-infective applications of metal oxide nanoparticles: a systematic review. *Wiley Interdisciplinary Reviews: Nanomedicine Nanobiotechnology,* 12(2), 1–36.

Abo-Zeid, Y., Ismail, N. S. M., McLean, G. R. & Hamdy, N. M. (2020). A molecular docking study repurposes FDA approved iron oxide nanoparticles to treat and control COVID-19 infection. *The European Journal of Pharmaceutical Sciences,* 153, 105465.

Adams, D., Garg, P. P., Suhr, O. B. & Vaishnaw, A. K. (2018). Patisiran, an RNAi therapeutic, for hereditary transthyretin amyloidosis. *The New England Journal of Medicine,* 379(1), 11–21.

Alphandéry, E. (2020). The potential of various nanotechnologies for corona virus diagnosis/treatment highlighted through a literature analysis. *Bioconjugate Chemistry,* 31(8), 1873–1882.

Antiochia, R. (2020) Nanobiosensors as new diagnostic tools for SARS, MERS and COVID-19: from past to perspectives. *Microchimica Acta*, 187:1–13

Cai, Q., Wang, R., Qiao, Z. & Yang, W. (2021). Single-digit Salmonella detection with the naked eye using bio-barcode immunoassay coupled with recombinase polymerase amplification and a CRISPR-Cas12a system. *Analyst,* 146, 5271.

Cao, G. & Wang, Y. (2004). Nanostructures and nanomaterials: synthesis, properties and applications. *Journal of the American Chemical Society*, 2, 94.

Chakraborty, D., Kumar, S., Chandrasekaran, N. & Mukherjee, A. (2020). Viral diagnostics and preventive techniques in the era of COVID-19: Role of nanoparticles. *Frontiers. Nanotechnology*, 2, 588795.

Cheng, X., Chen, G. & Rodriguez, W. R. (2009). Micro-and nanotechnology for viral detection. *Anaytical and Bioanalytical Chemistry*, 393, 487–501.

Chu, D. K., Pan, Y., Cheng, S. M., Hui, K. P., Krishnan, P. & Liu, Y. (2020). Molecular diagnosis of a novel corona virus (2019-nCoV) causing an outbreak of pneumonia. *Clinical Chemistry*, 66(4), 549–555.

Cordaro, A., Neri, G., Sciortino, M. T., Scala, A. & Piperno, A. (2020). Graphene-based strategies in liquid biopsy and in viral diseases diagnosis. *Nanomaterials*, 10(6), 1–18.

Corman, V. M., Landt, O., Kaiser, M., Molenkamp, R., Meijer, A., Chu, D. K., Bleicker, T., Brünink, S., Schneider, J., Schmidt, M. L., Mulders, D. G., Haagmans, B. L., Veer, B., van den Brink, S., Wijsman, L., Goderski, G., Romette, J. L., Ellis, J., Zambon, M., Peiris, M., Goossens, H., Reusken, C., Koopmans, M. P. & Drosten C. (2020). Detection of 2019 novel coronavirus (2019- nCoV) by real-time RT-PCR. *Eurosurveillance*, 25(3), 2000045

Dharmendra, K. M. & Rishabha, K. S. P. (2020). Corona virus: A review of COVID-19. *The Eurasian Journal of Medicine and Oncology*, 4, 8–25.

Draz, M. S. & Shafee, H. (2018). Applications of gold nanoparticles in virus detection. *Theranostics*, 8(7), 1985.

Du, T., Zhang, J., Li, C., Song, T., Li, P., Liu, J. Wang, S. (2020). Gold/Silver hybrid nanoparticles with enduring inhibition of coronavirus multiplication through multisite mechanisms. *Bioconjugate Chemistry*, 31(11), 2553–2563.

Foudeh, A. M., Didar, F. T., Veres, T. & Tabrizian, M. (2012). Microfluidic designs and techniques using lab-on-a-chip devices for pathogen detection for point-of-care diagnostics. *Lab Chip*, 12, 3249–3266.

Gowri, A., Kumar, A. & Anand, B. S. S. (2018). Recent advances in nanomaterials based biosensors for point of care (PoC) diagnosis of COVID-19: A mini review. *Trends in Analytical Chemistry*, 137, 116205.

Gutierrez, L., Li, X., Wang, J., Nangmenyi, G., Economy, J., Kuhlenschmidt, T. B. & Nguyen, T. H. (2009). Adsorption of rotavirus and bacteriophage MS2 using glass fiber coated with hematite nanoparticles. *Water Research*, 43(20), 5198–5208.

Ha, Y., Ko, S., Kim, I., Huang, Y., Mohanty, K., Huh, C. & Maynard, J. A. (2018). Recent advances incorporating superparamagnetic nanoparticles into immunoassays. *ACS Applied Nano Materials*, 1, 512–521.

Huang, C., Wen, T., Shi, F., Zeng, X. Y. & Jiao, Y. J. (2020). Rapid detection of igm antibodies against the SARS-CoV-2 virus via colloidal gold nanoparticle-based lateral-flow assay. *ACS Omega*, 5(21), 12550-12556.

Huang, L., Ding, L., Zhou, J., Chen, S., Chen, F., Zhao, C. & Liu, G. L. (2021). One-step rapid quantifcation of SARS-CoV-2 virus particles *via* low-cost nanoplasmonic sensors in generic microplate reader and point-of-care device. *Biosensors and Bioelectronics*, 171, 112685

Huang, Z., Hu, S., Xiong, Y., Wei, H., Xu, H., Duan, H. & Lai, W. (2019). Application and development of super paramagnetic nanoparticles in sample pre treatment and immune chromatographic assay. *Trends in Analytical Chemistry*, 114 (2019), 151-170.

Iannazzo, D., Pistone, A., Ferro, S., De Luca, L., Monforte, A. M., Romeo, R. & Pannecouque, C. (2018). Graphene quantum dots based systems as HIV inhibitors. *Bioconjugated Chemistry*, 29(9), 3084-3093.

Jamshidi, M., Lalbakhsh, A., Talla, J., Peroutka, Z., Hadjilooei, F. & Lalbakhsh, P. (2020). Artificial intelligence and COVID-19: Deep learning approaches for diagnosis and treatment. *Institute of Electrical and Electronics Engineers Access,* 8, 109581–109595

Jeremiah, S. S., Miyakawa, K., Morita, T., Yamaoka, Y. & Ryo, A. (2020). Potent antiviral effect of silver nanoparticles on SARS-CoV-2. *Biochemical and Biophysical Research Communications,* 533(1), 195–200.

Kim, H., Lee, S., Seo, H. W., Kang, B., Moon, J., Lee, K. G., Yong, D., Kang, H., Jung, J., Lim, E. K., Jeong, J., Part, H. G., Ryu, C. M. & Kang, T. (2010). Clustered regularly interspaced short palindromic repeats-mediated surface-enhanced Raman scattering assay for multidrug-resistant bacteria. *ACS Nano,* 14, 17241–17253.

Kokkinos, C. (2019). Electrochemical DNA biosensors based on labeling with nanoparticles. *Nanomaterials,* 9(10), 1361.

Kostarelos, K. (2020). Nanoscale nights of COVID-19. *Nature Nanotechnology*, 15(5), 343–344.

LaBauve, A. E., Rinker, T. E., Noureddine, A., Serda, R. E., Howe, J. Y., Sherman, M. B. & Negrete, O. A. (2018). Lipid-coated mesoporous silica nanoparticles for the delivery of the ML336 antiviral to inhibit encephalitic alphavirus infection. *Scientific Reports*, 8(1), 1–13.

Laksanasopin, T., Guo, T. W., Nayak, S., Sridhara, A. A., Xie, S. & Olowookere, O. O. (2015). A smartphone dongle for diagnosis of infectious diseases at the point of care. *Science Translational Medicine,* 4(7), 273.

Loeffelholz, M. J. & Tang, Y. W. (2021). Detection of SARS-CoV-2 at the point of care. *Bioanalysis*. 13(15), 1213-1223.

McKaya, G. (2020). Potential role of nitric oxide (NO) and silver/silver nanoparticles in the treatment of COVID-19 infections. *Journal of Biomedical Science*, 2(4).

Michael, H., Alan, L. G. & Serge, C. (2014). Nanomaterials for biosensing applications: A review. *Frontiers in Chemistry,* 2.

Moitra, P., Alafeef, M., Dighe, K., Frieman, M. B. & Pan, D. (2020). Selective naked-eye detection of SARS-CoV-2 mediated by N gene targeted antisense Oligonucleotides capped plasmonic nanoparticles. *ACS Nano,* 14, 7617–7627.

Nagaoka, H., Sato, Y., Xie, X., Hata, H., Eguchi, M., Sakurai, N. & Ohnishi, N. (2011). Coupling stimuli-responsive magnetic nanoparticles with Antibody-Antigen detection in immunoassays. *Analytical Chemistry*, 83, 9197-9200.

Nicogossian, A. (2012). In the news. *World Med Health Policy*, 4(1), 2020.

Ozin, G. A., Arsenault, A. C. & Cademartiri, L. (2009). Nanochemistry: A chemical approach to nanomaterials. *Royal Society of Chemistry,* 431.

Pandey, A., Nikam, A. N., Mutalik, S. P., Fernandes, G., Shreya, A. B. & Padya, B. S. (2020) Architectured therapeutic and diagnostic nanoplatforms for combating SARS-

CoV-2: Role of inorganic, organic, and radioactive materials. *ACS Biomaterials Science and Engineering,* 7(1), 31–54.

Paunovic, J., Vucevic, D., Radosavljevic, T., Mandic-Rajcevic, S. & Pantic, I. (2020). Iron-based nanoparticles and their potential toxicity: focus on oxidative stress and apoptosis. *Chemico-Biological Interact, 16,* 108935.

Ranjan, P., Singhal, A., Yadav, S., Kumar, N., Murali, S., Sanghi, S. K. & Khan, R. (2021). Rapid diagnosis of SARS-CoV-2 using potential point-of-care electrochemical immunosensor: toward the future prospects. *International Reviews of Immunology,* 40(1–2), 126–142.

Raval, B., Srivastav, A. K., Gupta, S. K., Kumar, U., Mahapatra, S. K., Gajjar, P. N. & Banerjee, I. (2020). Synthesis of exfoliated multilayer graphene and its putative interactions with SARS-CoV-2 virus investigated through computational studies. *Journal of Biomolecular Structure and Dynamics,* 40(2), 712-721.

Šafařík, I. & Šafaříková, M. (1999). Use of magnetic techniques for the isolation of cells. *Journal of Chromatography B: Biomedical Sciences and Applications*, 722(1–2), 33-53.

Sago, C. D., Lokugamage, M. P., Paunovska, K., Vanover, D. A., Monaco, C. M., Shah, N. N., Gamboa, C. M., Shah, N. N., Gamboa Castro, M., Anderson, S. E., Rudoltz, T. G., Lando, G. N., Munnilal Tiwari, P., Kirschman, J. L., Willett, N., Jang, Y. C., Santangelo, P. J., Bryksin, A. V. & Dahlman, J. E. (2018). High-throughput *in vivo* screen of functional mRNA delivery identifies nanoparticles for endothelial cell gene editing. *Proceedings of the National Academy of Sciences,* 115(42), E9944-E9952.

Sánchez-Cano, A., Ruiz-Vega, G., Vicente-Gómez, S., de la Serna, E., Sulleiro, E., Molina, I., Sánchez-Montalvá, A., Baldrich, E. & Baldrich, E. (2021). Development of a fast chemiluminescent magneto-immunoassay for sensitive *Plasmodium falciparum* detection in whole blood. *Analytical Chemistry,* 93, 12793–12800.

Seo, G., Lee, G., Kim, M. J., Baek, S. H., Choi, M., Ku, K. B., Lee, C. S., Jun, S., Park, D., Kim, H. G., Kim, S. J., Lee, J. O., Kim, B. T., Park, E. C. & Kim, S. I. (2020). Rapid detection of COVID-19 causative virus (SARS-CoV-2) in human nasopharyngeal swab specimens using field-effect transistor-based biosensor. *ACS Nano,* 14(4), 5135–5142.

Sivasankarapillai, V. S., Madaswamy, S. L. & Dhanusuraman, R. (2021). Role of nanotechnology in facing SARS-CoV-2 pandemic: solving crux of the matter with a hopeful arrow in the quiver. *Sensors International,* 2, 100096.

Sivasankarapillai, V. S., Pillai, A. M., Rahdar, A., Sobha, A. P., Das, S. S., Mitropoulos, A. C., Mokarrar, M. H. & Kyzas, G. Z. (2020). On facing the SARS-CoV-2 (COVID-19) with combination of nanomaterials and medicine: possible strategies and frst challenges. *Nanomaterials* 10(5), 852.

Speroni, F., Elviri, L., Careri, M. & Mangia, A. (2022). Magnetic particles functionalized with PAMAM-dendrimers and antibodies: a new system for an ELISA method able to detect Ara h3/4 peanut allergen in foods. *Analytical and Bioanalytical Chemistry*. 397, 3035–3042.

Srivastava, M., Srivastava, N., Mishra, P. & Malhotra, B. D. (2021). Prospects of nanomaterials-enabled biosensors for COVID-19 detection. *Science of the Total Environment,* 754, 142363

Tansil, N. C. & Gao, Z. (2006). Nanoparticles in biomolecular detection. *Nano Today,* 1, 28–37.

Vashist, S. K. (2017). Point-of-care diagnostics: Recent advances and trends. *Biosensors,* 7(4), 62.

Vermisoglou, E., Panacek, D., Jayaramulu, K., Pykal, M., Frebort, I., Kolar, M., Hajduch, M., Zboril, R & Otyepka, M. (2020). Human virus detection with graphene-based materials. *Biosensors and Bioelectronics*, 166, 112436.

Wang, L. & Lin, J. (2020). Recent advances on magnetic nanobead based biosensors: from separation to detection. *Trends in Analytical Chemistry*, 128(2020), 115915.

Wu, F., Mao, M., Cai, L., Lin, Q., Guan, X., Shi, X. & Ma, L. (2022). Platinum-decorated gold nanoparticle-based microfluidic chip immunoassay for ultrasensitive colorimetric detection of SARS-CoV-2 nucleocapsid protein *ACS Biomaterials Science and Engineering.* 8(9), 3924–3932.

Wu, F., Zhao, S., Yu, B., Chen, Y. M., Wang, W., Song, Z. G., Hu, Y., Tao, Z. W., Tian, J. H., Pei, Y. Y., Yuan, M. L., Zhang, Y. L., Dai, F. H., Liu, Y., Wang, Q. M., Zheng, J. J., Xu, L., Holmes, E. C. & Zhang, Y. Z. (2020). A new coronavirus associated with human respiratory disease in China. *Nature,* 579(7798), 265–269.

Xiang, J., Yan, M., Li, H., Liu, T., Lin, C. & Huang, S. (2020). Evaluation of enzyme-linked immunoassay and colloidal gold- immunochromatographic assay kit for detection of novel coronavirus (SARS-Cov-2) causing an outbreak of pneumonia (COVID-19). *MedRxiv*, 20028787.

Xiao, S. Y., Wu, Y. & Liu, H. (2020). Evolving status of the 2019 novel coronavirus infection: Proposal of conventional serologic assays for disease diagnosis and infection monitoring. *The Journal of Medical Virology,* 92, 464–467.

Xu, C., Akakuru, O. U., Zheng, J. & Wu, A. (2019). Applications of iron oxide-based magnetic nanoparticles in the diagnosis and treatment of bacterial infections. *Frontiers in Bioengineering and Biotechnology,* 7, 141.

Yuan, X., Yang, C., He, Q., Chen, J., Yu, D. & Li, J . (2020). Current and perspective diagnostic techniques for COVID-19. *ACS Infectious Diseases,* 6(8), 1998–2016.

Zhang, H., Penninger, J. M., Li, Y., Zhong, N. & Slutsky, A. S. (2020). Angiotensin-converting enzyme 2 (ACE2) as a SARS-CoV-2 receptor: molecular mechanisms and potential therapeutic target. *Intensive Care Medicine,* 46(4), 586–590.

# Chapter 5

# Recent Advancement in the Major Risk Factors and Treatment of SARS-CoV-2: A New Paradigm of Medicine in the Strategic Combating of the COVID-19 Pandemic

**Mansi Srivastava**[1]
**Siddhartha Dan**[2,*]
**Shruti Jain**[3]
**Prem Shankar Mishra**[4]
**and Abid Ali Sheikh**[5,†]

[1]Department of Bioscience and Biotechnology, Banasthali Vidyapith, Banasthali, Rajasthan, India
[2]Department of Biotechnology, Dr. B. R. Ambedkar National Institute of Technology, Jalandhar, Punjab, India
[3]Institute of Bioinformatics and Applied Biotechnology, Bengaluru, Karnataka, India
[4]Department of Pharmacy, School of Medical and Allied Sciences, Galgotias University, Greater Noida, Uttar Pradesh, India
[5]Training Official Scientific, National Institute of Biologicals, Noida, Uttar Pradesh, India

* Corresponding Author's Email: siddharthadan7@gmail.com.
† Corresponding Author's Email: abidalis2007@gmail.com.

In: Therapeutic Advances in Human Health and Diseases
Editors: Sushil Kumar Upadhyay, Manoj Singh and Anil Kumar Sharma
ISBN: 979-8-89113-304-4

## Abstract

The current study looked at people who were at high risk of morbidity and mortality as a result of SARS-CoV-2 infection and who improved or had a moderate clinical course after taking doxycycline. Despite its safety, we would not recommend using doxycycline in the treatment of COVID-19+ people unless they are under the care and supervision of a physician. The benefits of ivermectin and doxycycline as potential COVID-19 treatments are now being evaluated by the Indian Council of Medical Research. Once fibrosis has developed, azithromycin may have antifibrotic and proapoptotic effects on primary fibroblasts. As a result, in the late fibroproliferative-fibrotic phase of ARDS (Acute respiratory distress syndrome), COVID-19, azithromycin may reduce lung fibrosis. Intranasally administered N-acetylcysteine has been shown to reduce neutrophils, lymphocytes, goblet cells, bacterial count, turbinate hypertrophy, nasal symptoms, and rhinorrhea in non-allergic chronic rhinitis with goblet cell metaplasia. N-mucolytic acetylcysteine's action, ability to restore surface ciliary activity at the nasal epithelium, and regulation of the inflammatory response, which is a crucial component of the nasal mucosa's immunological defense system, are all credited with the advantages. In acute recurrent rhinosinusitis, a nasal douche containing flunisolide and N-acetylcysteine has been linked to a less stuffy nose, decreased severity of symptoms and rhino sinus signs as measured by endoscopy, improved cytological grading of neutrophil and eosinophil cells, fewer exacerbations, and increased mucociliary motility. Montelukast, a cysteinyl leukotriene receptor antagonist, may be utilized to treat COVID-19 infection, and the possibility of slowing the progression of severe COVID-19 will be examined. This cutting-edge therapy method requires input from the COVID-19 community in order to improve it, such as better protecting our patients who are already vulnerable owing to corona. While information has flowed freely throughout the pandemic, results from ongoing and future clinical trials are still needed to better understand the interactions between different medicinal medicines in the context of COVID-19 infections.

**Keywords:** SARS-CoV-2, ivermectin, doxycycline, azithromycin, n-acetylcysteine, montelukast

## 1. Introduction

The Coronavirus disease-2019 (COVID-19) outbreak started in Wuhan, China. The cause of this revolution was identified as the severe acute respiratory syndrome coronavirus 2 (SARS-CoV-2). Smooth tissues like the muzzle, lips, and nose are where the virus thrives. SARS-COV-2, single-stranded RNA viruses with a genome of 26–32 kb and a diameter of 65–125 nm, cause infection. Initially, the virus was dubbed the 2019 new coronavirus by Chinese researchers. The need for appropriate medical therapy for a new COVID-19 infection is urgent. SARS is a unique respiratory disease caused by viral infections that is still malignant. Drugs that have recently been available have been able to moderately handle indications, but no specific treatment or treatment has been assigned. Early discovery of a revolution is critical for all states' defense. Viral entry inhibitors, replication inhibitors, protease inhibitors, heterocyclic antivirals, drug delivery systems, and biological therapeutic medications are among the upcoming drugs that are considered to be directly relevant, as well as new therapeutic drugs. The current difficulty should be viewed as an incredible chance to remind us of our globalized society, which requires a multi-interdisciplinary technique incorporating cross-national disciplines of knowledge, as demonstrated in other scientific situations. It will be vital to promote interactions and increase team diversity. Obtaining novel and significant scientific solutions. From this perspective, nanotechnology is essentially a field in which scientists from a wide range of backgrounds have collaborated to solve a wide range of problems. Medicine is needed now more than ever to establish new foundations for tackling the recent global public health hazard, such as the emergence of likely new challenges in infectious diseases and rethinking a more sustainable future based on science (Upadhyay et al., 2021).

## 2. Risk Factors

### 2.1. Smoking

COVID-19 mainly causes respiratory tract infection because the commonly known receptor for SARS-CoV-2 is ACE2 (angiotensin-converting enzyme -2) (Brake et al., 2020) is expressed on the surface of alveolar epithelial cells (Glowacka et al., 2010). Smoking is injurious to health and makes smokers more vulnerable to bacterial and viral infections which leads to pulmonary and other severe respiratory diseases (Lawrence et al., 2019) as exposure to tobacco smoke causes inflammation in the lungs, increased mucosal inflammation, increased permeability in epithelial cells, mucus overproduction, impaired mucociliary clearance expression of inflammatory cytokines also increased, etc. (Strzelak et al., 2018).

All over the world different case studies were studied and the impact of smoking on the severity of COVID-19 was reported details of a few of them are mentioned in this review. Zhang et al. (2020) studied 140 COVID-19-positive patients, out of which 58 patients were severe and the %age of past smokers in these patients was 4% and current smokers was 2%. The 82 patients were non-serious and the %age of past smokers was 3% and current smokers were 0%. Guan et al. (2019) studied 1099 COVID-19 patients (the largest case study till now) out of which 173 were severe 5.2% were former smokers 16.9% were a current smoker and 926 were nonsevere in which 1.3% were a former smoker and 12.6% were a current smoker. Zhou et al. (2020) studied 191 COVID-19 patients out of which 54 died in the hospital of which 9% were current smokers and 137 returned back to home of which 4% were current smokers. Liu et al. (2019) studied 78 COVID-19 patients out of which patients suffering adverse outcomes have 27.8% proportion of patients with a history of smoking whereas patients that show improvement or stabilization in their condition have only 3% proportion of patients with a history of smoking. Chen et al. (2020) studied 274 COVID-19 patients, out of which 113 were non- survivors in which 6% were current smoker and 2% were former smoker and 161 were survivors in which 3% were current smoker and 3% were former smoker.

Mo et al. (2020) studied 155 COVID-19 patients out of which 85 were severe patients in which 4.7% were current smoker and 70 were non severe patients in which 2.9% were current smokers. Shi et al. (2020) studied 487 COVID-19 patients out of which 49 were severe patients in which 12.2% were current smokers and 438 were non severe patients in which 7.8% patients were current smokers. Colombi et al. (2020), studied 236 COVID-19 patients out of which 108 patients required ICU care and the %age of current smoker and former smoker was 15% and 3% respectively. In the remaining 128 patients no ICU care was required and the %age of current smoker and former smoker in this case was 2% and 8% respectively (Colombi et al., 2020).

During the course of study, we found two papers whose data for the impact of smoking on the severity of COVID-19 in patients were completely opposite from the data obtained by different other papers. Yang et al. (2020) studied 52 critically ill COVID-19 patients (adult patients), out of which 32 were non-survivor patients in which the proportion of smokers was 0% and 20 were survivor patients in which 10% were smokers. Another study studied 41 COVID-19 patients, out of which 13 required ICU care but none of them were current smoker whereas in the remaining 28 patients no ICU care was required, still 7% patients were current smokers. This variation in the results could be due to the small sample size included in the study (Huang et al., 2020). Therefore, a firm conclusion between the severity of COVID-19 and the smoking status of patients could not be stated (WHO, 2020) but it can be predicted that smoking most likely increases the severity of the disease (Vardavas et al., 2020).

## 2.2. Heart Failure/Cardiovascular Disease and COVID-19

On the prevalence of SARS-CoV-2 in patients with pre-existing heart failure, only little information is available. Despite a less than 1% pattern prevalence of constant chronic heart failure in the combinatorial analysis of 799 SARS-CoV-2 patients hospitalized in Wuhan, China, heart failure was identified as an inconvenience in 49% of patients who died and the recovered 3% of patients (Chen et al., 2020). Heart failure was seen in 52% of patients who died and 12% of patients who recovered in a study of 191 patients treated in two different medical centers in Wuhan (Zhang et al., 2020). The occurrence of acute heart failure was not recorded in certain hospitalized patients with COVID-19, but increased natriuretic peptide was found, particularly in patients with heart failure evidence. NT-proBNP levels were substantially lower in patients without high troponin ranges than in patients with elevated troponin ranges (139 vs. 1689 pg/ml) in the above-mentioned series of 416 hospitalized patients (Shi et al., 2020).

In SARS-CoV-2 hospitalized patients, cardiovascular disorders and their risk factors are quite prevalent. In a study of 191 patients hospitalized in Wuhan, comorbidities comprised 30% hypertension, 19% diabetes mellitus, and 8% coronary heart disease (Zhang et al., 2020). Patients with a history of heart failure may experience an abrupt decompensation as a result of COVID-19 dysregulation (Fried et al., 2020). The frequency of cardiovascular disorders and heart disease in general varies greatly from one group to the next. As a result, there is a broad group of prevalent cardiovascular illnesses in people with COVID-19. The majority of China's (Chen et al., 2020, Madjid et al., 2020; Wang et al., 2020; Xiong et al., 2020; Zhang et al., 2020) rates have been reported to be between 4.2% and 25%. Patients admitted to intensive care units (Chen et al., 2020) who died have a higher %age. According to one study, 22.7% of all fatal case patients have pre-existing cardiac and heart-related disorders, with a case fatality rate of 10.5%.

There is substantial evidence of a link between the hazard and severity of COVID-19 contamination and the hazard and severity of cardiovascular diseases (CVD) hazard variables of hypertension, diabetes, and cardiovascular illnesses (Dan et al., 2020). The importance of the link is reflected in the ensuing observational investigations. The link between standard cardiac and heart-associated disease and hospital fatalities was examined among patients hospitalized with SARS-CoV-2 using an inspection database from 169 emergency clinics in Asia, Europe, and North America (Mehra et al., 2020). Of a total of 8910 COVID-19 patients, 94.21% (8395 patients) survived and were released, while 5.78% (515) died in the hospital. In comparison to no contamination, baseline cardiovascular illness was independently linked to a higher risk of in-hospital (medical clinic) death (10.2% vs. 5.2%; chances proportion 2.70; 95% CI 2.08-3.51). According to the Chinese Center for Disease Control and Prevention, 72,314 cases (44,672) had been confirmed through February 11, 2020 (Chow et al., 1975). The overall mortality rate was 2.3%. The CFR was 14.8% among individuals who were Octogenarians or older. When all other factors were equal, a history of coronary heart disease (CHD) was accessible in 4.2% of lethal cases, but not in 22.7%. CHD had a 10.5% case fatality rate. Another study looked at 1099 cases from 30 different regions of China (Chow et al., 1975; Dan et al., 2020; Mehra et al., 2020).

A primary outcome was defined as dead or ICU admission and mechanical ventilation in 15.7% of the cases, while a secondary goal was defined as dead or ICU admission and mechanical ventilation in 6.1% of the cases. The prevalence of coronary heart disease (non-critical disease vs. critical disease, 1.8% vs. 5.8%, and primary endpoint vs. no primary endpoint, 9% vs. 2%) was consistently higher in patients with critical illness vs. non-critical illness, and patients with primary endpoint vs. no primary endpoint. There were strong inseparable connections with the outcome of death for coronary heart illnesses in 191 individuals from Wuhan province diagnosed before January 31, 2020 (24% vs. 1%, < 0.0001) (Zhang et al., 2020).

Frailty (86.7%), headache (80.0%), fever (73.3%), cough (66.7%), and eating problems were the most common symptoms during COVID-19's initial episode (73.3%). Headache (93.3%), frailty (91.1%), fever (71.1%), and chest pain were the most common symptoms of COVID-19's second wave (71.1%). Frailty and headache were thought to be the reason for the increased severity in each wave of the current pandemic. The patient's age has a significant impact on the prevalence and severity of symptoms (Piroth et al., 2021; Upadhyay et al., 2021). In terms of symptom prevalence and severity, the clinical findings of the illness differed significantly from the first to the second episode (Jain et al., 2020; Khan et al., 2021). The later symptoms of headache, anorexia, diarrhea, and stomach discomfort failed to show a significant link between the first and second waves of infection. However, among infected persons with reduced immunity, the otolaryngologic symptoms had the highest association values between episodes (Ata et al., 2020; Rath et al., 2020; Elshazli et al., 2021; Singh et al., 2021; Upadhyay et al., 2021). The second episode's duration (15.7 days) was judged to be shorter than the first one (17.0 days) (Srivastava et al., 2021).

## 2.3. Diabetes

Diabetes mellitus is a common disease, a survey in the United States says that 34.2 million or 10.5% of the total population have diabetes mellitus and it significantly increases the susceptibility towards covid-19 the possible reason could be that people suffering from diabetes mellitus have less efficient Tcells, higher affinity towards cellular binding and efficient virus entry, decreased virus clearance, presence of CVD and increased susceptibility to hyper inflammation and cytokine storm syndrome (Muniyappa et al., 2020). It has also been studied that diabetes increases the expression of ACE2 receptors due to which susceptibility to COVID-19 infection can increase (Rao et al., 2020). COVID-19 patients having diabetes may suffer severe outcomes. This can be predicted as an early analysis from Wuhan, China reported that approximately 20% of patients with diabetes required an intensive care unit (Lim et al., 2021) and recent data from Italy reported that more than two-thirds of COVID-19 patients having diabetes died (Remuzzi et al., 2020). Targher et al. (2020) compared the covid-19 patients having diabetes with the patients not have diabetes. They observed that patients having diabetes are more likely to be older, obese, and hypertensive. In fact, they had lower lymphocyte count, lower albumin and HDL-cholesterol levels, high neutrophil count, D-dimer, and higher liver enzymes. SARS-CoV-2 infects circulating immune cells and increases apoptosis of lymphocytes (CD3, CD4, and CD8 T cells), leading to lymphocytopenia (Guan et al., 2020). As MERS-CoV binds to the receptor-binding domain of human dipeptidyl peptidase IV (DPP-IV), a transgenic mouse model expressing this DPP-IV receptor on pulmonary alveolar cells has been used to study the effect of diabetes in worsening disease severity, showing an association of diabetes with greater weight loss and greater pulmonary inflammation, with macrophage infiltrates similar to those seen clinically in the disease (Kulcsar et al., 2019).

## 2.4. Cancer

Cancer itself is a dangerous disease that not only makes patients' immunity weak but also lowers the courage to fight. In this scenario, if a cancer patient gets infected with COVID-19 then the severity of the disease increases manifold. This can be said as data from China have shown that cancer patients having COVID-19 are at greater risk (approx 3.5 times) of suffering severe outcomes such as the requirement of mechanical ventilation or ICU then normal patients (Liang et al., 2020). Cancer patients require anticancer therapy from time to time and Zhang et al. (2020) studied that cancer patients undergoing therapy when infected with COVID-19 are at four times higher risk of experiencing severe outcomes as compared to those who undergone therapy before 14 days of COVID-19 infection (HR=4.079, 95% CI 1.086–15.322, p= 0.037).

A study was made in which 28 COVID-19-infected cancer patients were included with a Median age 65.0. Lung cancer was the most frequent cancer type (*n* = 7; 25.0%) followed by esophageal cancer (n = 4, 14.3%) and breast cancer (n = 3, 10.7%) (Zhang et al., 2020). Zhang et al. (2020) studied the outcomes of cancer patients with COVID-19 on active anticancer therapy and reported more than fourfold higher likelihood of experiencing severe events in those who received therapy in the preceding 14 days of COVID-19 diagnosis (HR=4.079, 95% CI 1.086–15.322, p= 0.037. Evidence suggests that patients who received surgery and concomitantly contracted COVID-19 were at much higher risk of severe clinical events than those who did not have surgery (Ng et al., 2020).

## 2.5. Pregnancy

Usually, pregnancy is a blessing but due to the current COVID-19 pandemic, has led to major concerns in pregnant women as pregnant women are at more risk for viral infections because in pregnancy there is partial immune suppression (Wastnedge et al., 2021). Accurate data on the risk of infection to pregnant women is not available (Liang et al., 2020), still, it is believed that pregnant women are at high risk of getting infected by COVID-19 and having complications during pregnancy (Villar et al., 2021). The common symptoms in pregnant women include fever, chest pain, shortness of breath, etc. which are not significantly different from other patients (Molteni et al., 2021). During this time one more major concern was that, if pregnant women get infected then the infection will transmit to the foetus or not. So, to estimate the scenario of transmission of disease from an infected mother to its neonate several studies were studied.

Chen et al. (2020) studied 9 confirmed COVID-19 pneumonia pregnant women. They were diagnosed with COVID-19 during the third semester of their pregnancy. All have caesarean delivery and 6 out of 9 have preterm delivery. Amniotic fluid, cord blood, and breastmilk samples were collected to test the presence of COVID-19 disease in newborns. All the newborns had negative results for the disease and the Apgar scores (APGAR: appearance, pulse, grimace, activity, and respiration) were 8-9 and 9-10 at 1 and 5 minutes respectively (Chen et al., 2020). Zhang et al. (2020) studied 9 confirmed covid-19 pregnant women giving birth to 10 newborns (1 twin). Symptoms begin to develop at different time spans. The 4 women showed symptoms before the delivery (1-6 days before), 2 women showed symptoms on the day of delivery and the remaining 3 showed symptoms after the delivery. Of the 7 women who have cesarean delivery and 2 show vaginal delivery and 6 out of 10 have preterm delivery (Zhang et al., 2020). Pharyngeal swab specimen was collected from 9 of the neonates from 1 and 9$^{th}$ day after delivery and all of them showed negative result for the disease. Zhang et al. (2020) studied 16 confirmed COVID-19 pregnant women and also compared the results with 45 pregnant women who were not infected. All 16 women were diagnosed during the third trimester of pregnancy and all had a cesarean delivery. A sample of throat swabs was collected from 10 infants to test the infection and all showed negative results. After comparing all the data of infected pregnant women and non-infected pregnant women they found that there is not much significant difference between the 2 groups of mothers in the occurrence of severe diabetes, preculture of the membrane, fatal distress, premature delivery, etc. in fact there was not much difference between 2 groups of newborns in weight, gestational age at delivery, parity, etc. (Zhang et al., 2020).

Liu et al. (2020) studied 3 confirmed cases of COVID-19 pregnant women. Case 1 was of a 34-year-old woman who showed symptoms during the third trimester of pregnancy and the delivery was cesarean delivery. Umbilical cord blood, plasma serum, and whole blood of the newborn were collected after 34 minutes of birth and the oropharyngeal swab was collected after one day and all results were negative. Case 2 was of a 34-year-old woman who showed symptoms during the third trimester of pregnancy and the delivery was cesarean delivery. Oropharyngeal swab, urine, whole blood, serum, and feces of the newborn was collected 27 minutes after birth and all results were negative. Case 3 was of a 30-year-old woman who showed symptoms during the third trimester of pregnancy and the delivery is vaginal delivery. Oropharyngeal swab, urine, serum, whole blood, and feces of the newborn was collected 2 and 3 days after delivery and all the results were negative. After delivery, all three 3 neonates were shifted to a sealed incubator with a separate air exchange system and no neonates were breast feed. At the time of delivery, efforts were made to minimize the contact of the baby with maternal blood (Liu et al., 2020).

## 3. Case Study of COVID-19

Six studies with 1527 patients were included in this analysis. The proportions of hypertension, cardia-cerebrovascular disease, and diabetes in patients with COVID-19 were 17.1%, 16.4%, and 9.7%, respectively. The incidences of hypertension, cardia-cerebrovascular diseases, and diabetes were about two folds, threefold, and twofold, respectively, higher in ICU/severe cases than in their non-ICU/severe counterparts (Li et al., 2020). Another study includes 191 patients, out of which 137 were discharged and 54 died in hospital. 91 (48%) patients had a comorbidity, with hypertension being the most common (58 [30%] patients), followed by diabetes (36 [19%] patients) and coronary heart disease (15 [8%] patients). death was higher in patients with diabetes or coronary heart disease (Remuzzi et al., 2020). A meta-analysis of eight studies including 46 248 patients with laboratory-confirmed COVID-19 indicated that those with the most severe disease were more likely to have hypertension (odds ratio 2.36 (95% confidence interval 1.46 to 3.83)), respiratory disease (2.46 (1.76 to 3.44)), and cardiovascular disease (3.42 (1.88 to 6.22) (Jordan et al., 2020). Of the 174 hospitalized patients with COVID-19, the median age was 59 years. The most common underlying comorbidities were chronic diseases, such as hypertension (24.7%) and diabetes (21.2%) (Guan et al., 2020; Zheng et al., 2020).

An inspection database from 169 emergency clinics in Asia, Europe, and North America was used to look into the link between standard cardiac and heart-related disorders and hospital fatalities among SARS-CoV-2 patients. In total, 94.21% (8395 patients) of COVID-19 patients survived and were discharged, while 5.78% (515) died in the hospital. Baseline cardiovascular sickness was independently connected to a greater probability of in-hospital (medical clinic) death when compared to no contamination (10.2% vs. 5.2%; chances proportion 2.70; 95% CI 2.08-3.51). Through February 11, 2020, the Chinese Center for Disease Control and Prevention had confirmed 72,314 cases (44,672). Overall, there was a 2.3% mortality rate. Individuals who were Octogenarians or older had a CFR (Case Fatality Rate) of 14.8%. When all other parameters were equal, 4.2% of deadly cases had a history of coronary heart disease (CHD), but 22.7% did not.

The case fatality rate for CHD was 10.5%. Another study examined 1099 cases from 30 different Chinese regions. In 15.7% of the cases, the primary outcome was death or ICU admission with mechanical ventilation, while in 6.1% of the cases, the secondary aim was death or ICU admission with mechanical ventilation. Patients with critical illness vs. non-critical illness (1.8% vs. 5.8%, and primary vs. no primary endpoint, 9% vs. 2%) had a greater prevalence of coronary heart disease (1.8% vs. 5.8%, and primary vs. no primary endpoint, 9% vs. 2%). In 191 Wuhan provincial residents diagnosed before January 31, 2020, there were substantial inseparable links with the outcome of death from coronary heart disease (24% vs. 1%, 0.0001).

During COVID-19's first episode, the most prevalent symptoms were frailty (86.7%), headache (80.0%), fever (73.3%), cough (66.7%), and feeding issues (73.3%). The most prevalent symptoms of COVID-19's second wave were headache (93.3%), fragility (91.1%), fever (71.1%), and chest pain (71.1%). The duration of the second episode (15.7 days) was deemed to be shorter than the first (17.0 days).

## 4. Medicines for Combating COVID-19

### 4.1. Doxycycline

SARS-CoV-2 is a novel coronavirus with few treatment options and no vaccination. Patients who test positive should self-quarantine and receive supportive care such as rest and hydration intake. Hospitalization is recommended for patients with severe disease or moderate disease with high-risk aspects, such as immunocompromised states (e.g., cancer therapy, chronic lung disease, diabetes, or extreme obesity). In a recent worldwide series, patients with lung cancer with COVID-19 infection had a high mortality rate of 33% (Garassino et al., 2020).

There's a lot of interest in repurposing already-approved drugs to treat COVID-19. For COVID-19+ patients, tetracycline and its derivatives (e.g., doxycycline) may provide a sensible and safe therapy option. Doxycycline is often used to treat bacterial infections and dermatologic diseases (such as acne vulgaris and rosacea) at a dose of 100 mg twice daily (Griffin et al., 2010). Tetracyclines have antiviral and anti-inflammatory effects, which may help to reduce the severity of a viral infection (Griffin et al., 2010; Fredeking et al., 2015; Rothan et al., 2015; Malek et al., 2020). Doxycycline has been shown to be effective against dengue and chikungunya virus infections in clinical trials (Rothan et al., 2015; Malek et al., 2020). Doxycycline may also alter a number of mechanisms that control viral replication (Kumar et al., 2008; Sargiacomo et al., 2020; Wu et al., 2020). Tetracyclines' pleiotropic properties are most likely due to their activities on atypical antibiotic molecular pathways (Griffin et al., 2010).

Doxycycline may prevent or alleviate the consequences of COVID-19 infection through a variety of modes of action. Doxycycline inhibits matrix metalloproteinases (MMPs), particularly MMP-9, which is thought to be necessary for initial viral entrance into the cell (Griffin et al., 2020). Interleukin (IL)-6 is inhibited by doxycycline, and both IL-6 and MMPs are essential regulators of the cytokine storm that is typically associated with severe viral pneumonitis (Kong et al., 2015; Phillips et al., 2017; Conforti et al., 2020). Doxycycline is a well-known ionophore that aids in the transport of zinc intracellularly, with higher cellular zinc concentrations inhibiting coronavirus replication *in vitro* (Velthuis et al., 2010; Griffin et al., 2020). Doxycycline inhibits nuclear factor (NF)-B (Santa-Cecília et al., 2016; Griffin et al., 2020), which may reduce the probability of viral entry by inhibiting the DPP4 cell surface receptor directly and reducing a hyperactive immune response after infection (Choi et al., 2017).

*In vivo,* nonantimicrobial, low-dose doxycycline has been observed to decrease CD147/EMMPRIN expression, which may be required for SARS-CoV-2 entrance into T cells (Emingil et al., 2008; Wang et al., 2020). Doxycycline has the ability to block papain-like proteinase (PLpro) and 3C-like primary protease (3CLpro), viral proteins that are both required for viral replication and lifecycle (Wu et al., 2020). In light of the foregoing, we provide a case series of four patients with COVID-19 infection and known high-risk pulmonary illness who were treated with conventional doxycycline doses for a period of 5 to 14 days. After discussing the potential risks and advantages with the patients and obtaining informed consent, they were started on doxycycline medication. In these four patients, no other antibiotics, antiviral medications, antimalarial medicines, zinc, or any other supplements thought to be helpful in SARS-CoV-2 treatment were used concurrently. These are the first cases that show a link between doxycycline and a potential reduction in the intensity of symptoms in COVID-19+ patients. In a short case series, it's difficult to prove a conclusive causal link between doxycycline treatment and faster recovery or lower morbidity from SARS-CoV-2 infection.

This study, we feel, provides a justification for launching bigger controlled trials investigating doxycycline usage in COVID-19+ patients. The individuals we studied had a variety of high-risk characteristics that were indicative of severe disease and a higher probability of death. Patients one and four were on treatment for advanced lung cancer, a category for whom COVID-19 infection had a death risk of more than 33% (Garassino and Teravolt, 2020). Inflammatory indicators such as CRP, transaminases, and CK (as seen in cases 1 and 4) are also linked to poor outcomes (Chen et al., 2020). High morbidity and mortality are also associated with advanced age and diffuse bilateral infiltrates (case 4) (Du et al., 2020). After several days of deterioration on azithromycin, Case 4 showed a temporal link between doxycycline delivery and clinical improvement. Patients with active pulmonary sarcoidosis, like in example 2, are also more susceptible to COVID-19 problems related to immunotoxicity, dysfunction, and dysregulation (Sweiss et al., 2020).

COVID-19 morbidity and death were significantly higher in the patients described. All of them improved, with the exception of one, who had bilateral pulmonary infiltrates that had resolved. None of the patients had a serious illness. The four patients in this case series received a typical antibiotic dose of doxycycline (100 mg twice daily or daily). Among the various tetracycline derivatives, doxycycline is distinctive in that it has a distinct dose split between its cellular cytotoxic/antimicrobial actions (>100mg) and its possible anti-inflammatory/antiviral/pro-ionophoric effects (40mg) (Kumar et al., 2008; Griffin et al., 2010; Fredeking et al., 2015; Conforti et al., 2020; Sargiacomo et al., 2020). This could be a key factor to consider when considering low-dose doxycycline (20 mg twice daily) as a COVID-19 preventive therapy. Doxycycline's potential efficacy against COVID-19 could be related to pleiotropic effects against the general pathways involved in viral infection, replication, and associated over-exuberant inflammatory response, as well as angiogenic effects (Griffin et al., 2010). Doxycycline has no known direct selectivity for SARS-CoV-2 suppression.

Doxycycline has been shown to have effect against recognized coreceptors DPP4/CD26 and coreceptor CD147/EMMPRIN, which are required for SARS-CoV entrance into T cells, even at sub microbial levels (Choi et al., 2017; Santa-Cecília et al., 2017; Wang et al., 2020). DPP4 (Dipeptidyl Peptidase IV) appears to have an NF- κB binding site, and inhibiting NF- κB reduces DPP4 expression (Choi, 2017). DPP4 expression is higher in elderly individuals and those with diabetes or pulmonary disease, which could explain why COVID-19 causes more morbidity and mortality (Sargiacomo et al., 2020). Finally, MMP-9 appears to be essential for virus infection to pass through the cell wall (Kong et al., 2015; Rothan et al., 2015). Doxycycline may be able to bind to PLpro after COVID-19 has infected the cell, which is responsible for proteolytic cleavage of the replicase polyprotein, which releases nonstructural proteins 1, 2, and 3 (Nsp1, Nsp2, and Nsp3), which are required for viral replication (Wu et al., 2020). It is projected to attach to 3CLpro or Nsp5, which is cleaved from polyproteins, causing subsequent cleavage of Nsp4-16 and mediating Nsp maturation, which is required for the virus lifecycle (Wu et al., 2020).

Doxycycline is an ionophore that binds divalent cations (including zinc) and increases zinc content in the cell by facilitating cell membrane transfer (Griffin et al., 2010; Velthuis et al., 2020). SARS-CoV-2 replication is inhibited by increased zinc levels. Inhibition of replicase protein processing and RNA-dependent RNA polymerase (RdRp) activity is thought to be the mechanisms (Velthuis et al., 2020). Finally, doxycycline may help avoid the cytokine storm that occurs after COVID-19 infection, which is thought to be caused by an overactive immune response to SARS-CoV-2. The direct suppression of NF-B by doxycycline is the main driver of its anti-inflammatory action (Santa-Cecília et al., 2016). The cytokine storm is driven by IL-6, which is directly regulated by NF-B (Brasier, 2010). Doxycycline may also cause apoptosis in senescent epithelial cells (Sargiacomo et al., 2020), which have been shown to express higher levels of DPP4/CD26, implying that viral replication is accelerated in these cells, which leads to induction of the cytokine storm. Finally, it was observed that four cases of individuals at high risk of morbidity and mortality from SARS-CoV-2 infection improved and/or had a mild clinical course after taking doxycycline. Despite the safety of doxycycline, we would not suggest its usage in the treatment of COVID-19+ individuals unless under the supervision and supervision of a physician. It's worth considering a larger randomized controlled trial (Yates et al., 2020).

## 4.2. Ivermectin

There are newer medications on the horizon that have been recommended despite having little experience and insufficient safety and efficacy data (Pal and Yadav, 2020). These modern alternatives are neither widely available nor inexpensive. We looked back at some of the old compounds and discovered that Ivermectin, which was first marketed as an anthelmintic, is an effective, safe, and economical COVID-19 preventive and treatment choice in Indian settings (Sinhaa et al., 2020). Ivermectin has recently been discovered to have potent antiviral activity (Sharun et al., 2020). It has the ability to swiftly convert RT-PCR negative (Caly et al., 2020). It can be utilized at any stage of COVID-19 infection, especially in the early viremic phase (Banerjee et al., 2020). It can be used with other drugs such as hydroxychloroquine, azithromycin, and doxycycline (Chowdhury et al., 2021).

Ivermectin is inexpensive, widely available, and free of serious adverse effects (Banerjee et al., 2020). This white paper aims to recommend Ivermectin, a powerful antiviral medicine, as a therapeutic option for COVID-19 prophylaxis and treatment in mild, moderate, and severe cases. **Ivermectin in the dose of 12 mg BD alone or in combination with other therapy for 5 to 7 days may be considered as safe therapeutic option for mild moderate or severe cases of COVID-19 infection. It is cost-effective especially when the other drugs are very costly and not easily available** and Ivermectin should be used sparingly for COVID-19 therapy.

Ivermectin's antiviral properties have only recently been found. In vitro, it has been shown to be effective against several flaviviruses (dengue fever, Japanese encephalitis, and tick-borne encephalitis virus) as well as the chikungunya virus. The same activity has now been tested in a variety of different viral illnesses. Its effectiveness in eradicating coronavirus in vitro has just been recognized (Gupta et al., 2020). In 48 hours, it decreases the viral load of SARS-CoV-2 by a factor of 5000 (Caly et al., 2020). Ivermectin was utilized in current clinical trials at doses ranging from 200 to 1200 mcg/kg body weight for 3–7 days, with encouraging outcomes in terms of symptomatology and viral load decrease.

### *4.2.1. Mechanism of Action of Ivermectin*

The nuclear-pore-complex sequestration of the SARS-CoV-2 viral nucleocapsid protein (NCP) into the host nucleus is an important stage in viral pathogenesis and resistance against the host immune response (Banerjee et al., 2020). Ivermectin inhibits host importin/transporter protein, which reduces SARS-CoV nucleocapsid protein (NCP) translocation (shuttling) from the cytoplasm to the nucleus, altering NCP, distribution disrupts viral propagation and survival (Caly et al., 2020). Ivermectin has been shown to be well-tolerated by most people. The majority of side effects have been minor and short-lived (Guzzo et al., 2002). In mice, rats, and rabbits, ivermectin has been demonstrated to be teratogenic. However, no suitable and well-controlled studies in pregnant women have been conducted. Because the safety of ivermectin in pregnancy has not been proved, it should not be used during pregnancy. Ivermectin; IVM (red block) inhibits and disrupts binding of thc SARS-CoV-2 S protein at the ACE-2 receptors (Zaidi and Dehgani-Mobaraki, 2021).

SARS-CoV-2 directly activates TLR-4 (Toll-like receptor 4) receptors, as well as LPS-mediated (lipopolysaccharide-mediated) activation (as seen in ICU settings), activating the NF-Kb pathway and MAP3 Kinases (Mitogen Activated Protein 3 kinases), resulting in increased intranuclear gene expression for proinflammatory cytokines and chemokines (responsible for cytokine storm) and NO release (responsible for blood vessel dilatation, fluid leak, low blood pressure, ARDS and sepsis). The activation of the NF-Kb and STAT-3 (Signal transducer and activator of transcription 3) pathways is crucial to the development and consequences of COVID-19. STAT-3 binds to PAK-1 and promotes the expression of IL-6. In the presence of t-PA, annexin A2 on the cell surface transforms plasminogen; PLG to plasmin. STAT-3 is activated and translocated to the nucleus by plasmin. STAT-3 activation activates hyaluronan synthase-2 in lung cells, resulting in hyaluronan deposition and diffuse alveolar damage, as well as hypoxia. STAT-3 also promotes TGF-beta, causing pulmonary fibrosis, which is a common feature of SARS-COV-2 lung pathology. Damaged type 2 cells produce PAI-1, and an existing hypoxic state leads PAI to be upregulated (through Hypoxic inducible factor-1) as well as direct STAT-3 stimulation. The simultaneous activation of STAT-3 and PAI-1 inhibits t-PA and urokinase-type plasminogen activators, resulting in the development of thrombi. In addition, the SARS-CoV-2 spike protein binds to CD147 on red blood cells, causing them to clump together. IVM then attaches to the SARS-CoV-2 Spike protein, preventing clumping. The direct activation of PD-L1 receptors on endothelial cells by STAT-3 may also contribute to T-cell lymphopenia in COVID-19.

IVM (Ivermectin) suppresses the NF-kb pathway and STAT-3 directly, as well as PAK-1 indirectly by increasing its ubiquitin-mediated degradation. Interferon regulatory genes and viral RNA-mediated activation of TLR-3 and TLR7/8-Myd88 transcription of interferon-regulator (IRF) family members are involved in a cell's natural antiviral response. This antiviral response must be blocked by limiting interferon production in order for a virus to develop an infection. Importin and KPNA proteins are involved in viral protein transport to the nucleus and subsequent IFN signaling. The SARS-CoV-2 proteins (ORF-3a, NSP-1, and ORF-6) directly disrupt IFN signaling, leading the virus to spread to the surrounding cells. IVM inhibits both importin a-b and KPNA-1 receptors (karyopherin subunit alpha 1 recetors), resulting in the release of natural antiviral IFN (Interferon). IVM also prevents viral replication by inhibiting viral RdRp. IVM Ivermectin, *ACE-2* angiotensin-converting-enzyme, LPS Lipopolysaccharide, *TLR* Toll-like receptor, t-PA tissue-like plasminogen activator, *PLG* Plasminogen, IMPab (IMP) Importin alpha-beta, Rdrp RNA dependant RNA polymerase, KPNA-1 (Karyopherin Subunit Alpha 1), NF-kB nuclear factor kappa-light-chain-enhancer of activated B cells, Map3Kinases Mitogen-activated Kinases, PAK-1 P21 Activated Kinase 1, STAT-3 Signal transducer and activator of transcription 3, PAI-1 Plasminogen activator inhibitor-1, HIF-1 Hypoxia-Inducible Factor.

### 4.3. Azithromycin

Azithromycin is a macrolide antibiotic that is used to treat a wide range of bacterial infections (Parnham et al., 2014). In addition to its antibacterial properties, this macrolide exhibits antiviral and immunomodulatory properties that could be useful in viral infections like COVID-19. The antiviral and immunomodulatory modes of action of azithromycin in the treatment of COVID-19 are depicted in Figure 1. SARS-CoV-2 binding to respiratory cells could be affected by azithromycin. Its intracellular accumulation resulted in a rise in pH, which could disrupt TGN (trans Golgi network) and lysosome functioning (Nujić et al., 2012; Poschet et al., 2020). Poschet et al. (2020) discovered that giving CF bronchial epithelial cells 100 μM for 1 hour and 1 μM of azithromycin for 48 hours increased TGN pH from 6.1 ± 0.2 to 6.7 ± 0.1. The authors speculated that the increased pH in TGN would affect hACE2 and other proteins' glycosylation (Poschet et al., 2020)]. Another direct antiviral mechanism of this macrolide has been proposed using molecular dynamic simulations. Given its similar volume and chemical properties to GM1, azithromycin produced a ganglioside-mimic. Because the SARS-CoV-2 spike protein has a ganglioside-binding site, azithromycin could prevent SARS-CoV-2 infection by binding to this site. This would prevent the viral spike protein from reaching gangliosides on the host plasma membrane, which are important in the pathogenesis of SARS-CoV-2 (Fantini eta al., 2020).

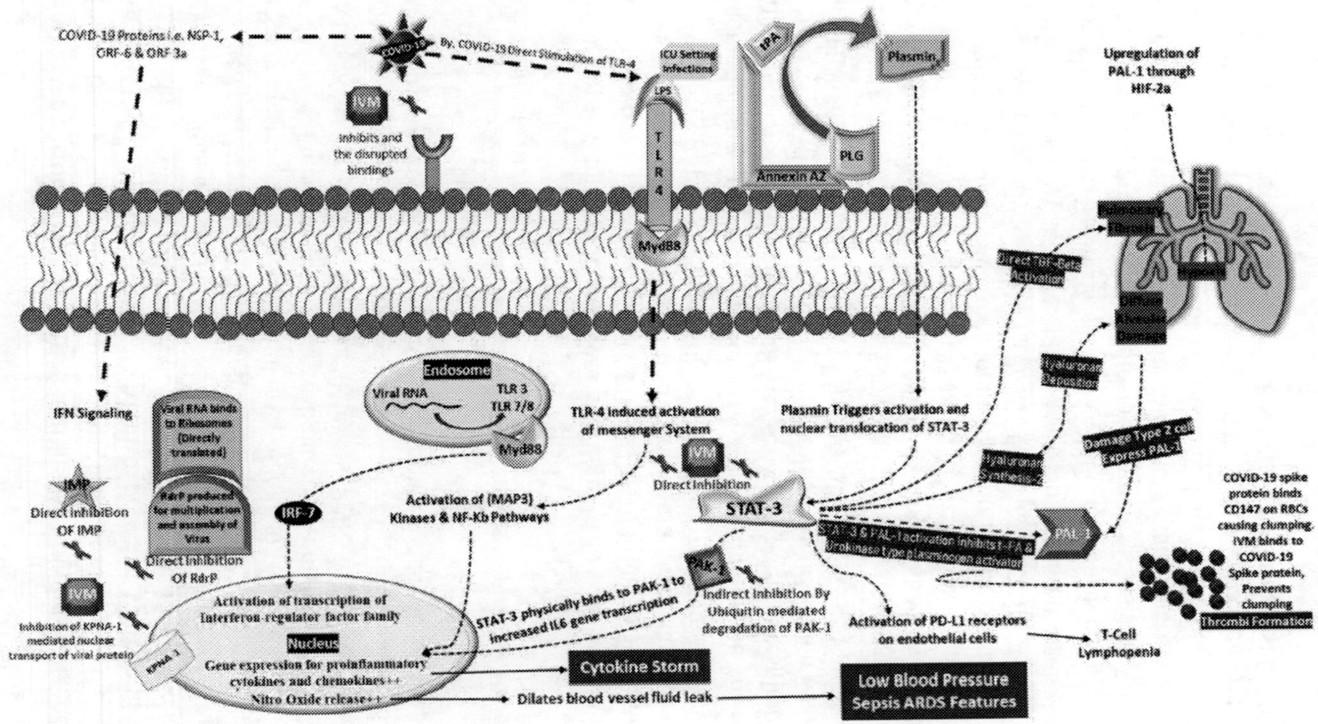


**Figure 1.** Ivermectin; IVM prevents and inhibits the SARS-CoV-2 S protein from binding to ACE-2 receptors. Activation pathways are shown by dotted lines, whereas inhibitory routes are represented by red dotted lines.

Furthermore, azithromycin may disrupt the connection between the spike protein and CD147, as well as CD147 expression (Ulrich and Pillat., 2020). The increase in lysosomal pH caused by azithromycin may affect endocytosis and the function of lysosomal proteases (cathepsins or furins), making the fusion process more difficult (Tyteca, et al., 2002; Nujić et al., 2012; Parnham et al., 2014; Poschet et al., 2020). Poschet et al. (2020) discovered that 100 M azithromycin might prevent excessive furin processing and activation. Because SARS-CoV-2 has been revealed to have a furin-like cleavage site in its spike protein, azithromycin's reduction in furin activation could inhibit SARS-CoV-2 from infecting human epithelial cells (Nitulescu et al., 2020; Poschet et al., 2020).

In infections of the lungs although it has been reported that it has a 37% oral bioavailability, the substantial tissue accumulation compensates for its sub-optimal absorption (Parnham et al., 2014). Azithromycin accumulates in epithelial cells, fibroblasts, lymphocytes, and alveolar macrophages, where concentrations might be 400 to 1,000 times greater than in serum (Parnham et al., 2014). Chemotactic drug delivery raises local drug concentrations even further, as stored azithromycin is released by blood phagocytes and other cells that migrate into infected and inflamed tissues (Parnham et al., 2014; Zheng et al., 2014). As a result, azithromycin has a half-life of 68-79 hours (Zhang et al., 2014). This medication has good lung tissue penetration and maintains drug concentrations for a long time (Danesi et al., 2003; Parnham et al., 2014; Zhang et al., 2014). A Cmax of 0.72-0.83 g/mL in bronchial washing and 8.93-9.13 g/mL in lung tissue was reported after taking 500 mg once a day (OD) for three days (Danesi et al., 2003; Damle et al., 2020). Peak concentrations in the epithelial lining fluid were 1.2-2.18 g/mL and 194 g/mL in alveolar macrophages after a single oral dose of 500 mg (Baldwin et al., 1990; Lucchi et al., 2008).

Azithromycin can be given as 500 mg or 250 mg OD for 3-5 days (Danesi et al., 2003). In viral infections, however, the appropriate dosage is uncertain. IDSA recommendations for community-acquired pneumonia (CAP) offer multiple regimens dependent on severity: outpatients should take 500 mg one day and 250 mg the next day for 3-5 days, whereas severe patients should take 500 mg OD for 5 days. 5 people were enrolled in the RECOVERY trial, which examined the impact of azithromycin in COVID-19, 500 mg OD during 10 days being studied (Horby et al., 2020).

Azithromycin has been demonstrated to have in vitro action against a wide range of viruses (Zika, Ebola, rhinovirus, enterovirus, influenza) with a wide range of 50% effective concentrations (EC50) depending on cell culture and multiplicity of infection (MOI) (Iannetta et al., 2017; Li, et al., 2019; Tran et al., 2019; Zeng et al., 2019; Damle et al., 2020). In the case of Zika virus, azithromycin was tested 12 hours before infection with a MOI of 0.1 in Vero, Huh7, A549, U87, and Hela cells, yielding an EC50 of 1.23-6.59 μM (Damle et al., 2020). In the case of Ebola, the experiment was carried out with Hela cells that had been pre-treated for 1-8 hours (MOI unknown) and had an EC50 of 0.69-2.79μM (Damle et al., 2020). In human bronchial epithelial cells with a MOI of 1.0, azithromycin was administered 24 hours before rhinovirus infection. Although the azithromycin EC50 was not measured in these conditions, rhinovirus replication was suppressed at 10 and 50 μM (Menzel at al., 2015; Damle et al., 2020). Zika and rhinovirus infections elevated virus-induced type I and III interferon responses, which reduced viral replication, suggesting that immunomodulatory activities, rather than antiviral efficacy, may be involved (Gielen et al., 2010; Schögler et al., 2015; Iannetta et al., 2017; Li, et al., 2019). Pre-treatment with azithromycin reduced viral load and alleviated hypothermia in mice with influenza A(H1N1) pneumonia (Tran et al., 2019).

Macrolides have been found to have antiviral efficacy against SARS-CoV-2 in vitro. In comparison to the control group, bafilomycin A reduced the entrance of pseudo virions by 99% (Ou et al., 2020). Azithromycin had an EC50 of 2.12 M, an EC90 of 8.65 M, and a 50% cytotoxic concentration > 40 M in Vero E6 cells with a MOI of 0.002, with a selectivity index of > 19 (Toure et al., 2020). On the other hand, another investigation in Vero E6 cells with a MOI of 0.25 azithromycin alone found no antiviral activity (Andreani et al., 2020). The combination of hydroxychloroquine at 5 mM and azithromycin at 5 mM and 10 mM, on the other hand, was found to be synergistic and suppressed viral replication considerably (Andreani et al., 2020). These disparities could be explained by the fact that the two trials had different MOIs. Because of the differences in MOI, cell lines, incubation durations, and analytical methodologies, caution is urged when interpreting these data (Damle et al., 2020). The aforementioned azithromycin treatment regimens could achieve therapeutic concentrations in the lungs, making them effective against SARS-CoV-2 (Andreani et al., 2020; Damle et al., 2020). Cmax/EC50 ratios of 91.5 in alveolar macrophages or 4.3 in lung tissue might be attained based on previously documented pharmacokinetic and *in vitro* results (Andreani et al., 2020; Damle et al., 2020). The authors of the Andreani et al. (2020) investigation concluded that the observed synergy with hydroxychloroquine was demonstrated at in vivo lung concentrations.

Azithromycin has immunomodulatory effects at many points in the inflammatory cascade, affecting cell activities and signaling pathways (Kanoh and Rubin, 2010; Zimmermann et al., 2018; Damle et al., 2020). By stabilizing the cell membrane, strengthening the transepithelial electrical barrier, and promoting the processing of the tight junction proteins claudins and junctional adhesion molecule-A in airway epithelial cells, macrolides can maintain cell integrity (Asgrimsson et al., 2006; Kanoh and Rubin, 2010; Arason et al., 2019). Even when not produced by bacteria, they can reduce mucus hypersecretion in vitro and in vivo, potentially improving mucociliary clearance (Kanoh and Rubin, 2010; Shimizu and Shimizu, 2012; Sligl et al., 2014). In addition, azithromycin relaxes precontracted airway smooth muscle cells directly (Parnham et al., 2014). By acting on inflammatory cells such as monocytes, macrophages, and fibroblasts *in vitro*, this macrolide can reduce the hypersecretion of pro-inflammatory cytokines and chemokines. IL-1β, IL-4, IL-5, IL-6, IL-8, IL-12, IFN-α, IP-10, TNF-, and GM-CSF have all been linked to its use (Kanoh and Rubin, 2010; Parnham et al., 2014; Zimmermann et al., 2018). Azithromycin altered alveolar macrophage polarization to the alternate activated anti-inflammatory M2 phenotype, resulting in reduced Th-1 cell responses (Parnham et al., 2014). It also boosted macrophage phagocytosis of apoptotic bronchial epithelial cells (Sligl et al., 2014).

Azithromycin has been demonstrated to inhibit CD4+ T-cell activation in lymphocytes (Ratzinger et al., 2014). Azithromycin, on the other hand, has been shown to stimulate the release of an anti-inflammatory cytokine (IL-10) involved in the healing of inflamed tissues (Kanoh and Rubin, 2010; Parnham et al., 2014). Azithromycin therapy reduced mortality in mice with pneumococcal pneumonia and viral bronchiolitis (Beigelman et al., 2010; Karlström et al., 2011). These results were discovered even in macrolide-resistant bacteria, implying that immunomodulatory characteristics, these advantages could be explained by aversion to cytokine storm, for example. Inflammatory cells (macrophages, lymphocytes, and neutrophils) were reduced in bronchoalveolar lavage and lung tissue by azithromycin (Beigelman et al., 2010). In addition, chemokines (G-CSF, CCL3/MIP-1, CCL4/MIP-1) and cytokines (IL-1, IL-6, IL-12, TNF-, and IFN-) were downregulated in the lungs (Beigelman et al., 2010).

*In vitro,* macrolides have been shown to reduce fibroblast proliferation, collagen synthesis, and transforming growth factor (TGF-β) levels in fibroblasts (Deretic and Timmins, 2020). Azithromycin significantly reduced fibrosis and restrictive lung function patterns in a mouse model of acute lung damage caused by bleomycin (Wuyts et al., 2010). Azithromycin may have antifibrotic and proapoptotic effects on primary fibroblasts once fibrosis has been established (Krempaska et al., 2020). As a result, azithromycin may decrease lung fibrosis in the late fibroproliferative-fibrotic phase of ARDS (Kawamura et al., 2018). Despite the lack of particular data, this macrolide has immunomodulatory capabilities that could be useful in the treatment of cancer.

### 4.4. N-acetylcysteine

Several clinical research on the impact of N-acetylcysteine on viral respiratory tract infections are now underway. A randomized controlled experiment found that taking N-acetylcysteine for a long time reduced the number of bouts of influenza and influenza-like sickness, the severity of the disease, and the length of time spent in bed due to respiratory disorders. In the N-acetylcysteine arm, only 25% of the virus-infected patients showed symptoms, compared to 79% in the placebo arm (De Flora et al., 1997). Benefits were also seen in individuals with community-acquired pneumonia, where plasma levels of malondialdehyde (an oxidative stress measure) and TNF- (an inflammatory mediator) were reduced and total antioxidant capacity was dramatically improved, among those treated with N-acetylcysteine (Zhang et al., 2018).

Furthermore, as compared to placebo, N-acetylcysteine resulted in a lower rate of ventilator-associated pneumonia. N-acetylcysteine-treated patients had a considerably shorter ICU stay, a faster time to hospital discharge, and a greater rate of complete recovery (Sharafkhah et al., 2018). In a clinical case study, oseltamivir and N-acetylcysteine combined therapy improved clinical outcomes in a woman with H1N1 influenza pneumonia, with clearing of pulmonary infiltrates, decreased need for oxygen supplementation, and lower C-reactive protein plasma levels (Lai et al., 2010).

However, the bulk of human studies involving N-acetylcysteine in COVID-19 infection were limited in scale, non-randomized, and lacked suitable comparator groups. 140 patients with severe COVID-19 infection and oxyhemoglobin saturation of less than 94% or respiratory rate greater than 24 breaths/minute were randomized to receive N-acetylcysteine 21,000 mg (approximately 300 mg/kg) or dextrose 5% for 20 hours in a single-center, randomized, double-blind, placebo-controlled trial conducted at the Emergency Department of a hospital in Brazil (placebo). In the 135 patients in the intention-to-treat population, 16 patients (24%) on placebo required endotracheal intubation and invasive mechanical breathing, compared to 14 patients (21%) in the N-acetylcysteine group (P=0.675). There were no changes in mechanical ventilation duration, death rate, ICU admission rate, ICU stay duration, or hospital stay (De Alencar et al., 2021).

A single-center, randomized, double-blind, placebo-controlled trial evaluating a combined metabolic cofactors supplementation encompassing L-serine, N-acetylcysteine, nicotinamide riboside, and L-carnitine tartrate in 309 adult patients with laboratory-confirmed COVID-19 infection found that the intervention group's mean recovery time was significantly shorter (5.7 vs 9.2 days, $P<0.0001$). On Day 14, serum alanine aminotransferase (P=0.032), lactate dehydrogenase (P<0.0001), and creatinine levels (P<0.0001) in the intervention group were significantly lower than on Day 0. Furthermore, on Day 14, patients who received metabolic cofactor supplementation had a larger magnitude of decrease in plasma levels of downregulated cytokines than those who received a placebo. On Day 14, the intervention group's plasma levels of cytokines linked to inflammatory reactions (CSF-1, IL-15RA, IL18, MCP-1, and TNF) were considerably lower than the placebo groups. Only two patients in the intervention group (2.8%) experienced a minor rash on the upper body as an adverse event (Wong et al., 2021).

In 40 patients with laboratory-confirmed COVID-19 infection, a multicenter, retrospective cohort research in Clinic Bascoy and ClnicaArvila Magna, Spain, compared the effectiveness of an ImmunoFormulation containing N-acetylcysteine to standard care. In the ImmunoFormulation cohort, 91% of patients recovered from the infection, compared to 47% in the control cohort ($P=0.006$). Patients with mild symptoms (11.22 vs. 28.00 days), moderate symptoms (17.57 vs. 28.00 days), and severe symptoms (17.57 vs. 28.00 days) had significantly shorter recovery times in the ImmunoFormulation cohort than in the control cohort (16.00 vs 25.42 days). Fever (2.25 vs 21.78 days), dry cough (4.38 vs 24.00 days), dyspnea (3.67 vs 20.00 days), headache (2.00 vs 26.50 days), diarrhea (5.25 vs 25.25 days), and weakness (1.92 vs 23.30 days) were all substantially shorter in the ImmunoFormulation cohort compared to the control group (all P0<05). Except for the loss of taste or smell (19.73 days), which was recognized as a long-term consequence of COVID-19, Immuno Formulation was associated with remission of all clinical symptoms within 2–5 days. There were no adverse medication reactions in any of the patients. In COVID-19 patients, Immune-formulation containing 560 mg N-acetylcysteine daily was an effective adjuvant therapy for the progression of symptomatology (Wong et al., 2021).

There has been no research that particularly examines the effect of N-acetylcysteine on COVID-19 infection *in vitro* or *in vivo*. Previous research on other viruses, such as influenza and respiratory syncytial virus, has suggested that N-acetylcysteine may be used in COVID-19. The capacity of N-acetylcysteine to synthesize glutathione, enhance T lymphocyte proliferative response, and modify the inflammatory pathway has shown potential. N-acetylcysteine, a glutathione precursor, has been proposed as a viable treatment method for preventing NF-B activation and addressing cytokine storm syndrome and respiratory distress in COVID-19 pneumonia patients (Horowitz et al., 2020). Through redox exchange processes, N-acetylcysteine combines with cystine in plasma, reducing it to cysteine and releasing diacetylcystine and N-acetylcysteine-cysteine, which then enters human erythrocytes and maintains glutathione synthesis (Whillier et al., 2009).

Additional research has revealed the effect of N-acetylcysteine on T-cell proliferation and IL-2 release, implying that intracellular thiols govern specific signaling pathways for a novel immunoregulatory target (Hadzic et al., 2005). In addition, *in vitro* stimulation of murine T-cells with N-acetylcysteine causes reactive oxygen species to be scavenged, as well as the expression of NFAT and nuclear translocation. N-acetylcysteine promotes Myc expression and CD98 production in Cd4cre-Gclc T-cells. Antigen-specific protection against viral infections requires intrinsic Gclc expression in T-cells. The antioxidative glutathione pathway is discovered to be critical for metabolic integration and reprogramming in T-cell-mediated inflammatory responses (Mak et al., 2017).

In this approach, high-dose N-acetylcysteine has been shown to replace decreased pulmonary glutathione levels while simultaneously improving lung function (Demedts et al., 2005). In chronic inflammatory illness, the medication also raises glutathione levels in peripheral blood T cells and inhibits the activation of the mammalian target of rapamycin (Lai et al., 2012). Given that severe COVID-19 shares common main risk factors with idiopathic pulmonary fibrosis, N-ability acetylcysteine to reduce the rate of decline in vital capacity and single-breath lung diffusion capacity for carbon monoxide suggests a viable treatment option for COVID-19 patients As a result, it is hypothesized that high-dose N-acetylcysteine can improve patient outcomes by enhancing innate and adaptive immunity by increasing glutathione reserves in T cells and modifying immune-system responses to reduce the severity of COVID-19 infection (Demedts et al., 2005; Lai et al., 2012; George et al., 2020). *In vitro* studies to test candidate therapeutic compounds in COVID-19 should use standardized assays, such as Vero cells, which can competently replicate and isolate the virus, whereas in vivo studies should use transgenic mice and Syrian hamsters, or cats and ferrets if larger experimental animals are preferred (Takayama, 2020).

It's worth noting that IL-6 is one of the key regulators of inflammation in COVID-19 (Rubin et al., 2021). In severe situations such as sepsis, acute respiratory distress syndrome, and COVID-19, increases in serum IL-6 concentrations have been observed (Jones and Hunter., 2021; McElvaney et al., 2021). Innate and adaptive immunity, efficient pathogen clearance, and physiological activities like acute-phase response control, hematopoiesis, lipid homeostasis, metabolism, and brain development all require IL-6 (Garbers et al., 2018). In essence, classical signaling facilitates IL-6's anti-inflammatory, pro-resolution, and antibacterial actions, whereas trans-signalling facilitates IL-6's pro-inflammatory activities (Jones and Jenkins., 2021). Targeting the pathogenic effects of IL-6-mediated inflammation should prevent the inadvertent elimination of the anti-inflammatory and pro-resolution properties of the protein. (McElvaney et al., 2021).

In patients with COVID-19, including those with acute hypoxemic respiratory failure, blocking IL-6 and the subsequent lowering of downstream effects on inflammation and the innate immune response may improve clinical outcomes (Angriman et al., 2021). Recent in vitro and in vivo evidence of N-potential acetylcysteine's role in IL-6 inhibition could spur more research into how the drug affects disease outcomes and how to maximize its benefits with concomitant pharmacotherapy to selectively inhibit the trans-signaling pathway through which IL-6 signals.

Adverse effects of oral and intravenous N-acetylcysteine therapy include diarrhea, nausea, vomiting, and mild-to-moderate hypersensitivity reactions such as urticaria, rash, angioedema, and asthma (Bethesda, 2012; Bateman et al., 2014). Antihistamines are useful for treating and avoiding the recurrence of anaphylactic reactions, and they are dose-related. Antihistamines should be used to treat urticaria, and N-acetylcysteine should be continued after the symptoms have subsided. Antihistamine, corticosteroid, or symptomatic treatment are required for angioedema and respiratory symptoms (Tarbox et al., 2018). In such circumstances, N-acetylcysteine should be stopped and restarted 1 hour after the antihistamine has been administered if there are no indications or symptoms of anaphylaxis (Bailey et al., 1998; Daoud et al., 2020). Patients who have a history of atopy (asthma and allergies) should take a prophylactic antihistamine 15 minutes before taking N-acetylcysteine to reduce the chance of adverse events (Schmidt and Dalhoff, 2001; Daoud et al., 2020).

There are currently six registered clinical trials assessing N-potential acetylcysteine's therapeutic efficacy against COVID-19 (Wong et al., 2021). The findings will support the use of N-acetylcysteine as an adjuvant therapy for COVID-19 depending on *in vitro* and early *in vivo* evidence. Study endpoints should appropriately include changes in SARS-CoV-2 associated blood cytokine levels, changes in peripheral-blood lymphocyte count and activation, improvement in clinical status, hospital length of stay, time to recovery, safety outcomes, and overall mortality, similar to clinical trials on other infectious respiratory illnesses. Although changed virus virulence, pathogenicity, and transmissibility have been recorded, SARS-CoV-2 variations appear to occur randomly in different geographical places around the world, they do not result in more severe infections than the original strain (Baric, 2020; Wong et al., 2021). Future trials in individuals infected with mutated SARS-CoV-2 strains may help validate or disprove the possibility of N-acetylcysteine as a therapy advantage.

It's worth noting that interactions between arthropods and coronaviruses are caused by molecular attraction forces between chitin found on the exoskeleton of mites on human skin (Demodecidae or Pyemotidae species) and lipids present on the viral envelope of SARS-CoV-2 (Tatu et al., 2021). Natural small molecules, such as cyclodextrins and phytosterols, may prevent viral lipid-dependent attachment to host cells, lowering the virus's infectivity (Baglivo et al., 2020). These natural chemicals are now available in a variety of dietary supplements (Baglivo et al., 2020). Their antiviral potential encourages more investigation into developing novel biomedical applications for the treatment and prevention of COVID-19. This suggests that N-acetylcysteine may play a role in preventing arthropod coronavirus contact and producing antimicrobial effects on *Demodex folliculorum* endosymbionts (Kubiak et al., 2018).

Ivermectin is a broad-spectrum anti-parasitic medicine that has anti-inflammatory and acaricidal effects on Demodex mites, as well as antiviral effectiveness against a variety of viruses (Caly et al., 2020). Downregulation of pro-inflammatory genes such as IL-8, TNF-, and cathelicidin LL-37, as well as downregulation of the ACE-2 receptor and viral entrance into respiratory epithelial and olfactory bulb cells, are all possible pathways (Chaccour et al., 2021). N-acetylcysteine can inhibit ivermectin-induced cell death due to reactive oxygen species formation as a free radical scavenger (Sharmeen et al., 2010), suggesting that their combination use may have benefits. Current clinical evidence, on the other hand, does not support the use of ivermectin for the treatment of COVID-19 since it does not significantly improve the time to symptom remission (López-Medina et al., 2021).

Patients with COVID-19 pneumonia may experience blood coagulation abnormalities, which include high fibrinogen and D-dimer levels as well as moderate thrombocytopenia (Connors and Levy, 2020; Levi et al., 2020), D-dimer levels that rise have been associated to a worse prognosis and a higher mortality rate (De Alencar et al., 2021). Neutrophil elastase activity affects D-dimer levels, lung inflammation, and pulmonary bleeding (De Alencar et al., 2021). As a result, suppressing elastase and neutrophil activation may be beneficial in COVID-19-related hemorrhagic or thrombotic consequences (De Alencar et al., 2021). When employed in high quantities, N-acetylcysteine has been shown to decrease elastase release and regulate neutrophil activity (De Alencar et al., 2021).

In cystic fibrosis patients with neutrophilic airway inflammation, high-dose N-acetylcysteine reduces the number of airway neutrophils actively producing elastase-rich granules (Tirouvanziam et al., 2006). Treatment with N-acetylcysteine can also slow the progression of elastase-induced lung emphysema, as seen by reduced airspace enlargements, partial recovery of expiratory flows, and normalization of lung collagen content (Rubio et al., 2004). These studies suggest that N-acetylcysteine may have a role in inflammation-mediated lung damage and blood coagulation problems in severe COVID-19 acetylcysteine's absorption and short plasma half-life have lately been resolved by novel formulations (Mursaleen et al., 2020). The incorporation of N-acetylcysteine into lipid- and polymer-based nanoparticles can improve muco-penetrating characteristics and thus medication efficacy in pulmonary and oral delivery (De Alencar et al., 2021).

The lipid nanoparticle approach, on the other hand, is constrained by N-low acetylcysteine's physicochemical stability and low-to-moderate encapsulation efficiency (De Alencar et al., 2021). A liposomal combination of azithromycin and N-acetylcysteine with co-encapsulated azithromycin and N-acetylcysteine was shown to have a synergistic impact against bacterial strains (Aljihani et al., 2020). The high cellular membrane permeability and targeting accuracy associated with such a delivery method suggest a possible role for N-acetylcysteine in antiviral medication co-formulation.

Recent research suggests that polymer-based nanoparticles containing N-acetylcysteine, such as N-acetylcysteine-loaded poly(lactic-co-glycolic acid), can help prevent acute lung injury by reducing the effects of reactive oxygen species and inflammation. With a smaller dose of N-acetylcysteine, the formulation distributes N-acetylcysteine directly to the lungs, resulting in enhanced pulmonary deposition and higher pulmonary concentrations (Karimi Zarchi et al., 2017). By prolonging drug release and particle retention, a polymer-based nanoparticle improves the pharmacokinetic and pharmacodynamic aspects of an encapsulated medication (Bailey and Berkland, 2009; Paranjpe and Müller-Goymann., 2014). Even though poly(lactic-co-glycolic acid) is one of the most widely used biodegradable polymers, its low drug loading necessitates a greater polymer load to facilitate dose delivery (Danhier et al., 2012). Biodegradable, water-soluble, biocompatible, biomimetic, and stable during storage are all characteristics of polymer-based nanoparticles. Additional targeting can be readily added to the surfaces. The danger of particle agglomeration and toxicity are both disadvantages (Mitchell et al., 2020).

N-acetylcysteine has been used intranasally to treat non-allergic chronic rhinitis with goblet cell metaplasia, with significant reductions in neutrophils, lymphocytes, goblet cells, bacterial count, turbinate hypertrophy, nasal symptoms, and rhinorrhea. The benefits are ascribed to N-mucolytic acetylcysteine's action, ability to restore surface ciliary activity at the nasal epithelium, and control of the inflammatory response, which is a key component of the nasal mucosa's immunological defense system (Maffezzoni et al., 2020). Similarly, nasal douche containing flunisolide (corticosteroid) and N-acetylcysteine has been linked to a less stuffy nose, reduced severity of symptoms and rhinosinus signs as measured by endoscopy, improved cytological grading of neutrophil and eosinophil cells, fewer exacerbations, and increased mucociliary motility in acute recurrent rhinosinusitis (Macchi et al., 2012).

Furthermore, a topical intranasal medication containing tuaminoheptane sulfate (vasoconstrictor) and N-acetylcysteine has a fast decongestant action, lowering resistance and increasing inspiratory flow (Cogo et al., 1996). In ragweed-sensitive patients, topical N-acetylcysteine administration in the nostrils was studied, and it was discovered that late-phase allergic response-mediated nasal symptoms can be minimized (Lane et al., 2009). In vivo, studies have shown that nasal application of N-acetylcysteine can reduce goblet cell loss and inflammation, as well as promote nasal mucosa wound healing and that combining N-acetylcysteine with a non-ionic surfactant (polyoxyethylene (C25) lauryl ether) can improve nasal bioavailability as a result of N-mucolytic acetylcysteine's activity (Wong et al., 2021). On top of the highly vascularized nasal cavity and huge surface area for drug absorption, evidence suggests that nasal route medication administration may be a potentially appealing technique for N-acetylcysteine (Wong et al., 2021).

## 4.5. Montelukast

Montelukast, a cysteinyl leukotriene (cysLT) receptor antagonist, may be used to treat COVID-19 infection, and the possibility of reducing severe COVID-19 progression will be discussed. COVID-19 has a wide range of clinical symptoms, from asymptomatic to acute respiratory distress syndrome and multi-organ failure. When the disease is severe, it can lead to pneumonia, respiratory failure, and mortality; acute complications in this scenario include acute lung damage, ARDS, sepsis, and shock. The excessive increase in proinflammatory cytokine levels is assumed to be the cause of this development (Rodriguez-Morales et al., 2020; Zhang et al., 2020).

Furthermore, COVID-19 binds to human ACE2 and enters the cell *via* angiotensin-converting enzyme (ACE) receptors, causing severe pneumonia and thus increasing mortality rates following infection (Fidan and Aydoğdu, 2020). Increased bradykinin and its bronchoconstrictor impact generate the cough that can develop with ACE inhibition, while montelukast, a specific LTD4 antagonist, inhibits bradykinin-induced airway hypersensitivity (Fidan and Aydoğdu, 2020). Although the exact mechanism of this impact is unknown, it is likely to be due to ACE receptors.

Respiratory failure, which is progressive and refractory to therapy, is the leading cause of COVID-19-related mortality (Fidan and Aydoğdu, 2020; Zhang et al., 2020). ARDS is an acute inflammatory lung injury that occurs frequently in these individuals and is caused by widespread alveolar injury induced by severe inflammation. It is a clinical disorder that is not well understood due to its complex pathophysiology. Leukocyte migration is induced by IL-6 and IL-8, tumor necrosis factor (TNF), and IL-1 produced in the early stages of the disease, as well as additional pro-inflammatory cytokines produced in the later stages of the disease. The activated leukocytes in the lungs then secrete reactive oxygen species and proteases, which cause damage to the capillary endothelium and alveolar epithelium.TNF-, IL-6, and IL-1b levels have been demonstrated to be reduced by montelukast medication in recent trials (Fidan and Aydoğdu, 2020; Rana et al., 2021). Montelukast has been shown to have a strong inhibitory impact on bradykinin-induced tracheal smooth muscle contractions, confirming the interaction between bradykinin and leukotriene mediators (Fidan and Aydoğdu, 2020).

Montelukast is an anti-inflammatory cysteinyl leukotriene (cysLT) receptor antagonist that has been shown to greatly reduce oxidative stress. CysLTs can also influence cytokine production. IL-4, IL-5, and IL-13 reduced protein expression in the lungs in response to high doses of i.v. administration of montelukast, which has an anti-inflammatory impact by suppressing T-helper type-2 cytokines. As a result, high-dose montelukast has been found to be beneficial as an anti-inflammatory drug in acute asthma (Wu et al., 2003). Furthermore, the usage of montelukast has been shown to reduce the frequency and severity of wheezing in patients with clinical episodic wheeze (wheezing after an upper respiratory tract infection caused by adenovirus, influenza, metapneumovirus, coronavirus). Montelukast does not appear to prevent viral infections in these patients, although it does appear to limit the upper respiratory tract (Brodlie., 2015; Fidan and Aydoğdu, 2020).

Montelukast has an influence on events emerging with ACE receptors, as well as an anti-inflammatory action with bradykinin and leukotriene antagonism, based on these findings; Because COVID-19 enters the cell *via* ACE receptors and causes death due to excessive inflammatory processes, montelukast was expected to have a limiting influence on the illness progression in COVID-19 infection. It shows that using it, possibly at large dosages, to lower the severity of the disease during the course of the disease or before the disease fully manifests in persons at risk could be useful. On these damages, montelukast's therapeutic benefits can be visible.

Atherogenic Vascular Inflammation and some severe COVID-19 problems are thought to be primarily attributable to the host (Zhang et al., 2020). They are impacted by age, gender, and comorbidities, particularly those associated with previous inflammatory vascular and pulmonary diseases. The cysLT are specifically engaged in the inflammatory phase of the atheromatous process, despite the fact that they have yet to be utilized in this indication. Antagonizing cysLT receptors reduces arterial spasm in human coronary arteries with atherosclerotic lesions significantly, but has no impact on healthy coronary arteries (Allen et al., 1993). According to a systematic evaluation of MK's anti-atheromatous capabilities in twenty-six animal and two human trials, all findings supported the efficacy of LKs and MK on the atheromatous process (Hoxha et al., 2018). As a result, LKs may lower COVID-19 mortality in atheromatous patients, providing protection that is (theoretically) proportional to the degree and severity of the lesions (Almerie et al., 2020).

Following reperfusion, the ischemia/reperfusion process causes downstream vascular lesions. Tissue hypoxia and hypoperfusion increase the likelihood of new endothelial lesions and ruptured atheroma plaque in individuals with severe atheromatous disease, leading to thrombosis and emboli. This could help to explain why COVID-19 is linked to an increased risk of arterial and venous thromboembolism, which affects about 30% of SARS-CoV-2-infected patients in intensive care units (Klok et al., 2020). In animal models of intestinal anastomosis (Sayin et al., 2020), skeletal muscles (Bilgiç et al., 2018), the spinal cord (Korkmaz et al., 2015), and even ovarian or testicular torsion/distortion, MK alleviates the ischemia/reperfusion phenomenon. An MK-coated coronary stent is now being developed (Barré et al., 2020).

Asthma, hyper-reactivity bronchitis, and post-infectious cough, for which LKs are commonly recommended, is a common and dangerous disorder that affects 7%–8% of the population, despite the fact that it is still underdiagnosed and undertreated (Barré et al., 2020). When MK is an asthmatic analog, it is helpful against cough regardless of functional respiratory characteristics (Miwa et al., 2018). MK, on the other hand, has not been found to be effective in the treatment of chronic post-infectious cough (Wang et al., 2020), despite a high level of subjective improvement in the placebo group in this trial (Wang et al., 2020). MK's effects on moderate symptomatic COVID-19 respiratory injury would be interesting to investigate (bronchospasms, cough, and chest pain). The need for speed in identifying prospective remedies has demanded greater research into a wide spectrum of potential therapeutic substances and their undesirable effects (Table 1) (Di Lorenzo et al., 2020).

**Table 1.** Undesirable effects of the drugs tested in COVID-19

| Drugs tested in COVID-19 | Side effects |
|---|---|
| Favipiravir | Most common: nausea, vomiting, diarrhea, abdominal pain, anorexia, headache, anemia, muscle and joint pain. |
| Remdesivir | Common: leukopenia and thrombocytopenia, abnormal liver function; confusion, aggressive behaviour, agitation, migraine, tremors, paresthesia, dysgeusia. |
| Lopinavir | Uncommon: muscle weakness, pancreas dysfunction, lethargy, convulsions, coma, hallucinations, ataxia, kidney failure |
| Ribavirin | Commonly used for the treatment of hepatitis C and for inflammatory lung diseases, such as bronchiolitis, this antiviral drug is always used in combination with other medicines, such as interferon alfa and peginterferon alfa and can be used both in the treatment of adult and in the treatment of pediatric patients. |
| Chloroquine/ hydroxychloroquine | Common: anorexia, weight loss, nausea, abdominal pain, diarrhea, vomiting, corneal changes; uncommon: affective lability, nervousness, headache, dizziness, accommodation disorders |
| | Rare: retinopathy with changes in pigmentation and visual field defects, edema and opacity dizziness, tinnitus, bundle branch block, atrioventricular block, abnormal liver function tests, hypoglycemia skin rash, graying of the hair, alopecia, rashes, tiredness, psoriasis not sensitive to light |

**Table 1.** (Continued)

| Drugs tested in COVID-19 | Side effects |
|---|---|
| Azithromycin | Most common: diarrhea.; Common: nausea, vomiting, abdominal pain, headache.; Uncommon: asthenia, irritability, dermatological disorders as rush skin, edema, urticaria; Rare: abnormal liver function |
| Anakinra | Most common: itching, erythema, pain, bruising, bleeding in the inoculation site, headache; common: abdominal pain, nausea, diarrhea |
| Tocilizumab | Most common: upper airway infections, hypercholesterolemia |
| | Common: pneumonia, cellulite, herpes zoster, abdominal pain, neutropenia, thrombocytopenia, abnormal liver function, gastrointestinal perforation, episodes of hypertension during drug infusion, headache, skin reactions |
| | Uncommon: hypothyroidism, stomach ulcers |
| Ivermectin | Common: dizziness, nausea, diarrhea, swelling of the joints, rapid heart beat |
| | Uncommon: loss of appetite, vomiting, constipation, weakness, drowsiness, swelling of the eyes, face, arms, hands, feet |
| Eculizumab | Most common: headache; Common: dizziness,diarrhea, abdominal pain, arthralgias, asthenia; Uncommon: back pain, abnormal liver function, kidney failure. |
| Emapalumab | Most common: infections, hypertension |
| Sarilumab | Most common: neutropenia; common: ALT elevation, injection site erythema |

*Frequency of adverse events: Most common ≥1/10; Common <1/10 - ≥ 1/100; Uncommon < 1/100->1/1000; Rare < 1/1000->1/10000.

## 4.6. Ruxolitinib

Ruxolitinib is an inhibitor of the Janus Kinase (Jak)-mediated signaling system, which has anti-inflammatory effects by inhibiting the production of cytokines (Verstovsek, 2013). Ruxolitinib is typically used in the field of hematology to treat splenomegaly or disease-related symptoms in adult patients with primary myelofibrosis. It's also licensed for treating adult polycythemiavera people who are resistant or intolerant to hydroxyurea. AIFA has also approved a compassionate use of Ruxolitinib in COVID-19 patients with respiratory failure who do not require invasive assisted ventilation (Mortara et al., 2021).

### 4.7. Colchicine

Colchicine is a chemical that can interfere with the inflammatory immunological response seen in COVID-19 patients. Colchicine is an anti-inflammatory medication that has been used for a long time to treat acute gouty arthritis attacks. It manages to suppress the release of cytokines, which are chemicals responsible for inflammation, such as IL-6. In Italy, a study has just begun (Di Lorenzo et al., 2020).

### 4.8. Heparin

The use of an old medicine, heparin, resulted in a 20% reduction in mortality among COVID-19 individuals with a significant rise in an indicator of the presence of blood clots. According to a study, the usage of heparin in COVID-19 individuals may have anticoagulant, anti-inflammatory, and maybe antiviral benefits. In the presence of a high value of D-dimer, a particularly critical marker for coagulopathy, fresh coronavirus infections have been linked to a high fatality rate. However, more research is needed to determine at what dosage the medicine might have antiviral capabilities. AIFA recently approved a research with enoxaparin (INHIXACOVID) (Di Lorenzo et al., 2020).

## Conclusion

To continue treating COVID-19 patients, we believe it is vital to change current therapy alternatives and develop a new therapeutic strategy. Finally, we provide four examples of people who were at high risk of SARS-CoV-2 infection-related morbidity and mortality and who improved and/or had a moderate clinical course after taking doxycycline. Despite its safety, we would not recommend using doxycycline in the treatment of COVID-19+ people unless they are under the care and supervision of a physician. A larger randomized controlled trial should be considered. The benefits of ivermectin and doxycycline as potential COVID-19 treatments are now being evaluated by the Indian Council of Medical Research. In a case series of Covid 19 patients treated with a combination of Ivermectin and Doxycycline, several observational studies in Bangladesh recently showed good results. The combination was evaluated by Dr. Tarek Alam of the Bangladesh Medical College. In a mouse model of acute lung injury caused by bleomycin, azithromycin dramatically reduced fibrosis and restrictive lung function. Once fibrosis has developed, azithromycin may have antifibrotic and proapoptotic effects on primary fibroblasts. As a result, azithromycin may reduce lung fibrosis in patients with ARDS who are in the late fibroproliferative-fibrotic stage. Despite the lack of specific data, COVID-19, a macrolide with immunomodulatory properties, could be effective in the treatment of cancer.

Intranasally administered N-acetylcysteine has been shown to reduce neutrophils, lymphocytes, goblet cells, bacterial count, turbinate hypertrophy, nasal symptoms, and rhinorrhea in non-allergic chronic rhinitis with goblet cell metaplasia. The action of N-mucolytic acetylcysteine, as well as its ability to restore surface ciliary activity at the nasal epithelium and regulation of the inflammatory response, which is a crucial component of the nasal mucosa's immunological defense system, are credited with the advantages. In acute recurrent rhinosinusitis, a nasal douche containing flunisolide (corticosteroid) and N-acetylcysteine has been linked to a less stuffy nose, decreased severity of symptoms and rhinosinus signs as measured by endoscopy, improved cytological grading of neutrophil and eosinophil cells, fewer exacerbations, and increased mucociliary motility. A topical intranasal medicine comprising tuaminoheptane sulfate (vasoconstrictor) and N-acetylcysteine also has a quick decongestant effect, decreasing resistance and enhancing inspiratory flow. Topical N-acetylcysteine injection in the nostrils was tested in ragweed-sensitive patients, and it was revealed that late-phase allergic response-mediated nasal symptoms can be reduced. *In vivo* studies have shown that nasal application of N-acetylcysteine can reduce goblet cell loss and inflammation, as well as promote nasal mucosa wound healing and that combining N-acetylcysteine with a non-ionic surfactant (polyoxyethylene (C25) lauryl ether) can improve nasal bioavailability as a result of the activity of N-mucolytic acetylcysteine. Evidence suggests that nasal route pharmaceutical delivery for N-acetylcysteine may be a potentially appealing strategy due to the highly vascularized nasal cavity and large surface area for drug absorption.

Montelukast, a cysteinyl leukotriene receptor antagonist, may be utilized to treat COVID-19 infection, and the possibility of slowing the progression of severe COVID-19 will be examined. The clinical signs of COVID-19 vary from asymptomatic to acute respiratory distress syndrome and multi-organ failure. Acute complications in this scenario include immediate lung damage, ARDS, sepsis, and shock; when the disease is severe, it can lead to pneumonia, respiratory failure, and death; acute complications in this scenario include acute lung damage, ARDS, sepsis, and shock. This development is thought to be caused by an excessive increase in proinflammatory cytokine levels. Furthermore, COVID-19 binds to human ACE2 and enters the cell through angiotensin-converting enzyme (ACE) receptors, resulting in severe pneumonia and an increase in infection-related mortality. Increased bradykinin and its bronchoconstrictor effect cause cough, while montelukast, a selective LTD4 antagonist, reduces bradykinin-induced airway hypersensitivity. Although the specific mechanism of this effect is uncertain, ACE receptors are most likely to blame. This development is thought to be caused by an excessive increase in proinflammatory cytokine levels. Furthermore, COVID-19 binds to human ACE2 and enters the cell through angiotensin-converting enzyme (ACE) receptors, resulting in severe pneumonia and an increase in infection-related mortality. Increased bradykinin and its bronchoconstrictor effect cause cough, while montelukast, a selective LTD4 antagonist, reduces bradykinin-induced airway hypersensitivity. Although the specific mechanism of this effect is uncertain, ACE receptors are most likely to blame.

## References

Aljihani, S. A., Alehaideb, Z. & Alarfaj, R. E. (2020). Enhancing azithromycin antibacterial activity by encapsulation in liposomes/liposomal-N-acetylcysteine formulations against resistant clinical strains of *Escherichia coli*. *Saudi Journal of Biological Sciences,* 27(11), 3065–3071.

Allen, S. P., Dashwood, M. R., Chester, A. H., Tadjkarimi, S., Collins, M. & Piper, P. J. (1993). Influence of Atherosclerosis on the Vascular Reactivity of Isolated Human Epicardial Coronary Arteries to Leukotriene C4. *Cardioscience*, 4(1), 47–54.

Almerie, M. Q. & Kerrigan, D. D. (2020). The association between obesity and poor outcome after COVID-19 indicates a potential therapeutic role for montelukast. *Medical Hypotheses,* 143, 109883.

Andreani, J., Le Bideau, M. & Duflot, I. (2020). In vitro testing of combined hydroxychloroquine and azithromycin on SARS-CoV-2 shows synergistic effect. *Microbial Pathogenesis,* 145, 104228.

Angriman, F., Ferreyro, B. L. & Burry, L. (2021). Interleukin-6 receptor blockade in patients with COVID-19: placing clinical trials into context. *Lancet Respiratory Medicine,* 9(6), 655-664.

Arason, A. J., Joelsson, J. P. & Valdimarsdottir, B. (2019). Azithromycin induces epidermal differentiation and multivesicular bodies in airway epithelia. *Respiratory Research,* 20(1), 1-19.

Asgrimsson, V., Gudjonsson, T. & Gudmundsson, G. H. (2006). Novel effects of azithromycin on tight junction proteins in human airway epithelia. *Antimicrobial Agents and Chemotherapy,* 50(5), 1805–1812.

Ata, F., Almasri, H., Sajid, J. & Yousaf, Z. (2020). COVID-19 presenting with diarrhoea and hyponatraemia. *BMJ case reports*, 13(6), e235456.

Baglivo, M., Baronio, M. & Natalini, G. (2020). Natural small molecules as inhibitors of coronavirus lipid-dependent attachment to host cells: a possible strategy for reducing SARS-COV-2 infectivity? *Acta Biomedica,* 91(1), 161–164.

Bailey, B. & McGuigan, M. A. (1998). Management of anaphylactoid reactions to intravenous N-acetylcysteine. *Annals of Emergency Medicine,* 31(6), 710–715.

Bailey, M. M. & Berkland, C. J. (2009). Nanoparticle formulations in pulmonary drug delivery. *Medicinal Research Reviews,* 29(1). 196–212.

Baldwin, D. R., Wise, R., Andrews, J. M., Ashby, J. P. & Honeybourne, D. (1990). Azithromycin concentrations at the sites of pulmonary infection. *European Respiratory Journal*, 3(8), 886–890.

Banerjee, K., Nandy, M., Dalai, C. K. & Ahmed, S. N. (2020). The battle against COVID 19 pandemic: what we need to know before we "test fire" Ivermectin. *Drug Research (Stuttg),* 70(8), 337–340.

Baric, R. S. (2020). Emergence of a Highly Fit SARS-CoV-2 Variant. *New England Journal of Medicine*. 383(27), 2684–2686.

Barré, J., Sabatier, J. M. & Annweiler, C. (2020). Montelukast drug may improve COVID-19 prognosis: A review of evidence. *Frontiers in Pharmacology*, 11, 1344.

Bateman, D. N., Dear, J. W. & Thanacoody, H. K. R. (2014). Reduction of adverse effects from intravenous acetylcysteine treatment for paracetamol poisoning: A randomised controlled trial. *Lancet*, 383(9918), 697–704.

Beigelman, A., Mikols, C. L. & Gunsten, S. P. (2010). Azithromycin attenuates airway inflammation in a mouse model of viral bronchiolitis. *Respiratory Research,* 11(1),1–11.

Bilgiç, M. İ., Altun, G., Çakıcı, H., Gideroğlu, K. & Saka, G. (2018). The protective effect of Montelukast against skeletal muscle ischemia reperfusion injury: An experimental rat model. *Ulusal Travma ve Acil Cerrahi Dergisi,* 24(3), 185–190.

Brake, S. J., Barnsley, K., Lu, W., Mc Alinden, K. D., Eapen, M. S. & Sohal, S. S. (2020). Smoking upregulates angiotensin-converting enzyme-2 receptor: a potential adhesion site for novel coronavirus SARS-CoV-2 (Covid-19). *Journal of Clinical Medicine, 9*(3), 841.

Brasier, A. R. (2010). The nuclear factor-kappaBinterleukin-6 signalling pathway mediating vascular inflammation. *Cardiovascular Research,* 86, 211–218.

Brodlie, M., Gupta, A., Rodriguez-Martinez, C. E., Castro-Rodriguez, J. A., Ducharme F. M. & McKean M. C. (2015). Leukotriene receptor antagonists as maintenance and intermittent therapy for episodic viral wheeze in children. *Cochrane Database Systematic Review*, 2015(10), CD008202.

Caly, L. Druce, J. D., Catton, M. G., Jans, D. A. & Wagstaff, K. M. (2020). The FDA-approved drug ivermectin inhibits the replication of SARS-CoV-2 in vitro. *Antiviral Research,* 178, 104787.

Caly, L., Druce, J. D., Catton, M. G., Jans, D. A. & Wagstaff, K. M. (2020). The FDA approved drug ivermectin inhibits the replication of SARS CoV-2 in vitro. *Antiviral Research,* 178, 104787.

Chaccour, C., Casellas, A. & Blanco-Di Matteo, A. (2021). The effect of early treatment with ivermectin on viral load, symptoms and humoral response in patients with non-severe COVID-19: a pilot, double-blind, placebo-controlled, randomized clinical trial. *Clinical Medicine*, 32.

Chen, T., Wu, D., Chen, H., Yan, W., Yang, D., Chen, G., Ma, K., Xu, D., Yu, H., Wang, H. & Wang, T. (2020). Clinical characteristics of 113 deceased patients with coronavirus disease 2019: Retrospective study. *British Medical Journal*, 368, m1295.

Chen, W., Zheng, K. I., Liu, S., Yan, Z., Xu, C. & Qiao, Z. (2020). Plasma CRP level is positively associated with the severity of COVID-19. *Annals of Clinical Microbiology and Antimicrobials*, 19(1), 1-7.

Choi, B., Lee, S., Kim, S. M., Lee, E. J., Lee, S. R., Kim, D. H., Jang, J. Y., Kang, S. W., Lee, K. U., Chang, E. J. & Song, J. K. (2017). Dipeptidyl peptidase-4 induces aortic valve calcification by inhibiting insulin-like growth factor-1 signaling in valvular interstitial cells. *Circulation,* 135(20), 1935–1950.

Chow, Y. W., Pietranico, R. & Mukerji, A. (1975). Studies of oxygen binding energy to hemoglobin molecule. *Biochemical and Biophysical Research Communications*, 66(4), 1424–1431.

Chowdhury, A. T., Shahbaz, M., Karim, M. R., Islam, J., Dan, G. & He, S. A. (2021). Comparative observational study on Ivermectin-Doxycycline and Hydroxychloroquine-Azithromycin therapy on COVID-19 patients. *Eurasian Journal of Medical Investigation*, 5(1), 63-70.

Cogo, A., Chieffo, A., Farinatti, M. & Ciaccia, A. (1996). Efficacy of topical tuaminoheptane combined with N-acetyl-cysteine in reducing nasal resistance. A double-blind rhinomanometric study versus xylometazoline and placebo. *Arzneimittelforschung*, 46(4), 385–388.

Colombi, D., Bodini, F. C., Petrini, M., Maffi, G., Morelli, N., Milanese, G., Silva, M., Sverzellati, N. & Michieletti, E. (2020). Well-aerated lung on admitting chest CT to predict adverse outcome in COVID-19 pneumonia. *Radiology*, 201433.

Conforti, C., Giuffrida, R., Zalaudek, I. & Di Meo, N. (2020). Doxycycline, a widely used antibiotic in dermatology with a possible anti-inflammatory action against IL-6 in COVID-19 outbreak. *Dermatologic Therapy,* 33(4), e13437.

Connors, J. M. & Levy, J. H. (2020). COVID-19 and its implications for thrombosis and anticoagulation. *Blood*, 135(23), 2033–2040.

Damle, B., Vourvahis, M., Wang, E., Leaney, J. & Corrigan, B. (2020). Clinical pharmacology perspectives on the antiviral activity of azithromycin and use in COVID-19. *Clinical Pharmacology and Therapeutics,* 108(2), 201-211.

Dan, S., Pant, M. & Upadhyay, S. K. (2020). The Case Fatality Rate in COVID-19 Patients with cardiovascular disease: Global health challenge and paradigm in the current pandemic. *Current Pharmacology Reports,* 6, 315–324.

Danesi, R., Lupetti, A., Barbara, C., Ghelardi, E., Chella, A.; Malizia, T., Senesi, S., Angeletti, C. A., Del Tacca, M. & Campa, M. (2003). Comparative distribution of azithromycin in lung tissue of patients given oral daily doses of 500 and 1000 mg. *Journal of Antimicrobial Chemotherapy,* 51(4), 939–945.

Danhier, F., Ansorena, E., Silva, J. M., Coco, R., Le Breton, A. & Préat, V. (2012). PLGA-based nanoparticles: an overview of biomedical applications. *Journal of Controlled Release,* 161(2), 505–522.

Daoud, A., Dalhoff, K. P. Christensen, M. B., Bøgevig, S. & Petersen, T. S. (2020). Two-bag intravenous N-acetylcysteine, antihistamine pretreatment and high plasma paracetamol levels are associated with a lower incidence of anaphylactoid reactions to N-acetylcysteine. *Clinical Toxicology,* 58(7), 698–704.

De Alencar, J. C. G., Moreira, C. D. L. & Müller, A. D. (2021). Double-blind, Randomized, Placebo-controlled Trial With N-acetylcysteine for Treatment of Severe Acute Respiratory Syndrome Caused by Coronavirus Disease 2019 (COVID-19). *Clinical Infectious Diseases,* 72(11), e736-e741.

De Flora, S., Grassi. C. & Carati. L. (1997). Attenuation of influenza-like symptomatology and improvement of cell-mediated immunity with long-term N-acetylcysteine treatment. *European Respiratory Journal,* 10(7), 1535–1541.

Demedts, M., Behr, J. & Buhl, R. (2005). High-Dose Acetylcysteine in Idiopathic Pulmonary Fibrosis. *New England Journal of Medicine,* 353(21), 2229–2242.

Deretic, V. & Timmins, G. S. (2020). Azithromycin and ciprofloxacin have a chloroquine-like effect on respiratory epithelial cells. *BioRxiv.*

Di Lorenzo, G., Di Trolio, R., Kozlakidis, Z., Busto, G., Ingenito, C., Buonerba, L., Ferrara, C., Libroia, A., Ragone, G., Ioio, C. D., Savastano, B., Polverino, M., De Falco, F., Iaccarino, S. & Leo, E. (2020). COVID 19 therapies and anti-cancer drugs: A systematic review of recent literature. *Critical Reviews in Oncology/Hematology,* 152, 102991.

Du, R. H., Liang, L. R., Yang, C. Q., Wang, W., Cao, T. Z., Li, M., Guo, G. Y., Du, J., Zheng, C. L., Zhu, Q. & Hu, M. (2020). Predictors of mortality for patients with COVID-19 pneumonia caused by SARS-CoV-2: A prospective cohort study. *European Respiratory Journal,* 55(5).

Elshazli, R. M., Kline, A., Elgaml, A., Aboutaleb, M. H., Salim, M. M., Omar, M., Munshi, R., Mankowski, N., Hussein, M. H., Attia, A. S., Toraih, E. A., Settin, A., Killackey, M., Fawzy, M. S. & Kandil, E. (2021). Gastroenterology manifestations and COVID-19 outcomes: A meta-analysis of 25,252 cohorts among the first and second waves. *Journal of Medical Virology,* 93(5), 2740–2768.

Emingil, G., Atilla, G., Sorsa, T. & Tervahartiala, T. (2008). The effect of adjunctive subantimicrobial dose doxycycline therapy on GCF EMMPRIN levels in chronic periodontitis. *Journal of Periodontology*, 79(3), 469–476.

Fantini, J., Chahinian, H. & Yahi, N. (2020). Synergistic antiviral effect of hydroxychloroquine and ACCEPTED MANUSCRIPT azithromycin in combination against SARS-CoV-2, *International Journal of Antimicrobial Agents,* 56(2), 106020.

Fidan, C. & Aydoğdu A. (2020). As a potential treatment of COVID-19: Montelukast. *Medical Hypotheses*, 142, 109828.

Fredeking, T. M., Zavala-Castro, J. E., González-Martínez, P., Moguel-Rodríguez, W., Sanchez, E. C., Foster, M. J. & Diaz-Quijano, F. A. (2015). Dengue Patients Treated with Doxycycline Showed Lower Mortality Associated to a Reduction in IL-6 and TNF Levels. *Recent Patents on Anti-Infective Drug Discovery*, 10(1), 51-58.

Fried, J. A., Ramasubbu, K., Bhatt, R., Topkara, V. K., Clerkin, K. J., Horn, E., Rabbani, L., Brodie, D., Jain, S. S., Kirtanc, A., Masoumi, A., Takeda, K., Kumaraiah, D., Burkhoff, D., Leon. M., Schwartz, A., Uriel, N. & Sayer, G. (2020). The variety of cardiovascular presentations of COVID-19. *Circulation,* 141(23), 1930-1936.

Garassino, M. & Teravolt (2020). Thoracic cancERs international coVid 19 cOLlaboraTion: First results of a global collaboration to address the impact of COVID-19 in patients with thoracic malignancies. Presented at the American Association for Cancer Research Annual Virtual Meeting, Philadelphia, PA.

Garbers, C., Heink, S., Korn, T. & Rose-John, S. (2018). Interleukin-6: Designing specific therapeutics for a complex cytokine. *Nature Reviews Drug Discovery,* 17(6), 395–412.

George, P. M., Wells, A. U. & Jenkins, R. G. (2020). Pulmonary fibrosis and COVID-19: The potential role for antifibrotic therapy. *Lancet Respiratory Medicine*. *8(8)*, 807–815.

Gielen, V., Johnston. S. L. & Edwards, M. R. (2010). Azithromycin induces anti-viral responses in bronchial epithelial cells. *European Respiratory Journal*, 36(3), 646–654.

Glowacka, I., Bertram, S., Herzog, P., Pfefferle, S., Steffen, I., Muench, M.O., Simmons, G., Hofmann, H., Kuri, T., Weber, F. & Eichler, J. (2010). Differential downregulation of ACE2 by the spike proteins of severe acute respiratory syndrome coronavirus and human coronavirus NL63. *Journal of Virology,* 84(2), 1198-1205.

Griffin, M. O., Fricovsky, E., Ceballos, G. & Villarreal, F. (2010). Tetracyclines: a pleitropic family of compounds with promising therapeutic properties. Review of the literature. *American Journal of Physiology-Cell Physiology*, 299(3), C539-548.

Guan, W. J., Liang, W. H., Zhao, Y., Liang, H. R., Chen, Z. S., Li, Y. M., Liu, X. Q., Chen, R. C., Tang, C. L., Wang, T., Ou, C. Q., Li, L., Chen, P. Y., Sang, L., Wang, W., Li, J. F., Li, C. C., Ou, L. M., Cheng, B. & Xiong, S. (2020). China Medical Treatment Expert Group for COVID-19. Comorbidity and its impact on 1590 patients with COVID-19 in China: a nationwide analysis. *European Respiratory Journal*, 55(5), 2000547.

Guan, W. J., Ni, Z. Y., Hu, Y., Liang, W. H., Ou, C. Q., He, J. X., Liu, L., Shan, H., Lei, C. L., Hui, D. S. & Du, B. (2020). Clinical characteristics of coronavirus disease 2019 in China. *New England Journal of Medicine,* 382(18), 1708-1720.

Gupta, D., Sahoo, A. K. & Singh, A. (2020). Ivermectin: potential candidate for the treatment of Covid 19. *Brazilian Journal of Infectious Diseases,* 24(4), 369–371.

Guzzo, C. A., Furtek, C. I., Porras, A. G., Chen C., Tipping, R., Clineschmidt, C. M., Sciberras, D. G., Hsieh, J. Y. & Lasseter, K. C. (2002). Safety, tolerability, and pharmacokinetics of escalating high doses of ivermectin in healthy adult subjects. *Journal of Clinical Pharmacology,* 42(10), 1122-1133.

Hadzic, T., Li, L., Cheng, N., Walsh, S. A., Spitz, D. R. & Knudson, C. M. (2005). The role of low molecular weight thiols in T lymphocyte proliferation and IL-2 secretion. *Journal of Immunology,* 175(12) 7965–7972.

Horby, P., Landray, M. & Haynes, R. (2020). Randomised Evaluation of Covid-19 Therapy (RECOVERY). *European Union Drug Regulating Authorities Clinical Trials Database,* pp. 1–35.

Horowitz, R. I., Freeman, P. R. & Bruzzese, J. (2020). Efficacy of glutathione therapy in relieving dyspnea associated with COVID-19 pneumonia: a report of 2 cases. *Respiratory Medicine Case Reports,* 30, 101063.

Hoxha, M., Lewis-Mikhael, A. M. & Bueno-Cavanillas, A. (2018). Potential role of leukotriene receptor antagonists in reducing cardiovascular and cerbrovascular risk: A systematic review of human. *Biomedicine and Pharmacotherapy*, 106, 956–965.

Huang, C., Wang, Y., Li, X., Ren, L., Zhao, J., Hu, Y., Zhang, L., Fan, G., Xu, J., Gu, X. & Cheng, Z. (2020). Clinical features of patients infected with 2019 novel coronavirus in Wuhan, China. *The Lancet*, 395(10223), 497-506.

Iannetta, M., Ippolito, G. & Nicastri, E. (2017). Azithromycin Shows Anti-Zika Virus Activity in Human Glial Cells. *Antimicrobial Agents and Chemotherapy*, 61(9), e01152-17.

Jain, V. K., Iyengar, K., Vaish, A. & Vaishya, R. (2020). Differential mortality in COVID-19 patients from India and western countries. *Diabetes and Metabolic Syndrome: Clinical Research and Reviews,* 14(5), 1037-1041.

Jones, S. A. & Hunter, C. A. (2021) Is IL-6 a key cytokine target for therapy in COVID-19? *Nature Reviews Immunology,* 21(6), 337–339.

Jones, S. A. & Jenkins, B. J. (2018). Recent insights into targeting the IL-6 cytokine family in inflammatory diseases and cancer. *Nature Reviews Immunology,* 18(12), 773–789.

Jordan, R. E., Adab, P. & Cheng, K. K. (2020). Covid-19: risk factors for severe disease and death. *British Medical Journal,* 368, 1-2, m1198.

Kanoh, S. & Rubin, B. K. (2010). Mechanisms of action and clinical application of macrolides as immunomodulatory medications. *Clinical Microbiology Reviews,* 23(3), 590-615.

Karimi Zarchi, A. A., Faramarzi, M. A., Gilani, K., Ghazi-Khansari, M., Ghamami, G. & Amani, A. (2017). N-acetylcysteine-loaded PLGA nanoparticles outperform conventional N-acetylcysteine in acute lung injuries in vivo. *International journal Polymeric Materials,* 66(9), 443–454.

Karlström, A., Heston. S. M. & Boyd, K. L. (2011). Toll-like receptor 2 mediates fatal immunopathology in mice during treatment of secondary pneumococcal pneumonia following influenza. *Journal of Infectious Diseases,* 204(9), 1358–1366.

Kawamura, K., Ichikado, K. & Takaki, M. (2018). Adjunctive therapy with azithromycin for moderate and severe acute respiratory distress syndrome: a retrospective, propensity score-matching analysis of prospectively collected data at a single center. *nternational Journal of Antimicrobial Agents,* 51(6), 918–924.

Khan, A., Zia, T., Suleman, M., Khan, T., Ali, S. S., Abbasi, A. A., Mohammad, A. & Wei, D. Q. (2021). Higher infectivity of the SARS-CoV-2 new variants is associated with K417N/T, E484K, and N501Y mutants: An insight from structural data. *Journal of Cellular Physiology,* 1–13.

Kircik, L. H., Del Rosso, J. Q., Layton, A. M. & Schauber, J. (2016). Over 25 years of clinical experience with ivermectin: An overview of safety for an increasing number of indications. *Journal of Drugs in Dermatology,* 15(3), 325–332.

Klok, F. A., Kruip, M. J. H. A., van der Meer, N. J. M., Arbous, M. S., Gommers, D. A. M. P. J. & Kant, K. M. (2020). Incidence of thrombotic complications in critically ill ICU patients with COVID-19. *Thrombosis Research,* 191, 145–147.

Kong, M. Y., Whitley, R. J., Peng, N., Oster, R., Schoeb, T. R., Sullender, W., Ambalavanan, N., Clancy, J. P., Gaggar, A. & Blalock, J. E. (2015). Matrix metalloproteinase-9 mediates rsv infection in vitro and in vivo. *Viruses.* 7(8), 4230-4253.

Korkmaz, K., Gedik, H. S., Budak, A. B., Yener, A. U., Kaya, E., Genc, S. B. & Cagli, K. (2015). Effect of Montelukast on Spinal Cord Ischemia-Reperfusion Injury. *Turkish Neurosurgery,* 25(5), 757–765.

Krempaska, K., Barnowski, S. & Gavini, J. (2020). Azithromycin has enhanced effects on lung fibroblasts from idiopathic pulmonary fibrosis (IPF) patients compared to controls. *Respiratory Research*, 21(1), 1-16.

Kubiak, K., Sielawa, H., Chen, W. & Dzika, E. (2018). Endosymbiosis and its significance in dermatology. *Journal of the European Academy of Dermatology and Venereology,* 32(3), 347–354.

Kulcsar, K. A., Coleman, C. M., Beck, S. E. & Frieman, M. B. (2019). Comorbid diabetes results in immune dysregulation and enhanced disease severity following MERS-CoV infection. *JCI Insight*, 4(20), e131774.

Kumar, N., Xin, Z. T., Liang, Y., Ly, H. & Liang, Y. (2008). NF-kappaB signaling differentially regulates influenza virus RNA synthesis. *Journal of Virology,* 82(20), 9880-9889.

Lai, K. Y., Ng, W. Y., Osburga Chan, P. K., Wong, K. F. & Chen, F. (2010). High-dose N-acetylcysteine therapy for novel H1N1 influenza pneumonia. *Ann Internal Medicine,* 152(10), 687–688.

Lai, Z. W., Hanczko, R. & Bonilla, E. (2012). N-acetylcysteine reduces disease activity by blocking mammalian target of rapamycin in T cells from systemic lupus erythematosus patients: a randomized, double-blind, placebo-controlled trial. *Arthritis and Rheumatology*, 64(9), 2937–2946.

Lane, C. J., Redding, D. R., Gonzalez, K. A., Cardenas, V. J., Boldogh, I. & Sur, S. (2009). Topical N-acetyl cysteine (NAC) Reduces Late Phase Nasal Symptoms Following Ragweed Challenge. *Journal of Allergy and Clinical Immunology,* 123(2), S53.

Lawrence, H., Hunter, A., Murray, R., Lim, W. S. & McKeever, T. (2019). Cigarette smoking and the occurrence of influenza-Systematic review. *Journal of Infection*, 79, 401–406.

Levi, M., Thachil, J., Iba, T. & Levy, J. H. (2020). Coagulation abnormalities and thrombosis in patients with COVID-19. *Lancet Haematology,* 7(6), e438–e440.

Li, B., Yang, J., Zhao, F., Zhi, L., Wang, X., Liu, L., Bi, Z. & Zhao, Y. (2020). Prevalence and impact of cardiovascular metabolic diseases on COVID-19 in China. *Clinical Research in Cardiology,* 109(5), 531-538.

Li, C., Zu, S. & Deng, Y. Q. (2019). Azithromycin protects against Zika virus infection by upregulating virus-induced type I and III interferon responses. *Antimicrobial Agents and Chemotherapy,* 63(12), e00394-19.

Liang, W., Guan, W., Chen, R., Wang, W., Li, J., Xu, K., Li, C., Ai, Q., Lu, W., Liang, H. & Li, S. (2020). Cancer patients in SARS-CoV-2 infection: a nationwide analysis in China. *Lancet Oncology*, 21(3), 335-337.

Lim, S., Bae, J. H., Kwon, H. S. & Nauck, M. A. (2021). COVID-19 and diabetes mellitus: from pathophysiology to clinical management. *Nature Reviews Endocrinology*, 17(1), 11–30.

Liu, W., Tao, Z. W., Wang, L., Yuan, M. L., Liu, K., Zhou, L., Wei, S., Deng, Y., Liu, J., Liu, H. G. & Ming Y. X. (2020). Analysis of factors associated with disease outcomes in hospitalized patients with 2019 novel coronavirus disease. *Chinese Medicine,* 133(9), 1032-1038.

López-Medina, E., López, P. & Hurtado, I. C. (2021). Effect of Ivermectin on Time to Resolution of Symptoms Among Adults With Mild COVID-19: a Randomized Clinical Trial. *Journal of the American Medical Association,* 325(14), 1426–1435.

Lucchi, M., Damle, B. & Fang, A. (2008). Pharmacokinetics of azithromycin in serum, bronchial washings, alveolar macrophages and lung tissue following a single oral dose of extended or immediate release formulations of azithromycin. *Journal of Antimicrobial Chemotherapy,* 61, 884–891.

Macchi, A., Terranova, P. & Castelnuovo, P. (2012). Recurrent acute rhinosinusitis: a single blind clinical study of N-acetylcysteinevsambroxol associated to corticosteroid therapy. *International Journal of Immunopathology and Pharmacology,* 25(1), 207–217.

Madjid, M., Safavi-Naeini, P., Solomon, S. D. & Vardeny, O. (2020). Potential effects of coronaviruses on the cardiovascular system: A review. *Journal of the American Medical Association and Cardiology*, 5(7), 831-840.

Maffezzoni, E., Notargiacomo, M., Agostini, S. & Gelardi, M. (2020). Efficacy of a nasal spray containing N-acetylcysteine in hypertonic solution in the treatment of nonallergic chronic rhinitis with goblet cell metaplasia. *Journal of Biological Regulators and Homeostatic Agents,* 34(6), 2345–2352.

Mak, T. W., Grusdat, M. & Duncan, G. S. (2017), Glutathione Primes T Cell Metabolism for Inflammation. *Immunity,* 46(4), 675–689.

Malek, A. E., Granwehr, B. P. & Kontoyiannis, D. P. (2020). Doxycycline as a potential partner of COVID-19 therapies. *ID Cases,* 21, e00864.

McElvaney, O. J., Curley, G. F., Rose-John, S. & McElvaney, N. G. (2021). Interleukin-6: Obstacles to targeting a complex cytokine in critical illness. *Lancet Respiratory Medicine,* 9(6), 643-654.

Mehra, M. R., Desai, S. S., Kuy, S., Henry, T. D. & Patel, A. N. (2020). Cardiovascular disease, drug therapy, and mortality in COVID-19. *New England Journal of Medicine,* 382(25), e102.

Menzel, M., Akbarshahi, H. & Uller, L. (2015). Azithromycin exhibits interferon-inducing properties in an experimental mouse model of asthma exacerbation. *European Respiratory Journal*, 8(19), 31601–31611.

Metlay, J. P., Waterer, G. W. & Long, A. C. (2019). Diagnosis and treatment of adults with community-acquired pneumonia. An official clinical practice guideline of the American Thoracic Society and Infectious Diseases Society of America. *American Journal of Respiratory and Critical Care Medicine,* 200(7), E45–E67.

Mitchell, M. J., Billingsley, M. M., Haley, R. M., Wechsler, M. E., Peppas, N. A. & Langer, R. (2020). Engineering precision nanoparticles for drug delivery. *Nature Reviews Drug Discovery,* 20(2), 101–124.

Miwa, N., Nagano, T., Ohnishi, H., Nishiuma, T., Takenaka, K. & Shirotani, T. (2018). An Open-Label, Multi-Institutional, Randomized Study to Evaluate the Additive Effect of a Leukotriene Receptor Antagonist on Cough Score in Patients with Cough-Variant Asthma Being Treated with Inhaled Corticosteroids. *Kobe Journal of Medical Sciences,* 64(4), 134–E139.

Mo, P., Xing Y., Xiao, Y., Deng, L., Zhao, Q., Wang, H., Xiong, Y., Cheng, Z., Gao, S., Liang, K. & Luo, M. (2020). Clinical characteristics of refractory COVID-19 pneumonia in Wuhan, China. *Clinical Infectious Diseases,* 16; ciaa270.

Molteni, E., Astley, C. M., Ma, W., Sudre, C. H., Magee, L. A., Murray, B., Fall, T., Gomez, M. F., Tsereteli, N., Franks, P. W., Brownstein, J. S., Davies, R., Wolf, J., Spector, T. D., Ourselin, S., Steves, C. J., Chan, A. T. & Modat, M. (2021). Symptoms and syndromes associated with SARS-CoV-2 infection and severity in pregnant women from two community cohorts. *Scientific Reports,* 11(1), 6928.

Mortara, A., Mazzetti, S., Margonato, D., Delfino, P., Bersano, C., Catagnano, F., Lauriola, M., Grosso, P., Perseghin, G., & Ippoliti, G. (2021). Compassionate use of ruxolitinib in patients with SARS-Cov-2 infection not on mechanical ventilation: Short-term effects on inflammation and ventilation. *Clinical and translational science*, 14(3), 1062–1068.

Muniyappa, R. & Gubbi, S. (2020). COVID-19 pandemic, corona viruses, and diabetes mellitus. *American Journal of Physiology-Endocrinology and Metabolism*, 318(5), 736-741.

Mursaleen, L., Noble, B., Chan, S, H. Y. & Somavarapu, S. (2020). N-AcetylcysteineNanocarriers Protect against Oxidative Stress in a Cellular Model of Parkinson's Disease. *Antioxidants*, 9(7), 600.

Ng, K., Poon, B. H., Kiat Puar, T. H., Shan Quah, J. L., Loh, W. J., Wong, Y. J., Tan, T. Y. & Raghuram, J. (2020). COVID-19 and the risk to health care workers: a case report. *Annals of Internal Medicine,* 172(11), 766-767.

Nitulescu, G. M., Paunescu, H., Moschos, S. A., Petrakis, D., Nitulescu, G., Ion, G., Spandidos, D. A., Nikolouzakis, T. K., Drakoulis, N. & Tsatsakis, A. (2020). Comprehensive analysis of drugs to treat SARS-CoV-2 infection: Mechanistic insights into current COVID-19 therapies. *International Journal of Molecular Medicine,* 46(2), 467-488.

Nujić, K., Banjanac, M., Munić, V., Polančec, D. & Eraković Haber, V. (2012). Impairment of lysosomal functions by azithromycin and chloroquine contributes to anti-inflammatory phenotype. *Cellular Immunology*, 279, 78–86.

Ou, X., Liu, Y. & Lei, X.(2020). Characterization of spike glycoprotein of SARS-CoV-2 on virus entry and its immune cross-reactivity with SARS-CoV. *Nature Communications,* 11(1), 1620.

Pal, R. & Yadav, U. (2020). COVID-19 pandemic in India: present scenario and a steep climb ahead. *Journal of Primary Care & Community Health,* 11, 1-4.

Paranjpe, M. & Müller-Goymann, C. C. (2014). Nanoparticle-mediated pulmonary drug delivery: a review. *International Journal of Molecular Sciences*, 15(4), 5852–5873.

Parnham, M. J., Haber, V. E., Giamarellos-Bourboulis, E. J., Perletti, G., Verleden, G. M. & Vos, R. (2014). Azithromycin: Mechanisms of action and their relevance for clinical applications. *Pharmacology & Therapeutics*, 143(2), 225-245.

Phillips, J. M., Gallagher, T. & Weiss, S. R. (2017). Neurovirulent murine coronavirus JHM.SD uses cellular zinc metalloproteases for virus entry and cell-cell fusion. *Journal of Virology*, 91, e01564-16.

Piroth, L., Cottenet, J., Mariet, A. M., Bonniaud, P., Blot, M. & Tubert-Bitter, P. (2021). Quantin, C. Comparison of the characteristics, morbidity, and mortality of COVID-19 and seasonal influenza: a nationwide, population-based retrospective cohort study. ***Lancet Respiratory Medicine*, 9(3), 251-259.**

Poschet, J., Perkett, E., Timmins, G., & Deretic, V. (2020). Azithromycin and ciprofloxacin have a chloroquinelike effect on respiratory epithelial cells. *BioRxiv.*

Rana, S., Dhiman, U., Parihar, R. D., & Upadhyay, S. K. (2021). *In silico* analysis of tumor necrosis factor (TNF) in *Homo sapiens*. *Biointerface Research in Applied Chemistry,* 12(1), 781-794.

Rao, S., Lau, A. & So, H. C. (2020). Exploring diseases/traits and blood proteins causally related to expression of ACE2, the putative receptor of SARS-CoV-2: A Mendelian randomization analysis highlights tentative relevance of diabetes-related traits. Diabetes Care. *Diabetes Care*, 43(7), 1416-1426.

Rath, D., Petersen-Uribe, A., Avdiu, A., Witzel, K., Jaeger, P., Zdanyte, M., Heinzmann, D., Tavlaki, E., Müller, K. & Gawaz, M. P. (2020). Impaired cardiac function is associated with mortality in patients with acute COVID-19 infection. *Clinical Research in Cardiology*, 109(12),1491–1499.

Ratzinger, F., Haslacher, H. & Poeppl, W. (2014). Azithromycin suppresses CD4 + T-cell activation by direct modulation of mTOR activity. *Scientific Reports,* 4(1),1–10.

Remuzzi, A. & Remuzzi, G. (2020). COVID-19 and Italy: what next? *The Lancet*, 395(10231), 1225-1228.

Rodriguez-Morales, A. J., Cardona-Ospina, J. A., Gutierrez-Ocampo, E., Villamizar-Pena, R., Holguin-Rivera, Y. & Escalera-Antezana, J. P. (2020). Clinical, laboratory and imaging features of COVID-19: A systematic review and meta-analysis. *Travel Medicine and Infectious Disease*, 34, 101623.

Rothan, H. A., Bahrani, H., Mohamed, Z., Teoh, T. C., Shankar, E. M., Rahman, N. A. & Yusof, R. A. (2015). combination of doxycycline and ribavirin alleviated chikungunya infection. *PLoS One*, 10(5), e0126360.

Rubin, E. J., Longo, D. L. & Baden, L. R. (2021). Interleukin-6 Receptor Inhibition in COVID-19 — Cooling the Inflammatory Soup. *New England Journal of Medicine,* 384(16), 1564–1565.

Rubio, M. L., Martin-Mosquero, M. C. Ortega, M. & Peces-Barba, G. (2004). Oral N-Acetylcysteine attenuates elastase-induced pulmonary emphysema in rats. *Chest*, 125(4), 1500–1506.

Santa-Cecília, F. V., Socias, B., Ouidja, M. O., Sepulveda-Diaz, J. E., Acuña, L., Silva, R. L., Michel, P. P., Del-Bel, E., Cunha, T. M. & Raisman-Vozari, R. (2016). Doxycycline suppresses microglial activation by inhibiting the p38 MAPK and NF-kB signaling pathways. *Neurotoxicity Research*, 29(4), 447-459.

Sargiacomo, C., Sotgia, F. & Lisanti, M. P. (2020). COVID-19 and chronological aging: senolytics and other anti-aging drugs for the treatment or prevention of corona virus infection? *Aging*, 12(8), 6511–6517.

Sayin, T., Cimen, S., Cimen, S., Bostanci, T., Akbaba, S. & Yildirim, Z. (2020). Colonic anastomosis can be protected from ischemia reperfusion injury with intra-peritoneal Montelukast treatment. *Asian Journal of Surgery*, 43(1), 130–138.

Schaller, M., Gonser, L. & Belge, K. (2017). Dual anti-inflammatory and anti-parasitic action of topical ivermectin 1% in papulopustular rosacea. *Journal of the European Academy of Dermatology and Venereology,* 31(11), 1907–1911.

Schmidt, L. E. & Dalhoff, K. (2001). Risk factors in the development of adverse reactions to N-acetylcysteine in patients with paracetamol poisoning. *British Journal of Clinical Pharmacology,* 51(1), 87–91.

Schögler, A., Kopf, B. S. & Edwards. M. R. (2015). Novel antiviral properties of azithromycin in cystic fibrosis airway epithelial cells. *European Respiratory Journal*, 45(2), 428-443.

Sharafkhah, M., Abdolrazaghnejad, A., Zarinfar, N., Mohammadbeigi, A., Massoudifar, A. & Abaszadeh, S. (2018). Safety and efficacy of N-acetyl-cysteine for prophylaxis of ventilator-associated pneumonia: A randomized, double blind, placebo-controlled clinical trial. *Medical Gas Research,* 8(1), 19–23.

Sharmeen, S., Skrtic, M. & Sukhai, M. A. (2010). The antiparasitic agent ivermectin induces chloride-dependent membrane hyperpolarization and cell death in leukemia cells. *Blood*, 116(18), 3593–3603.

Sharun, K., Dhama, K., Patel, S. K., Pathak, M. Tiwari, R., Singh, B. R., Sah, R., Bonilla-Aldana, D. K., Rodriguez-Morales, A. J. & Leblebicioglu, H. (2020). Ivermectin, a new candidate therapeutic against SARS-CoV-2/COVID-19. *Annals of Clinical Microbiology and Antimicrobials,* 9(1), 23.

Shi, S., Qin, M., Shen, B., Cai, Y., Liu, T., Yang, F., Gong, W., Liu, X., Liang, J., Zhao, Q., Huang, H., Yang. B. & Huang, C. (2020). Association of cardiac injury with mortality in hospitalized patients with COVID-19 in Wuhan, China. *Journal of American Medical Association Cardiology*, 5(7), 802-810.

Shi, Y., Yu, X., Zhao, H., Wang, H., Zhao, R. & Sheng, J. (2020). Host susceptibility to severe COVID-19 and establishment of a host risk score: findings of 487 cases outside Wuhan. *Critical Care,* 24(1), 1-4.

Shimizu, T. & Shimizu, S. (2012). Azithromycin inhibits mucus hypersecretion from airway epithelial cells. *Mediators of Inflammation,* 265714.

Singh, D. & Yi, S. V. (2021). On the origin and evolution of SARS-CoV-2. *Experimental and Molecular Medicine,* 53, 537–547.

Sinhaa, S., Sehgalb, A. & Sehgala, R. (2020). Ivermectin: Is it to Be a potent therapeutic option for COVID-19? *Clinical Infection and Immunity,* 5(2), 51-53.

Sligl, W. I., Asadi, L. & Eurich, D. T. (2014). Macrolides and mortality in critically Ill patients with community-acquired pneumonia: A systematic review and meta-analysis. *Critical Care Medicine,* 42(2), 420–432.

Srivastava, S., Banu, S., Singh, P., Sowpati, D. T. & Mishra, R. K. (2021). SARS-CoV-2 genomics: An Indian perspective on sequencing viral variants. *Journal of Biosciences,* 46(1), 1-4.

Strzelak, A., Ratajczak, A., Adamiec, A. & Feleszko, W. (2018). Tobacco smoke induces and alters immune responses in the lung triggering inflammation, allergy, asthma and other lung diseases: a mechanistic review. *International Journal of Environmental Research and Public Health*, 15(5).

Sweiss, N. J., Korsten, P., Syed, H. J., Syed A., Baughman, R. P., Yee, A. M. F., Culver, D. A., Sosenko, T. Azuma, A., Bonella, F., Costabel, U., Drake, W. P.. Drent, M., Lower, E. E., Israel-Biet, D., Mostard, R. L. M., Nunes, H., Rottoli, P., Spagnolo, P., Wells, A. U., Wuyts, W. A. & Judson, M. A. (2020). When the game changes: guidance to adjust sarcoidosis management during the COVID-19 pandemic. *Chest*, 158(3), 892-895.

Takayama, K. (2020). In Vitro and Animal Models for SARS-CoV-2 research. *Trends in Pharmacological Sciences,* 41(8), 513–517.

Tarbox, J. A., Bansal, A. & Peiris, A. N. (2018). Angioedema. *Journal of the American Medical Association,* 319(19), 2054.

Targher, G., Mantovani, A., Wang, X. B., Yan, H. D., Sun, Q. F., Pan, K. H., Byrne, C. D., Zheng, K. I., Chen, Y. P., Eslam, M. & George, J. (2020). Patients with diabetes are at higher risk for severe illness from COVID-19. *Diabetes and Metabolism Journal,* 46(4), 335-337.

Tatu, A. L., Nadasdy, T. & Nwabudike, L. C. (2021). Chitin-lipid interactions and the potential relationship between Demodex and SARS-CoV-2. *Dermatologic Therapy,* 34(3), e14935.

Tirouvanziam, R., Conrad, C. K., Bottiglieri, T., Herzenberg, L. A., Moss, R. B. & Herzenberg, L. A. (2006). High-dose oral N-acetylcysteine, a glutathione prodrug, modulates inflammation in cystic fibrosis. *Proceedings of the National Academy of Sciences USA,* 103(12), 4628–4633.

Tonnesen, P., Marott, J. L., Nordestgaard, B., Bojesen, S. E. & Lange, P. (2019). Secular trends in smoking in relation to prevalent and incident smoking-related disease: A prospective population-based study. *Tobacco Induced Diseases,* 17.

Touret, F., Gilles, M. & Barral, K. (2020). In vitro screening of a FDA approved chemical library reveals potential inhibitors of SARS-CoV-2 replication. *Scientific Reports,* 10(1), 1-8.

Tran, D. H., Sugamata, R. & Hirose, T. (2019). Azithromycin, a 15-membered macrolide antibiotic, inhibits influenza A(H1N1)pdm09 virus infection by interfering with virus internalization process. *Journal of Antibiotics,* 72(10), 759–768.

Tyteca, D., Van Der Smissen, P., Mettlen M, Van Bambeke, F., Tulkens, P. M., Mingeot-Leclercq, M. P., Courtoy, P. J. (2002). Azithromycin, a lysosomotropic antibiotic, has distinct effects on fluid-phase and receptor-mediated endocytosis, but does not impair phagocytosis in J774 macrophages. *Experimental Cell Research,* 281(1), 86–100.

Ulrich, H. & Pillat, M. M. (2020). CD147 as a target for COVID-19 treatment: Suggested effects of azithromycin and stem cell engagement. *Stem Cell Reviews and Reports*, 16, 434-440.

Upadhyay, S. K., Dan, S., Girdhar, M. & Rastogi, K. (2021). Recent advancement in SARS-CoV-2 diagnosis, treatment, and vaccine formulation: a new paradigm of nanotechnology in strategic combating of COVID-19 pandemic. *Current Pharmacology Reports,* 1-14.

Upadhyay, S. K., Singh, R., Babita, K. G. & Singh, G. (2020). The outbreak and challenges of novel coronavirus (COVID-19): The global pandemic emergency of early 2K20 and Indian scenario. *International Journal of Biology, Pharmacy and Allied Sciences,* 9, 1173–1199.

Upadhyay, S. K., Dan, S., Girdhar, M. & Rastogi, K.(2021). Recent advancement in SARS-CoV-2 diagnosis, treatment, and vaccine formulation: A new paradigm of nanotechnology in strategic combating of COVID-19 pandemic. *Current Pharmacology Reports,* 7, 1-14.

Vardavas, C. I. & Nikitara, K. (2020). COVID-19 and smoking: A systematic review of the evidence. *Tobacco Induced Diseases,* 18.

Velthuis A. J. W., Van den Worm, S. H. E., Sims A. C., Baric, R. S., Snijder, E. J. & Van Hemert, M. J. (2010). Zn2+ inhibits coronavirus and arterivirus RNA polymerase activity in vitro and zinc ionophores block the replication of these viruses in cell culture. *PLOS Pathogens*, *6*, e1001176.

Verstovsek, S. (2013). Ruxolitinib: An oral Janus kinase 1 and Janus kinase 2 inhibitor in the management of myelofibrosis. *Journal of Postgraduate Medicine*, 125(1):128-135.

Villar, J., Ariff, S., Gunier, R. B., Thiruvengadam, R., Rauch, S., Kholin, A., Roggero, P., Prefumo, F., Do Vale, M. S., Cardona-Perez, J. A., Maiz, N., Cetin, I., Savasi, V., Deruelle, P., Easter, S. R., Sichitiu, J., Soto Conti, C. P., Ernawati, E., Mhatre, M., Teji, J.S., Liu, B., Capelli, C., Oberto, M., Salazar, L., Gravett, M. G., Cavoretto, P. I., Nachinab, V. B., Galadanci, H., Oros, D., Ayede, A. I., Sentilhes, L., Bako, B., Savorani, M., Cena, H., García-May, P. K., Etuk, S., Casale, R., Abd-Elsalam, S., Ikenoue, S., Aminu, M. B., Vecciarelli, C., Duro, E. A., Usman, M. A., John-Akinola, Y., Nieto, R.; Ferrazi, E., Bhutta, Z. A., Lager, A., Kennedy, S. H. & Papageorghiou, A. T. (2021). Maternal and neonatal morbidity and mortality among pregnant women with and without COVID-19 infection: The INTERCOVID multinational cohort study. *Journal of Americam Medical Association Pediatrics,* 175(8), 817–826.

Wang, B., Hu, B., Hu, C., Zhu, F., Liu, X., Zhang, J., Wang, B., Xiang, H., Cheng, H., Xiong, Y., Zhao, Y., Li, Y., Wang, X. & Peng, Z (2020). Clinical characteristics of 138 hospitalized patients with 2019 novel coronavirus-infected pneumonia in Wuhan, China. *Journal of the American Medical Association,* 323(11), 1061–1069.

Wang, X., Xu, W., Hu, G., Xia, S., Sun, Z., Liu, Z., Xie, Y., Zhang, R., Jiang, S. & Lu, L. (2020). SARS-CoV-2 infects T lymphocytes through its spike protein-mediated membrane fusion. *Cell Molecular Immunology. 17(8)*, 1-3.

Wang, Y., Tian, J. & Liu, J. (2020). Suppressive effect of leukotriene antagonists on capsular contracture in patients who underwent breast surgery with prosthesis: A meta-analysis. *Plastic and Reconstructive Surgery,* 145, 901–911.

Wastnedge, E., Reynolds, R. M., Van Boeckel, S. R., Stock, S. J., Denison, F. C., Maybin, J. A. & Critchley, H. (2021). Pregnancy and COVID-19. *Physiological Reviews,* 101(1), 303–318.

Whillier, S., Raftos, J. E., Chapman, B. & Kuchel, P. W. (2009). Role of N-acetylcysteine and cystine in glutathione synthesis in human erythrocytes. *Redox Report,* 14(3), 115–124.

WHO (2020). Report of the WHO-China Joint Mission on Coronavirus Disease 2019 (COVID-19). Accessed on March 19, 2020. https://www.who.int/docs/default-source/coronaviruse/who-china-joint-mission-on-covid-19final-report.pdf.

Wong, K. K., Lee, S. W. H. & Kua, K. P. (2021). N-Acetylcysteine as Adjuvant Therapy for COVID-19 – A Perspective on the Current State of the Evidence. *ournal of Inflammation Research,* 14, 2993-3013.

Wu, A. Y., Chik, S. C., Chan, A. W., Li, Z., Tsang, K. W. & Li, W. (2003). Anti-inflammatory effects of high-dose montelukast in an animal model of acute asthma. *Clinical & Experimental Allergy,* 33(3), 359-66.

Wu, C., Liu, Y., Yang, Y., Zhang, P., Zhong, W., Wang, Y., Wang, Q., Xu, Y., Li, M., Li, X., Zheng, M., Chen, L. & Li, H. (2020). Analysis of therapeutic targets for SARS-CoV-2 and discovery of potential drugs by computational methods. *Acta Pharmaceutica Sinica B*, 10, 766–788.

Wuyts,W. A., Willems, S. & Vos, R. (2010). Azithromycin reduces pulmonary fibrosis in a bleomycin mouse model. *Experimental Lung Research,* 36(10), 602–614.

Xiong, T. Y., Redwood, S., Prendergast, B. & Chen, M. (2020). Coronaviruses and the cardiovascular system: acute and long-term implications. *European Heart Journal,* 41(19), 1798-1800.

Yang, X., Yu, Y., Xu, J., Shu, H., Liu, H., Wu, Y., Zhang, L., Yu, Z., Fang, M., Yu, T. & Wang, Y. (2020). Clinical course and outcomes of critically ill patients with SARS-CoV-2 pneumonia in Wuhan, China: A single-centered, retrospective, observational study. *Lancet Respiratory Medicine*, 8(5), 475-481.

Yates, P. A., Newman, S. A., Oshry, L. J., Glassman, R. H., Leone, A. M. & Reichel, E. (2020). Doxycycline treatment of high-risk COVID-19-positive patients with comorbid pulmonary disease. *Therapeutic Advances in Respiratory Disease,* 14, 1-5.

Zaidi, A. K., & Dehgani-Mobaraki, P. (2021). The mechanisms of action of Ivermectin against SARS-CoV-2: An evidence-based clinical review article. *Journal of Antibiotics,* 1–13.

Zeng, S., Meng, X. & Huang, Q. (2019). Spiramycin and azithromycin, safe for administration to children, exert antiviral activity against enterovirus A71 in vitro and in vivo. *International Journal of Antimicrobial Agents,* 53(4), 362–369.

Zhang, H., Penninger, J. M., Li, Y., Zhong, N. & Slutsky, A. S. (2020). Angiotensin-converting enzyme 2 (ACE2) as a SARS-CoV-2 receptor: molecular mechanisms and potential therapeutic target. *Intensive Care Medicine,* 46, 586–590.

Zhang, J. J., Dong, X., Cao, Y. Y., Yuan, Y. D., Yang, Y. B. & Yan, Y. Q. (2020). Clinical characteristics of 140 patients infected with SARS-CoV-2 in Wuhan, China. *Allergy*, 75(7), 1730-1741.

Zhang, J. J., Dong, X., Cao, Y. Y., Yuan, Y. D., Yang, Y. B., Yan, Y. Q., Akdis, C. A. & Gao, Y. D. (2020). Clinical characteristics of 140 patients infected with SARS-CoV-2 in Wuhan, China. *Allergy*, 75(7), 1730-1741.

Zhang, L., Zhu, F., Xie, L., Wang, C., Wang, J., Chen, R., Jia, P., Guan, H. Q., Peng, L., Chen, Y. & Peng, P. (2020). Clinical characteristics of COVID-19-infected cancer patients: A retrospective case study in three hospitals within Wuhan, China. *Annals of Oncology,* 31(7), 894-901.

Zhang, Q., Ju, Y., Ma, Y. & Wang, T. (2018). N-acetylcysteine improves oxidative stress and inflammatory response in patients with community acquired pneumonia: A randomized controlled trial. *Medicine*. 97(45), e13087–e13087.

Zhang, X., Tan, Y., Ling, Y., Lu, G., Liu, F. & Yi, Z. (2020). Viral and host factors related to the clinical outcome of COVID-19. *Nature*, 583(7816), 437–440.

Zheng, S., Matzneller, P., Zeitlinger M. & Schmidt, S. (2014). Development of a population pharmacokinetic model characterizing the tissue distribution of azithromycin in healthy subjects. *Antimicrobial Agents and Chemotherapy,* 58(11), 6675–6684.

Zheng, Z., Peng, F., Xu, B., Zhao, J., Liu, H., Peng, J., Li, Q., Jiang, C., Zhou, Y., Liu, S., Ye, C., Zhang, P., Xing, Y., Guo, H. & Tang, W. (2020). Risk factors of critical and mortal COVID-19 cases: A systematic literature review and meta-analysis, *Journal of Infection,* 81(2), e16–e25.

Zhou, F., Yu, T., Du, R., Fan, G., Liu, Y., Liu, Z., Xiang, J., Wang, Y., Song, B., Gu, X. & Guan, L. (2020). Clinical course and risk factors for mortality of adult inpatients with COVID-19 in Wuhan, China: a retrospective cohort study. *The lancet*, 395(10229), 1054-1062.

Zimmermann, P., Ziesenitz, V. C. & Curtis, N. (2018). The immunomodulatory effects of macrolides-A systematic review of the underlying mechanisms. *Frontiers in Immunology,* 9, 302.

## Chapter 6

# Coronavirus Disease (SARS-CoV-2) Associated Mucormycosis (Zygomycosis): Stochastic Assemblages, Causes, Cures and Epidemiology

**Mohit Pant**[1]
**Siddhartha Dan**[2,3]
**Samyak Nag**[4]
**Lajpreet Kaur**[5]
**Rashmi Pandey**[6]
**Himanshu Ojha**[5,*]
**and Mallika Pathak**[7,†]

[1]Department of Pharmacovigilance, Parexel International Pvt. Ltd., Mohali, Punjab, India
[2]Department of Biotechnology, I. K. Gujral Punjab Technical University, Jalandhar, Punjab, India
[3]Department of Biotechnology, Dr. B. R. Ambedkar National Institute of Technology, Jalandhar, Punjab, India
[4]Amity Institute of Pharmacy, Amity University, Noida, Uttar Pradesh, India
[5]CBRN Protection and Decontamination Research Group, Division of CBRN Defence, Institute of Nuclear Medicine and Allied Sciences, DRDO, Timarpur, Delhi, India
[6]Guru Gobind Singh Indraprastha University, Dwarka, Delhi, India
[7]Department of Chemistry, Miranda House, University of Delhi, Delhi, India

---

[*] Corresponding Author's Email: himanshu@inmas.drdo.in.
[†] Corresponding Author's Email: mallika.pathak@mirandahouse.ac.in.

In: Therapeutic Advances in Human Health and Diseases
Editors: Sushil Kumar Upadhyay, Manoj Singh and Anil Kumar Sharma
ISBN: 979-8-89113-304-4

## Abstract

Invasive fungal infection (IFI), for instance, mucormycosis is generally caused due to many species of saprophytic fungi and prevails in patients with different co-morbidities, for instance, diabetes and including organ transplantation and appears in very rare cases and emerged to be fatal fungal infection. The second wave of severe acute respiratory syndrome coronavirus 2 (SARS-CoV-2) epidemics has revealed increased cases of bacterial and fungal co-infections prevalent in SARS-CoV-2 patients, for example, pulmonary aspergillosis associated with SARS-CoV-2. This chapter presented various cases of mucormycosis, for example, individuals recovering from SARS-CoV-2 who underwent a fresh heart transplant for the management of severe heart failure. Several reported cases developed upper respiratory and systemic symptoms in the transplanted heart after two months and were reported positive in RT-PCR for SARS-CoV-2 diagnosis. Cutaneous mucormycosis has emerged in individuals after three months of recovery from SARS-CoV-2. This review paper also described in advance the properly reported mucormycosis cases prevailing in SARS-CoV-2 patients and demonstrated the significant mechanism of action by which eventually SARS-CoV-2 can incline to invasive fungal infections in patients suffering from diabetes mellitus, neutropenia and under the improper dosage regimen of corticosteroids for managing the severe case of SARS-CoV-2. Mucormycosis prevailing in SARS-CoV-2 patients should be characterized to identify the correlation between these diseases. Physicians should be watchful to investigate and proper action to be enforced for mucormycosis in SARS-CoV-2 infected patients. The antifungal drug Amphotericin-B deoxycholate is the first choice of treatment and liposomal dosage forms are preferred because of reduced nephrotoxicity. There are some cases of patients who are intolerant to amphotericin liposomal preparation therefore; posaconazole should be clinically investigated as an ideal substitute course of action. Iron internalization novel inhibitors in *Rhizopus oryzae* might disturb the fungus's potential for enforcing angio-invasive growth. This crucial function of iron internalization during *R. oryzae* infection also strengthens the assurance of utilizing novel iron chelators, for instance, deferasirox and lipid polyene like caspofungin to boost the survival outcomes in mucormycosis patients.

**Keywords:** SARS-CoV-2, mucormycosis, invasive fungal infection, epidemiology, antifungal drugs

## 1. Introduction

Aspergillosis and Mucormycosis were found infrequent, hazardous fungal infections with mortality rates over 50% regardless of antifungal therapy and surgical epithelialization (Ibrahim et al., 2012; Falcone et al., 2011). *Rhizopus arrhizus*, causing all 70% of mucormycosis is also closely related to several clinical (pulmonary, cutaneous, rhino-orbital-cerebral, and gastric) in adults (Ibrahim et al., 2012). The fungal infection is known for its destructive pathogenic nature, peculiarized by seizure beyond tissue planes and speedy tissue demolition (Ibrahim and Kontoyiannis, 2013). The considerable threat factors for the life-threatening fungal disease i.e., Mucormycosis involve unconstrained Ketoacidosis, Stem cell and solid organ emigrate, Diabetes mellitus, Haematological malignancy, Iron reduction is accomplished with chelation therapy with $C_{25}H_{48}N_6O_8$ (Deferoxamine) and cortisone-like medicines usage (Ibrahim and Kontoyiannis, 2013). The investigation of mucormycosis is made by spotting the ingenious fungal structure by histopathological analysis of tissue prototypes from patients currently on treatment with mistrust signals and symptoms (Ibrahim and Kontoyiannis, 2013).

In general, initial therapy of mucormycosis requires advance traumatic surgical drafting of the contaminated tissue, which involves the administration of liposomal amphotericin B (L-AmB) or amphotericin B deoxycholate (AmB) (Ibrahim and Kontoyiannis, 2013). *Aspergillus fumigatus* is responsible for more than 70% of all cases of mediated aspergillosis (Cicek et al., 2017). Aggressive aspergillosis usually occurs in immunosuppressed sufferers undergoing chronic corticosteroid therapy for prolonged neutropenia from malignancy (Falcone et al., 2011; Cicek et al., 2017). Recognition of demonstrated, expected, or potentially invasive aspergillosis is determined by host status and a mixture of explanation and mycological findings (Ascioglu et al., 2002).

The optimal therapy of aspergillosis is the introduction of or isavuconazole or voriconazole (Falcone et al., 2011; Cicek et al., 2017). Both infections have been identified as a secondary obstacle of SARS-CoV-2 (Coronavirus disease 2019), especially among negatively unwell patients in the concentrated care unit (ICU) (Lai, 2020; Thompson et al., 2020; Machado et al., 2021). Reports have shown that up to 35% of these sufferers develop pulmonary aspergillosis related to prior corticosteroid consumption and are open to high mortality (Delliere et al., 2020; Lai, 2020; Thompson et al., 2020; Machado et al., 2021). In contrast, the prevalence of spreading pulmonary mucormycosis following SARS-CoV-2 is rare, with only two cases currently reported (Pasero et al., 2020; Zurl et al., 2021). To our understanding, we observed the first case of possible mucormycosis combined with probable pulmonary aspergillosis in a male with SARS-CoV-2 in the intensive care unit (ICU) (Johnson et al., 2021).

Saprophytic fungi present in the environment such as most commonly occurring *Rhizopus, Mucor, Rhizomucor, Aposphysomyces, Cunninghamella, Licitheimia* (*Absidia*), *Saksenaea*, are found to be responsible for the generation of invasive fungal infection characterized as Mucormycosis (earlier known as Zygomycosis) (Roden et al., 2005). This could be presented through six diverse clinical reports including the rhinocerebral, pulmonary, cutaneous, gastro-intestinal, disseminated, and miscellaneous (Spellberg et al., 2005). The cutaneous type is the third most prevalent manifestation after the former two and additionally it is observed in 19% of mucormycosis patients (Roden et al., 2005). Factors that could be proven to be risky for the infection will include solid organ transplant recipients (SOTRs), prolonged and severe neutropenia, hematologic malignancies, stem cell transplantations, poorly controlled diabetes mellitus (DM), major trauma, neonatal prematurity, prolonged use of corticosteroids, illicit intravenous drug intake, deferoxamine therapy, malnutrition, and potential nosocomial sources (Roden et al., 2005; Petrikkos et al., 2012; Rammaert et al., 2012). Out of all invasive fungal infections, mucormycosis comprises 2-6% of the total infections (Pappas et al., 2010; Rammaert et al., 2012). It was reported by the multi-center prospective TRANSNET, that by the end of one annum, the collective rate of Spreading in solid organ transplant recipients was 0.07% (Pappas et al., 2010).

Severe-acute-respiratory syndrome caused by SARS-CoV-2 (novel coronavirus), coronavirus disease, the current ongoing COVID-19 pandemic has recorded over 110 million cases along with 2.4 million decreases across the world. Furthermore, several COVID-19 patients have been observed and diagnosed with diverse bacterial and fungal infections (Lansbury et al., 2020). The authors herein describe a heart transplant recipient who had developed a cutaneous mucormycosis infection after COVID-19. This review gives insights into the literature proximate to the incidence of mucormycosis after COVID-19, and additionally explores the potential mechanisms (Khatri et al., 2021). Primarily diagnosed in immunosuppressive patients such as cases of uncontrolled diabetes, prolonged corticosteroid usage, and hematologic malignancies; mucormycosis has been found to be a rare infection (Werthman-Ehrenreich, 2021) (Figure 1).

Due to the hospitalization conditions, treatment inclusive of corticosteroids and often antibiotics, or pre-existing co-morbidities, patients with severe COVID-19 infection are more prone to develop the secondary fungal infection as the co-infection. Ever since the initiation of the pandemic a superimposed *Aspergillus* infection has been reported with the COVID-19 infection (Koehler et al., 2020; Mohamed et al., 2020). Contrastingly, fewer data records have been found associated with mucormycosis of that of COVID-19 cases. A rare case of severe COVID-19 infection associated with invasive pulmonary mucormycosis has been discussed.

Reports of critical cases of COVID-19 pneumonia indicate the very often occurrence of secondary infections related to invasive pulmonary aspergillosis (Koehler et al., 2020; Mohamed et al., 2020). In contrast, isolated cases of Mucor infection have been seen in COVID-19 patients. A study describes the case of a 60-year-old patient, who has ongoing treatment of diabetes and contoured with the rhino-orbital mucor infection which was diagnosed with nasal biopsy culture (Mehta and Pandey, 2020). This patient died of shock as the eventual cytokine storm developed (Mehta and Pandey, 2020). One more case documented by Werthman-Ehrenreich is of a 33-year-old diabetic woman in ketoacidosis along with the co-occurrence of COVID-19 pneumonia, who has been further diagnosed with rhino-orbital cerebral mucormycosis through biopsy. She was ultimately moved to intensive care by reason of the neurological involvement of extensive fungus and also the poor prognosis (Werthman-Ehrenreich, 2021).

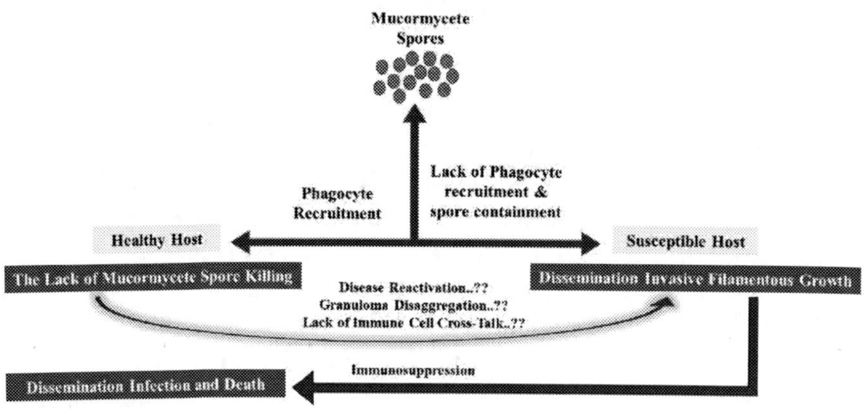


**Figure 1.** Mucormycosis in healthy and immunosuppressive patients and its effect.

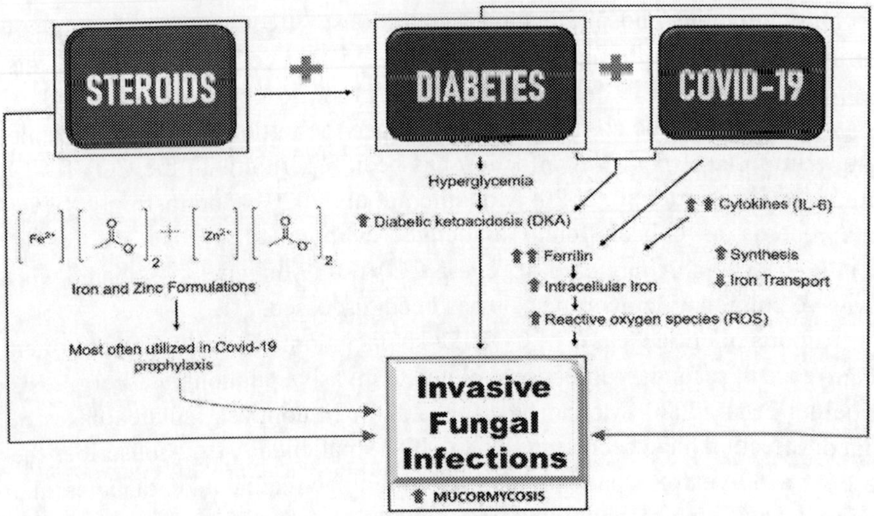


**Figure 2.** Impact of immunocompromised condition patients and medicine on invasive fungal infections.

Furthermore, Placik et al., (2020) reported the case of a 49-year-old COVID-19 patient who developed tension pneumothorax with a bronchopleural fistula. For the repairment of the fistula, a cardiothoracic surgery has been performed a thoracotomy along with which an observation led to empyema which grew *Rhizopus* species on culture. This patient also departed due to illness (Placik et al., 2020). The IFI Mucormycosis if not diagnosed simultaneously with COVID-19 infection, then it has a mortality rate of 40-60% (Cornely et al., 2019). Further in cases wherein these two infections are found to be co-occurring then the mortality rate reaches 100% as per the review literature so far. Though diabetes is the greatest risk factor for mucor infection to occur, along with these several other immunosuppressive conditions also lead to this infection. The Rhino-cerebral infection is commonly observed in diabetic patients whereas with other immunosuppressive patients, pulmonary mucormycosis is diagnosed (Jeong et al., 2017). The patients due to their uncontrolled diabetes, hospitalization conditions, and corticosteroid intake as treatment became more prone to invasive fungal infections (Figure 2).

Mucorales infections are being identified by the angio-invasion and prompt progression which leads to thrombosis and prevalent tissue necrosis. Pulmonary mucor infection expresses persistent fever, cough, and dyspnoea, whereas rhino-cerebral exhibits headache, fever, sinus congestion, unilateral facial swelling, and dark lesions on the nasal bridge and inner mouth. Being determined by the severity of the infection, several nonspecific image findings can be observed of mucormycosis such that they can be exhibited as a solitary nodule, lobar consolidation, or a cavitary lesion. In the study by Hammer et al., (2018) CT features of pulmonary mucormycosis in 30 patients with definite or probable disease were researched. They observed that a reverse halo sign, which is a GGO surrounded by a condensed merging of crescentic shape has been found in 67% of their patients. Additionally, it was found that 53% of patients had a large perilesional halo while 87% had the peripheral distribution of their lung lesions (Hammer et al., 2018).

Conversely, the CT finding can alone not diagnose pulmonary mucormycosis because some reports such that of reverse halo sign may also be found in the cases of invasive aspergillosis and COVID-19 infection. The patient's chest CT exhibited diffuse GGO and multiple cavitary lesions; being nonspecific and probably due to her multi-organ infection. Likewise, the assays that can be performed in clinical laboratories including the beta-D glucan and the serum galactomannan antigen could prove to determine the fungal infection but are not allied to Mucorales. Therefore, the diagnosis linked to mucormycosis entails manifold techniques consisting of clinical laboratory testing, radiographic or histological observations, along fungal culture analysis. The fungal cultures of mucormycosis do not show any typical growth which could be an essential parameter to note in order to obtain a proper diagnosis.

The treatment of voriconazole, micafungin, and liposomal amphotericin B has been given to the patient due to multi-organ culture growth. Antagonistic source control in addition to surgical debridement is the basis of disease management. In cases where surgical debridement is not possible in the context of higher mortality risk, such as in the case of this study, the higher dose of liposomal amphotericin B is the standard care. The patient had been on liposomal amphotericin B (in conc. 5 mg/kg/day) treatment initially, yet higher doses (in conc. of 10 mg/kg/day) have been found related to an increase in the response to treatment (Lanternier et al., 2015). The combination of amphotericin B with either posaconazole or echinocandins is not yet suggested by any sort of treatment guidelines. Contrastingly, research on mice has shown improved survival when injected with the combination of these.

Ibrahim et al., (2008) worked on mice wherein they induced neutropenia or DKA along with the infection of mucormycosis. They observed improved survival in the mice treated with micafungin or anidulafungin with liposomal amphotericin B in comparison to any monotherapy with only the agent

(Ibrahim et al., 2008). In addition, a demonstrative study on 41 patients which rhino-cerebral mucormycosis compared the effects of polyene (amphotericin B lipid complex, liposomal amphotericin B, or amphotericin B deoxycholate) plus caspofungin therapy versus polyene monotherapy on survival time. It was reported that greater outcomes and improved survival times at 30 days post-discharge were a result of combination therapy (Reed et al., 2008). The patient under study had also been treated with combination therapy in the hope of improving survival chances because surgical debridement was not involved.

Propagation of mucormycosis has touched its peak during the COVID-19 pandemic which demonstrates its acuteness and significant deadly fungal infection originated by fungi associated with the mucoraceae family (Mohindra et al., 2007). The existence of these fungi has been observed in soil, fruit, and faeces, and can be enforced for culturing through the utilization of mucosa derived from nasal and buccal of healthy volunteers (Goel et al., 2009). The feature of this pathogen was revealed to be an asexual spore-generating fungus that may be enforced for infection in the oral and nasal cavities by the process of inhalation. The prevalence of a normal immune system ejected the spores by the action of phagocytic leukocytes (Goel et al., 2009). Transformation of the pathogen in individuals is generally enforced into hyphae with pre-influenced features, for instance, uncontrolled diabetes mellitus, which happened precisely in the prevalence of ketoacidosis, probability of malignancy, for instance, lymphoma and leukemia, transplantation of organ, renal failure, organ transplantation, rheumatologic disorders by utilizing immunosuppressive moieties, for instance, sustained utilization of corticosteroids for longer duration, AIDS, chronic sinusitis and extensive burn (Viterbo et al., 2011; Afroze et al., 2017). Leukocytes presented minimum effectiveness on the fungi in the form of hyphae and the differentiation of pathogens can be enforced more conveniently during co-morbid situations (Afroze et al., 2017). The proliferation of organs generally initiated and permeated the walls of vessels of the infected area and emerged as the consequence of ischemia, thrombosis, and necrosis (Goel et al., 2009). The fungal infection may generally escalate into the paranasal sinuses and then permeate into spaces of the orbital and intracranial region by direct expansion or through the bloodstream (Figure 3) (Afroze et al., 2017). This pathogenesis is termed rhino orbito-cerebral mucormycosis and is the most common type of human mucormycosis (Goel et al., 2009).

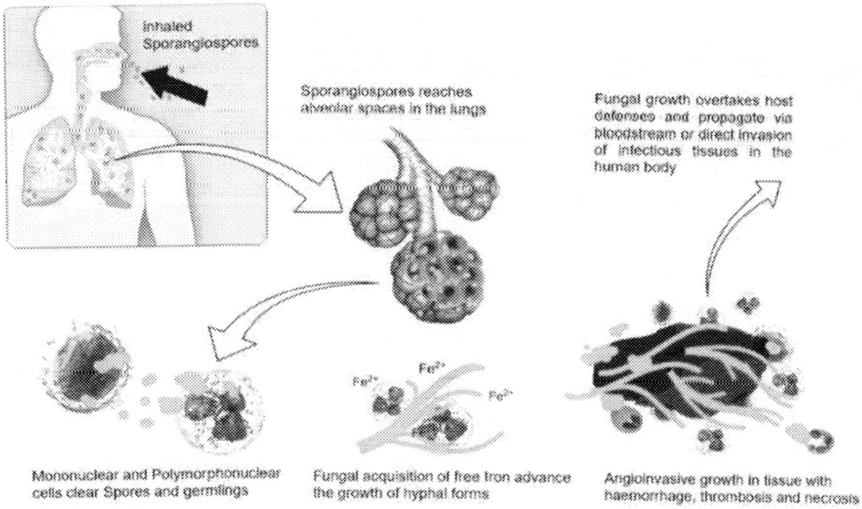


**Figure 3.** Pathway of fungal infection: Direct expansion and bloodstream permeation leading to paranasal sinuses, orbital, and intracranial spaces.

The pulmonary, cutaneous, gastrointestinal, and distributed characteristics of mucormycosis are unconventional demonstrations of this infection (Mignogna et al., 2011). Some investigations reported that there is enough evidence of superimposition or coinfection of mucormycosis in COVID-19 patients (Chen et al., 2020). The studies showcased that T lymphocytes, for instance, CD4 and CD8 revealed to be minimal in severe COVID-19, and levels of IL-2 R, IL-6, IL-10, and TNF-α are significantly elevated in these cases (Chen et al., 2020). There is an absence of evidence for COVID-19 emerging as a pre-influenced feature for cases like rhino-orbital or rhino-orbitocerebral mucormycosis. There is evidence in the case study that revealed that COVID-19 and the corresponding corticosteroid therapy without completing the dosing interval presented the only pre-influencing features that made the patient susceptible to rhino-orbitocerebral mucormycosis. This evidence may demonstrate that the existence of COVID-19 for the minimum duration of corticosteroid therapy can predispose the patient to mucormycosis.

Another case study reported that COVID-19 and the corresponding corticosteroid therapy without completing the dose interval presented the case of shoot up in blood glucose levels and then followed by the case of rhino-orbital mucormycosis. Headache, facial pain and paraesthesia, inflammation, periorbital and nasal swelling, proptosis, eyelid drooping, external and internal ophthalmoplegia, blackish necrosis of palate and nasal mucosa, and visual loss emerged evidently as the most common symptoms prevailing in the case of rhino-orbitocerebral mucormycosis (Mohindra et al., 2007). This fungal disease generally propagates on the mucosal layer of the nasal and buccal cavity extending throughout to paranasal sinuses (Afroze et al., 2017). The fungus is generally initiated into the orbital space through the region of lamina papyracea. The loss of vision generally emerges from the optic nerve participation or vessels reaching the retina. Engagement of intracranial space can be enforced directly through the region of orbital orifices and sinus walls or can be enforced through systemic circulation.

There is other evidence of cavernous sinus thrombosis as the fatal problem that enforced the damage to the cranial nerves, namely, III, IV, V1, V2, and VI (McCarthy et al., 2014). Diagnosis is very crucial regarding proper investigation analysis and imaging, i.e., CT and MRI emerged as most significant to estimate the mucormycosis progression (Mohindra et al., 2007). The imaging detection of the infected area can reveal engaged paranasal sinus opacifications, alterations of intraorbital tissue signal in the presence or absence of focal mass, bone destruction of sinus walls, cavernous sinus filling defect, intracranial focal mass, and the meningeal signal variation (Mohindra et al., 2007; Afroze et al., 2017). Validation of the mucormycosis is enforced by the blackish necrotic tissue's estimation in the engaged region evident by histopathology. The histological stains that detect the mucor structure comprise hematoxylin and eosin, Gomori methenamine silver (GMS), and Periodic acid-Schiff (PAS) (Goel et al., 2009). The investigation through histopathologic studies reveals relatively wide non-septate hyphae with branches at right angle, inflammation of granulomatous necrosis, and vasculitis synergized with the existence of mucor hyphae prevailed within the vascular wall and lumen (Mignogna et al., 2011). Both cases comprise unilateral complete internal and external ophthalmoplegia.

One of the Case studies revealed the bilateral loss of vision but the absence of significant proptosis or periorbital inflammation. The imaging of enrolled patients demonstrated that the density of infections enforced increased posteriorly, precisely in the posterior air cells of the ethmoidal and sphenoidal sinuses, and close to the orbital apex. The MRI of the brain also presented the fungal infection progression into the region of the anterior cranial fossa. Another case revealed potential unilateral proptosis, vision loss, and orbital inflammation. The imaging report revealed the engagement of left sphenoidal, ethmoidal, and maxillary sinuses. Mucormycosis has been confirmed by the implementation of Endoscopic sinus surgery and investigation by histopathological analyses certified mucormycosis in both investigational cases. The deadly fungal injection, rhino-orbitocerebral mucormycosis during the cases of engagement in the brain revealed shoot in mortality up to 50-85% (Prabhu et al., 2018).

The survival rates of mucormycosis rely on advanced diagnosis, eliminating basic pre-influence features, for instance, aggressive necrotic tissue autolysis, and appropriate systemic antifungal agents (Goel et al., 2009). Pre-influencing features, for instance, corticosteroid medication should be terminated, and immediate control of blood sugar should be enforced. Liposomal amphotericin B should be the gold standard drug for mucormycosis treatment and effectively ameliorates the rate of survival (McCarthy et al., 2014). The oral antifungal drug posaconazole has been enforced as a concomitant therapy post-treatment of mucormycosis by amphotericin B (Greenberg et al., 2006). Daily uniformly necrotic tissue autolysis from paranasal sinuses is essential to antagonize the mucormycosis progression (Mohindra et al., 2007). The sinus irrigation and the engaged focus area with diluted amphotericin B are suggested (Mohindra et al., 2007). There should be an endorsement of orbital exenteration in the prevalence of focal mass or necrotic tissues reported in most studies (Mohindra et al., 2007). In their case, pre-influencing features were controlled, prescription of IV amphotericin B was enforced, and daily autolysis of the paranasal sinus and irrigation with diluted amphotericin B were performed. It is very pathetic that patients from Case I studies have shown high mortality because of the mucormycosis progression and has been spread into intracranial space. The mortality rate in their Case 2 studies was absent and has been treated by proper medical intervention and time-to-time grafting and epithelialization of the paranasal sinuses (Veisi et al., 2021).

Corticosteroid therapy generated a rhino-orbital and/or rhino-orbitocerebral mucormycosis risk in patients of COVID-19 and become more vulnerable during the presence of concomitant risk, for instance, the presence of DM. Orbital pain, vision changes, and orbital inflammation should be enforced for investigation in COVID-19 patients. The progression of the infection into intracranial space may emerge to be dangerous (Veisi et al., 2021).

## 2. Pharmacokinetic Challenges of Treatment for Mucormycosis

Clinical investigation of antifungal intervention is very crucial for mucormycosis treatment and enforced for the past ten years which presented the crucialness as the perfect scenario of antifungal intervention to boost survival. Caillot et al., (1997) and (Greene et al., (2007) observed that treatment applied during the period of initial recommended radiographic implementation of invasive pulmonary aspergillosis, is, the halo sign, was correlated with a better effective approach of treatment along with significant response and survival as compared to patients who have been intervened with antifungal medication enforced by the utilization of computed tomographic imaging outcomes that majorly lasted for 7–10 days. Postponement in treatment permits an unrestricted proliferation of angio-invasive fungal including thrombotic necrosis of neighboring tissue that restricts life-saving drug delivery to the infection areas (Berenguer et al., 1995; Shibuya et al., 2004; Ben-Ami et al., 2009).

The quick onset rate of growth of most Mucorales *in vivo* presented a great opportunity for significant mucormycosis treatment i.e., Widespread can be applied before angiogenesis and for aspergillosis patients. The importance of diagnosis and advanced treatment at regular time intervals was demonstrated in a retrospective study of 70 leukemia patients with documented evidence of mucormycosis. It postpones the intervention of amphotericin B-based dosage forms by 5 days was related to a twofold boost in mortality at the duration of 12 weeks after diagnosis (Chamilos et al., 2008). Likewise, the latest retrospective investigation conducted by Lass-Florl and colleagues presented that 84% of patients carrying pulmonary zygomycosis were experiencing insignificant medication during the time of diagnosis which was manifested by microscopic examination (Lass-Florl et al., 2007).

Hence, treatment regimens at the time of early phases of the infection should prioritize the implementation of expected drugs and investigate their pharmacokinetics, for instance, liposome amphotericin B formulations in the presence or absence of echinocandins to rapidly pack the drug in infected tissue and eventually proliferation of fungus will be hindered and the risk of further angioinvasion is reduced. At the time of stabilization of infection, much preference can be kept on the suitability of oral interventional drugs with boosted safety profiles, for instance, pharmacokinetic parameters of posaconazole can be enforced for optimization through cautious clinical investigation of diet optimization, gastrointestinal disturbances, and therapeutic drug monitoring. Therefore, the implementation of posaconazole for the primary treatment of mucormycosis persist in investigational and ought to be enforced with the plethora of cautions, receivable to the reporting of uncertain characteristic in many experimental investigations of mucormycosis propagation (Saoulidis et al., 2011).

## 3. New Drug Targets for Mucormycosis

Figure 4 designated the process of management of mucormycosis and rapid treatment identification with its classification such as antifungal medications, surgical incision, and rectification of comorbid conditions like hyperglycemia, ketosis, acidosis, and other metabolic deformity.

The process of genome sequencing has been enforced for *R. oryzae* has generated data for enforcing significant strategies for boosting antifungal function. Synthesis of chitin would emerge to be site-specific for drug action which should be implemented against *Rhizopus*. Since the 1970s, the antagonist action on the synthesis of chitin has been discovered and investigated properly, for instance, polyoxins and nikkomycins revealed their progression as significant therapeutic interventions and that has been restricted by their very low uptake in whole fungal cells and the differential susceptibilities of CHS gene products to the antagonist action of these antifungals (Hector, 1993). Emerged limitations might be precisely problematic for Mucorales, provided the condition of equivalent and highly excessive nature of synthesis of chitin in these fungi (Ma et al., 2009).

*In vitro* studies confirmed that investigated amalgamation of micafungin and the chitin synthesis inhibitor, for instance, nikkomycin Z, which investigative reported the synergistic interactions for isolates of *A. fumigatus*, but not enforced for *R. oryzae* (Chiou et al., 2001; Dannaoui et al., 2009). Although *in vitro* was reported synergistic interactions. Therefore, amphotericin B or triazoles, for instance, posaconazole, itraconazole, or ravuconazole are amalgamed with a calcineurin inhibitor, for instance, cyclosporine against several Mucorales members (Dannaoui et al., 2009). Concomitantly targeting of the cell wall, cell membrane, and pathways of signal transduction engaged in fungal homeostatic retaliation. For example, PKC (protein kinase C) or the CaN (calcineurin) pathway can emerge as a crucial plan of action for boosting the activity of drugs in this exceptionally compatible pathogen.

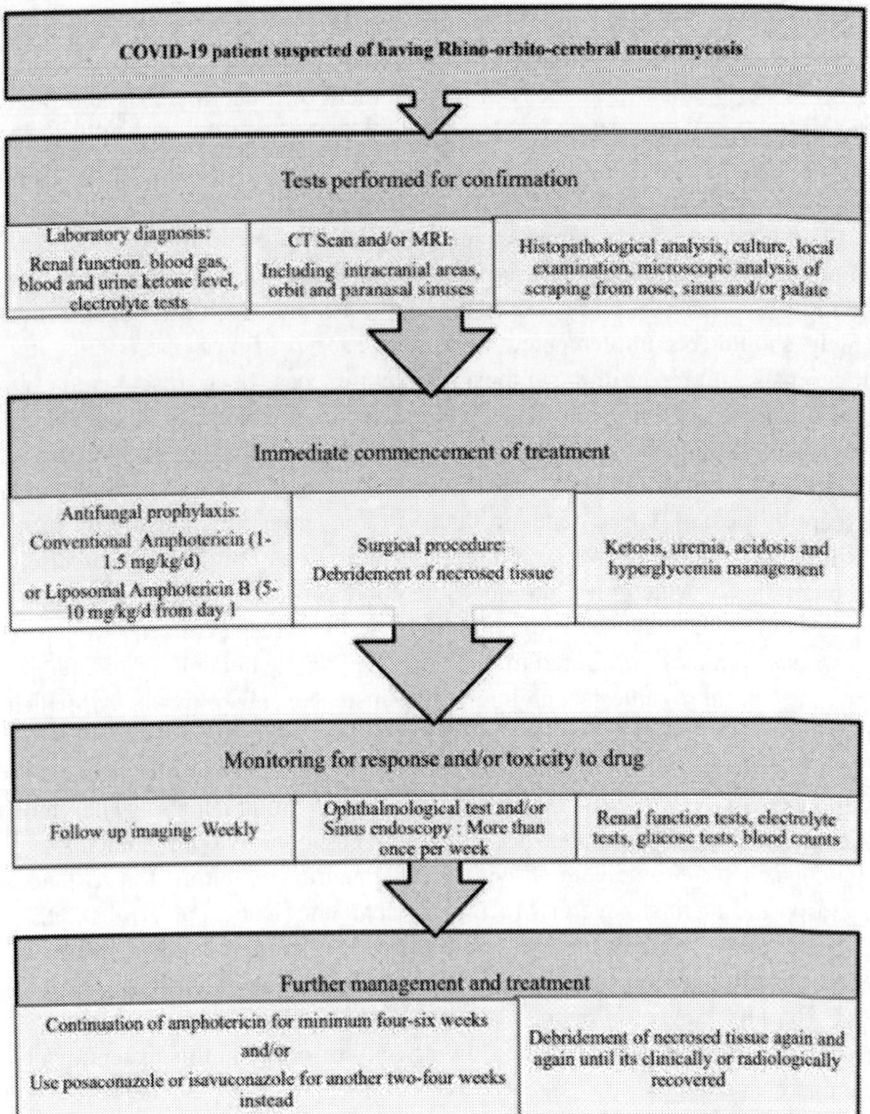


**Figure 4.** Sequential explanation for mucormycosis management in COVID-19 patients.

**Table 1.** Pre-clinical and clinical investigation of combination therapy for treatment of mucormycosis

| Combination Therapy | Description | References |
|---|---|---|
| Liposome amphotericin B(LAmB) synergized with granulocyte-macrophage colony-stimulating factor | It showcases effectiveness in a murine model of invasive mucormycosis | Rodriguez et al., 2009 |
| Caspofungin and LAmB | Propagated mucormycosis in diabetic ketoacidosis (DKA) prevailing in mice synergistically boosted survival differentiated with placebo. It effectively boosted the survival of rhino-orbitocerebral patients. | Spellberg et al., 2005 |
| LAmB and micafungin or anidulafungin | It boosted survival in mice prevailing neutropenic and DKA with propagated mucormycosis. | Ibrahim et al., 2012 |
| LAmB and deferasirox | *In vitro* investigation revealed the fungicidal activity of deferasirox for clinical isolates of Mucorales. It significantly boosted the survival in DKA mice and enhanced the survival of rhinocerebral mucormycosis patients who are showcasing continuous brain stem disease despite monotherapy of LAmB. | Spellberg et al., 2012 |
| LAmB and Echinocandins | It is accessible as an intravenous formulation. It showcased significant improvement in survival in DKA mice but the absence of clinical studies | Spellberg et al., 2012 |
| Posaconazole and Isavuconazole | *In vitro* investigation of Posaconazole and isavuconazole revealed significant activity against clinical isolates of Mucorales Absence of significant improvement survival data in DKA mice and absence of clinical data. Unavailability of intravenous formulation. | Rodriguez et al., 2008; Spellberg et al., 2012 |
| A triple combination of LAmB, deferasirox, and caspofungin | Triple therapy can be augmented after establishing the superiority of dual therapy as compared to monotherapy. It significantly improved survival and lowered the load on infected tissue with mucormycosis in DKA mice as compared to dual drug combination and placebo. | Roux et al., 2010; Spellberg et al., 2012 |
| Echinocandins and deferasirox | *In vitro* investigation revealed the fungicidal activity of deferasirox for clinical isolates of Mucorales. It significantly boosted the survival of DKA mice. It has safety issues and an absence of intravenous dosage forms | Soummer et al., 2008; Spellberg et al., 2012 |

**Abbreviations** - LAmB: Liposome amphotericin B & DKA: Diabetic ketoacidosis.

Genomic sequencing investigation of *R. oryzae* further ensured the remarkable significance of free iron for enforcing pathogenesis and boosting attacking pathogen growth (Ma et al., 2009). In contrast to other microbes, *R. orzyae* presented the absence of genes for enzyme non-ribosomal peptide synthases which present the conventional siderophores i.e., hydroxamate siderophores. Rather, *R. oryzae* depends precisely on rhizoferrin, which is unsuccessful in obtaining serum-bound iron (De Locht et al., 1994) and hence relies on free iron or the enzyme iron reductases influence i.e., rFTR1 and enzyme heme oxygenases to enhance the internalization of iron from the hemoglobin of the host. Iron internalization novel inhibitors in *R. oryzae* might disturb the fungus's potential for enforcing angio-invasive growth. This crucial function of iron internalization during *R. oryzae* infection also strengthens the assurance of utilizing novel iron chelators, for instance, deferasirox and lipid polyene like caspofungin to boost the survival outcomes in mucormycosis patients (Table 1). There are a lot of concerns that need to be addressed regarding associated drugs for administration, including the optimal dose, dosage frequency, and duration or course of these advanced therapies for mucormycosis (Lewis et al., 2001).

The deadly COVID-19 infection has been correlated with an extensive diversity of disease models which generally varies from a mild cough to life-threatening or fatal pneumonia (Mehta and Pandey, 2020). Multiple manifestations and complications have been enforced for documentation, and novel cases are emerging and reported every day as we gather more detailed information regarding the novel COVID-19 pandemic.

Mucormycosis or zygomycosis which is also termed phycomycosis, was reported for the first time in 1885 by Paltauf, it is an unconventional and violent fungal infection that eventually influences patients by modifying their immunological system (Paltauf, 1885). It is the most common form of destructive fungal disease and revealed rhinocerebral manifestation (Arnáiz-García et al., 2009). However, it has a minimum rate of incidence which may reach up to 1.7 per million population and several cases have been observed and eventually lead to a remarkable enhancement of incidence in the current scenario of the unprecedented COVID-19 pandemic (Werthman-Ehrenreich, 2021).

SARS-CoV-2 is also accountable for generating lower respiratory tract infection and eventually led to acute respiratory distress syndrome (ARDS), which somewhat resembles SARS-CoV and MERS (Wang et al., 2020). Apart from the dispersed alveolar destruction and emerged with severe exudates at inflammatory areas, patients infected with COVID-19 have consequences of immunosuppression which led to a reduction in $CD4^+$ T and $CD8^+$ T cells at every time (Yang et al., 2020). There was course of SARS-CoV infection expanded in 2003, the fungal infection cases ranged from 14.8-27%, which eventually emerged as the major reason for mortality for severe ARDS patients, and data was found that mortality from the ARDS was a maximum of 73.7% (Li and Pan, 2003; Zhang et al., 2003; Yin et al., 2004). Investigations have revealed that SARS-CoV and SARS-CoV-2 are affiliated to identical species and have identical rates with similar biological and clinical features (Peeri et al., 2020). These incidences in 2003 are very crucial for physicians to enforce attention and get aware of the high chances of the enhanced incidence rate of fungal infections in those patients who are infected or recovered from COVID-19, which is identical to the detection and observation of cases of mucormycosis patients.

Many incidental investigational case reports have been published earlier, but a firm connection between COVID-19 and enhanced fungal infections can be established. In September 2020, Mehta and Pandey presented rhino-orbital mucormycosis case in one patient, who was suffering from COVID-19 (White et al., 2020). In the same month, Werthman-Ehrenreich published one more similar case (Werthman-Ehrenreich, 2021).

White *et al.,* (2020) investigated 135 adults infected with COVID-19 and presented a rate of incidence of 26.7% for invasive fungal infections (White et al., 2020). Song *et al.,* (2020) investigated the correlation between COVID-19 and invasive fungal sinusitis, and eventually demonstrated that many patients who are infected by or recovered from COVID-19 are at enhanced risk of harboring invasive fungal infections and in such cases, the author subsequently presented a management algorithm (Yin et al., 2004). A recently published review reported that 8% of patients who are infected by or recovered from COVID-19, and at the time of hospital admission they harbored bacterial or fungal infections, with extensive utilization of broad-spectrum antibiotics and steroids (Rawson et al., 2020).

There could be many significant causes for this correlation, for instance, immunosuppression emergence by COVID-19 infection, or may be the irrational steroids and broad-spectrum antibiotics utilization in COVID-19 management, which eventually led to the emergence or worsening of a pre-existing fungal disease. The National Institute of Health in coordination with the Randomised Evaluation of COVID-19 Therapy ('RECOVERY') Collaborative Group suggested only steroid utilization in patients who are dependent on ventilators or supplemental oxygen, however, should be avoided in milder cases (Horby et al., 2021). The guidelines precisely describe the enhanced risk of emerging a secondary infection (NIH, 2019).

Mucor has been categorized as a saprophytic fungus and the extensive prevalence of its spore in nature, and also been observed in food, soil, air, and decomposing organic material (Ballester et al., 2012). The minimum significance of virulence may prevail in the nasal mucosa of healthy people (Elinav et al., 2009). The immunocompromised patient can develop the fungus in the region of paranasal sinuses and expand intracranially including other neighboring structures such as the orbit. Paranasal sinuses observed with non-contrast computed tomography are generally the primary choice of evaluation. The gadolinium-boosted magnetic resonance imaging is being adopted during the reckoning of intra-orbital or intracranial extension. Focal bony abrasion and expansion of the extra sinus are strongly recommended for the diagnosis (Ballester et al., 2012).

After the authentication of diagnosis, surgical incision of the inflamed region must be enforced very quicky. Surgery solely has been presented to be healing; however, belligerent commenced surgical procedure has been revealed to boost the rate of survival (Elinav et al., 2009; Goldstein et al., 2009). The antifungal drug Amphotericin-B deoxycholate is the first choice of treatment and liposomal dosage forms are preferred because of reduced nephrotoxicity. There are some cases of patients who are intolerant to amphotericin liposomal preparation; therefore, posaconazole should be clinically investigated as an ideal substitute course of action (Goldstein et al., 2009; Scheckenbach et al., 2010). Prognosis revealed to be disappointing even with belligerent surgery and intravenous LAmB and mortality rates were reported to be 33.3-80%, reaching the maximum of 100% in highly transmissible infections (Jung et al., 2009; Scheckenbach et al., 2010).

## 4. Components of an Outbreak Investigation

### 4.1. Verify the Diagnosis and Define a Case

Among transplant patients, the most widely accepted and used case definition was developed for invasive fungal infections to be used in clinical trials by the European Organization for Research and Treatment of Cancer (EORTC) and the National Institute of Allergy and Infectious Diseases Mycoses Study Group (MSG) (De Pauw et al., 2008). For example: In histopathologic findings out of 169 MSG/EORTC probable and proven cases, 160 were positive for mucoromycete hyphae. Of a total of 169 cases, only 52 (31%) were identified without histopathology and did not accompany positive culture.

## 4.2. Cutaneous Mucormycosis Case Definition

With the pieces of evidence of mucormycosis, cutaneous infections case definitions included soft tissue infections such as positive fungal culture and observation of broad pauci-septae hyphae having to branch on microscopy at right angles, primarily at skin lesions periphery (Castrejón-Pérez et al., 2017; Hartnett et al., 2019) (Table 2).

**Table 2.** Defining the cases for invasive mucormycosis, in compliance with the National Institute of Allergy and Infectious Diseases Mycoses Study Group (MSG) and European Organization for Research and Treatment of Cancer (EORTC)

| **Confirmed Invasive Mucormycosis:** Presence confirmed by pathology and/or culture of sterile material | |
|---|---|
| Microscopic confirmation | Cytopathologic, histopathologic, or direct microscopic investigation of a specimen generated by the technique of needle aspiration or biopsy in which hyphae are featured to be seen escorted by proof of associated tissue damage/vascular invasion. Mucormycete-specific microscopic examinations may include:<br>• Broad, pauciseptate hyphae<br>• Large angle of branching, approaching right angles<br>• Irregular branching<br>• Angioinvasion<br>• • Intravascular thrombosis. |
| Cultural confirmation | Recovery of a mold by enforcing specimen culturing generated by a sterile method from a sterile and clinically normal or radiologically abnormal site consonant with an infectious disease progression. Pathogenic ascomycete genera include but are not limited to *Cunninghamella, Mucor, Rhizomucor, Rhizopus, Lichtheimia, Apophysomyces, Saksenaea, Cokeromyces*. |

**Table 2.** (Continued)

| | |
|---|---|
| **Probable Invasive Mucormycosis**: Probable disease requires a host factor, a clinical criterion, and a mycological criterion, in the absence of confirmed non-mucormycete mold (e.g., *Aspergillus*). | |
| Host Factors | New history of neutropenia i.e., 10 days temporally connected to the onset of fungal disease<br><br>• Delivery of allogeneic stem cell transplant<br>• Sustained use of corticosteroids (mean minimum dose of 0.3 mg/kg/day of prednisone equivalent for >3 weeks)<br>• Treatment with other recognized T cell immunosuppressants, for instance, TNF-alpha blockers, specific monoclonal antibodies, cyclosporine, or nucleoside analogs during the past 3 months<br>• Inherited severe immunodeficiency, for instance, chronic granulomatous disease or severe combined immunodeficiency. |
| **Clinical Benchmark** | |
| Lower respiratory tract disease | Presence of one of the following three signs on CT:<br><br>1. Dense, well-circumscribed lesion(s) with or without a halo sign<br>2. Air-crescent sign<br>3. Cavity. |
| Tracheobronchitis | Tracheobronchial ulceration, nodule, pseudomembrane, plaque, or eschar seen on bronchoscopic analysis |
| Sinonasal infection | Imaging showing sinusitis plus at least one of the following three signs:<br><br>1. Acute localized pain (including radiating to the eye)<br>2. Nasal ulcer with black eschar<br>3. Extension from the paranasal sinus across bony barriers, including into the orbit. |
| CNS infection | One of the following two signs:<br><br>1. Focal lesion on imaging<br>2. Meningeal enhancement on MRI or CT. |
| Mycological criteria | Mold in sputum, bronchoalveolar lavage fluid, bronchial brush, or sinus aspirate samples indicated by one of the following:<br><br>1. Presence of fungal elements indicating a mold<br>2. Recovery from the culture of a mold. |
| **Possible Invasive Mucormycosis:** Possible disease requires a host factor and a clinical criterion from **Probable Invasive Mucormycosis** above. | |

### 4.3. Laboratory Confirmation

Inpatient specimens and mucormycetes's laboratory confirmation is the central part of all the above-mentioned case definitions, and laboratory capacity for mycology varies by hospital. Species identification of mucormycetes will be difficult and in clinical laboratories misidentifications occur, although mycology expertise will be able to identify species of suspected mucromycete cultures. The cultures will be sent out to laboratories for reference diagnostic, where limited capacity is present. Identification of mucormycetes can be done by polymerase chain reaction (PCR) in formalin-fixed paraffin- embedded biopsy having histopathologic pieces of evidence at CDC of fungal hyphae (Gholinejad-Ghadi et al., 2018; Reich et al., 2018). For a fee, PCR is also performed on tissue and tissue blocks in some institutes. However, the PCR technique is highly dependent on the abundance, quality, and source of specimen. In risk patients, in serum for the detection of mucormycete DNA, PCR testing is very useful in some analysis, having faster detection and the results with culture are consonant and by PCR mucormycetes species are identified in tissues (Millon et al., 2013; Legrand et al., 2016).

### 4.4. Hospital Trends in Mucormycosis and Other Mold Infections

Since mucormycosis is intermittent even among patients having the highest risk, the examination is defensible, when it is uncertain whether a rise in the number of contaminations signifies a genuine outburst, especially if cases seem to group on place or time or among patients who share different contacts. For instance, a rise from two to four cases each year at a solitary clinic could be a result of the possibility or could indicate that in the facility a new source of mucormycetes is present, which leads to the number of infections.

### 4.5. Seasonality Trends

Mucormycosis infections may have some seasonal outlines that are investigated in some studies. There are two studies from Israel, three from the eastern Mediterranean (Talmi et al., 2002; Shpitzer et al., 2005), and one from Lebanon (Al-Ajam et al., 2006), found that most of the infections of mucormycosis during August over December, at reached its peak at end of the hot and dry summer season. A study found that per 10,000 patients-days there are 5.7 invasive mold infections in summer as compared to spring having 1.3 per 10,000 during 2012-2015 (Sivagnanam et al., 2017). Season plays a very crucial role in investigating a bunch of infections, however small sample size of cases over a prolonged period of time at any provided hospital makes interpretation difficult regarding the cruciality of seasonality The investigators who noticed bunching over time are more likely to mention or publish seasonality as a risk other than those which do not.

## 4.6. Involvement of Key Partners and Notifications

For the investigation of mucormycosis, a multidisciplinary team is required. The team includes people with expertise in case finding, clinical expertise, infection control, and environmental assessment. To a suspected outbreak, an effective response requires close collaboration and early communication among facility maintenance, environmental services, infection prevention, construction, infectious disease, nursing, media relations, and hospital administration. During the investigation of an outbreak of mucormycosis in the beginning, we assembled a meeting with representatives from each of the groups. In count, patients in hospitals should be notified who develop mucormycosis as an alleged result of an infection regulator break, should also notify patients at increased risk during mucormycosis outbursts that are likely to be associated with healthcare (Dudzinski et al., 2010) by notifying patients of recognized infection regulator breaks that upsurge the risk of harm or injury, even if there is a low chance of patient harm.

At four hospitals in Massachusetts, it was found in a recent study that there is no increase in malpractice claims following the implantation of a communication and resolution program in which hospitals and patients are communicated about adverse effects and when it's appropriate, they took the responsibility (Kachalia et al., 2018). For additional assistance, hospitals should consult their public health department, communications expert, and legal counsel. Timely notification of patients and hospital staff can:

1. If they show any concerning symptoms, it encourages patients to seek early care and potentially leads to timely diagnosis
2. In community and hospital, it provides the opportunity to avoid exposure to mold and to educate patients

3. Remind visitors, clinicians, and patients about the importance of infection regulator intrusions; through transparency, build public and patient trust.

Key details that should be collected on a line list for each patient include (Hartnett et al., 2019):

1. The age of each patient
2. Admission date(s), as well as discharge dates for previous hospitalizations within several months of suspected onset
3. Outpatient visits and prior admissions
4. Underlying conditions and patient risk factors (e.g., prolonged neutropenia, diabetes mellitus, hematopoietic stem cell transplant, and hematologic diseases)
5. Immunosuppressive medications (e.g., cancer chemotherapy, corticosteroids, other immunotherapy and biologics)
6. Symptoms and signs of fungal infection, with approximate dates of onset
7. Histopathology specimen collection date(s) and findings
8. Specimen source, species, and culture date(s)
9. Antifungal medications are given with dates and indication (Treatment and prophylaxis)
10. Room and unit assignments with dates
11. Invasive disease versus colonization by EORTC/MSG definition or clinician determination
12. Lines, procedures, surgeries, and devices
13. Outcomes, including date of discharge or death.

## 5. Epidemic Curve

An epidemic curve is most useful because infections of mucormycosis are rare when cases from previous years are included. This curve is helpful in differentiating proven cases from the cases that are possible and probable. In the vulnerable population of patients, the initial symptoms and signs of mucormycosis are common and non-specific because it will be difficult to assign the infection onset date. The date regarding extracting the information of receiving the first diagnostic specimen was more reliable during the feasibility of medical records as an information source (Llata et al., 2011). The state-wise cases of mucormycosis are summarized in Table 3 (Rochna et al., 2021).

On 7th June 2021, **the** following data was collected as described in following (Rocha et al., 2021):

1. 28,252 Mucormycosis cases have been reported till above mentioned date.
2. Maharashtra and Gujarat are reported to be the worst affected among the other 26 states for mucormycosis cases. The number of mucormycosis cases reported in Maharashtra emerged to be the highest having a tally of 6,329 followed by Gujarat having a tally of 5,486 mucormycosis cases.
3. Mucormycosis has been developed in 86% of COVID-19 recovered patients and another reported 62.3% have pre-existing medical conditions of diabetes.

**Table 3.** State-wise cases of mucormycosis in India in May 2021

| Date | Cases | 21 May, 2021 | 22 May, 2021 |
|---|---|---|---|
| Maharashtra | Total cases | 1,500 | 2,000 |
| | Death | 90 | |
| Gujarat | Total cases | 1,163 | 2281 |
| | Death | 61 | |
| Madhya Pradesh | Total cases | 575 | 720 |
| | Death | 31 | |
| Haryana | Total cases | 268 | 250 |
| | Death | 8 | |
| Delhi | Total cases | 203 | 197 |
| | Death | 1 | |
| Uttar Pradesh | Total cases | 169 | 112 |
| | Death | 8 | |
| Bihar | Total cases | 103 | 56 |
| | Death | 2 | |
| Chhattisgarh | Total cases | 101 | 87 |
| | Death | 1 | |
| Karnataka | Total cases | 97 | 500 |
| | Death | 0 | |
| Telangana | Total cases | 90 | 350 |
| | Death | 10 | |

On 28th June 2021, the following data has been collected as described in the following (Rocha et al., 2021):

1. The total tally of mucormycosis cases reported till above mentioned date is 40,845 cases and revealed its nature as rhinocerebral in 31,344 infected patients and the mortality of infected patients has been updated as 3,129.
2. Mucormycosis has been developed in 85.5% of COVID-19-recovered patients and another reported 64.11% have a pre-existing medical condition of diabetes and those infected by improper dosage regimen of steroids stand at 64.11% till above mentioned date.
3. 32% of mucormycosis cases have been reported in the age group of 18-45 years, followed by 42% of mucormycosis cases in the age group of 45-60 years, however, 24% of geriatric patients have been infected with mucormycosis.

## 6. Summary and Future Perspectives

Acute respiratory distress syndrome emerges from severe viral pneumonia, for instance, influenza and COVID-19 which raises the need for ventilatory support, corticosteroids administration, and other concomitant medications to prevent severe inflammation of airways (Dan et al., 2020; Upadhyay et al., 2021; Dan et al., 2022). Corticosteroid medication has both benefits and adverse reactions in terms of treating viral pneumonia and exposing the patient to secondary bacterial and invasive fungal infections (IFIs) i.e., mucormycosis by influencing morbidity and mortality. Mucormycosis is a fatal fungal infection with an enhanced belligerent disposition for increased chances of spreading which is correlated with an impoverished prognosis due to delayed diagnosis and therapeutic management. Conventionally, uncontrolled diabetes mellitus (DM) and other immunosuppressive circumstances, for instance, corticosteroid medication are familiar risk elements for mucormycosis.

Consideration of pathology of the lung, immune dysfunctions, and corticosteroid medication exposed severe viral pneumonia patients to IFIs, for instance, aspergillosis and mucormycosis. The amalgamation of corticosteroid medication and DM can enforce immunosuppression and hyperglycemia which enhance the risk elements of mucormycosis in a sensitive individual. Antifungal medication emerged to be a life-rescuing clinical intervention in the eradication of mucormycosis, and liposomal amphotericin B dosage form is the suggested first-choice treatment. Posaconazole and isavuconazole are precious drugs during conditions of intolerance or poor metabolism. The guidelines also suggest the parallel approach of surgical grafting and antifungal intervention, along with questionable efficacy persist on combination therapy of antifungals. However, antifungal combination intervention in the treatment of mucormycosis presented astonishing efficacy results in patients suffering from diabetes and leukemia. The reliance on invasive methods to extract biological specimens from clinically complicated tissues for the diagnosis of mucormycosis and the panic condition regarding airborne SARS-CoV2 transmission at the time of aerosol formulation methods in oral and maxillofacial surgery at unprecedented pandemic COVID-19 worsened the situation which enforced the urgency of prompt mucormycosis diagnosis.

## Conclusion

Mucormycosis emerged to be the intersection of two consequences, for instance, COVID-19 and comorbidities like poorly managed DM during the pandemic times. There are well-documented cases of differentiation between CAPA (COVID-19-associated pulmonary aspergillosis) and CAMCR (COVID-19-associated mucormycosis). Physicians should be vigilant enough and should understand, diagnose, and manage CAMCR prevailing in an extremely ill patient with COVID-19 and DM, during the clinical condition of rhino-orbital or rhino-cerebral. Craniofacial pain in the absence of swelling may emerge as neuropathic pain in patients suffering from DM synergizing with COVID-19 and in the absence of facial asymmetry or necrosis should not demonstrate mucormycosis in these patients. However, the impact of preventive antifungal combination medication persists without being clinically proven. The management of hyperglycemia appears to be crucial for the prevention and eradication of mucormycosis. Similarly, to other immunosuppressive conditions, for instance, severe viral pneumonia which eventually becomes prominent by additional risk factors exposes the individuals to secondary IFIs, for instance, mucormycosis and IAM (influenza-associated mucormycosis). An extensive literature review has been enforced and presented that the IAM has emerged commonly from pulmonary mucormycosis whereas, alternative types of mucormycosis, for instance, gastrointestinal, pulmonary, and diffused mucormycosis were observed in CAM. Still after boosted medical intervention, CAM emerged to be significantly fatal. Extensive research is crucial to investigate several poor prognostic elements in CAM and the way forward of reducing their influence on morbidity and mortality. Clinicians should be vigilant enough to diagnose mucormycosis in COVID-19-infected patients. Extensive and continuous research should be enforced to investigate the significant correlation between these two deadly infections.

## References


Afroze, S. N., Korlepara, R., & Rao, G. V. (2017). Mucormycosis in a diabetic patient: a case report with an insight into its pathophysiology. *Contemporary Clinical Dentistry*, 8, 662-666.

Al-Ajam, M. R., Bizri, A. R., Mokhbat, J., Weedon, J., & Lutwick, L. (2006). Mucormycosis in the Eastern Mediterranean: a seasonal disease. *Epidemiology and Infection*, 134(2), 341-346.

Arnáiz-García, M. E., Alonso-Peña, D., González-Vela, M. C., García-Palomo, J. D., Sanz-Giménez-Rico, J. R., & Arnáiz-García, A. M. (2009). Cutaneous mucormycosis: report of five cases and review of the literature. *Journal of Plastic, Reconstructive and Aesthetic Surgery*, 62, 434-441.

Ascioglu, S., Rex, J., De Pauw, B., Bennett, J., Bille, J., & Crokaert, F. (2002). Defining opportunistic invasive fungal infections in immunocompromised patients with cancer and hematopoietic stem cell transplants: an international consensus. *Clinical Infectious Disease*, 34, 7-14.

Ballester, D. G., González-García, R., García, C. M., Ruiz-Laza, L., & Gil, F. M. (2012). Mucormycosis of the head and neck: report of five cases with different presentations. *Journal of Cranio-Maxillofacial Surgery*, 40(7), 584-591.

Ben-Ami, R., Luna, M., Lewis, R. E., Walsh, T. J., & Kontoyiannis, D. P. (2009). A clinicopathological study of pulmonary mucormycosis in cancer patients: extensive angioinvasion but limited inflammatory response. *Journal of Infection*, 59, 134-138.

Berenguer, J., Allende, M. C., & Lee, J. W. (1995). Pathogenesis of pulmonary aspergillosis. Granulocytopenia versus cyclosporine and methylprednisolone-induced immunosuppression. *American Journal of Respiratory and Critical Care Medicine*, 152, 1079-1086.

Caillot, D., Casasnovas, O., & Bernard, A. (1997). Improved management of invasive pulmonary aspergillosis in neutropenic patients using early thoracic computed tomographic scan and surgery. *Journal of Clinical Oncology*, 15, 139-147.

Castrejón-Pérez, A. D., Welsh, E. C., Miranda, I., Ocampo-Candiani, J., & Welsh, O. (2017). Cutaneous mucormycosis. *Anais Brasileiros de Dermatologia*, 92, 304-311.

Chamilos, G., Lewis, R. E., & Kontoyiannis, D. P. (2008). Delaying amphotericin B-based frontline therapy significantly increases mortality among patients with hematologic malignancy who have zygomycosis. *Clinical Infectious Diseases*, 47, 503-509.

Chen, G., Wu, D., & Guo, W. (2020). Clinical and immunological features of severe and moderate coronavirus disease 2019. *Journal of Clinical Investigation*, 130, 2620-2629.

Chen, N., Zhou, M., & Dong, X. (2020). Epidemiological and clinical characteristics of 99 cases of 2019 novel coronavirus pneumonia in Wuhan, China: a descriptive study. *The Lancet*, 395, 507-513.

Chiou, C. C., Mavrogiorgos, N., Tillem, E., Hector, R., & Walsh, T. J. (2001). Synergy, pharmacodynamics, and time-sequenced ultrastructural changes of the interaction between nikkomycin Z and the echinocandin FK463 against Aspergillus fumigatus. *Antimicrobial Agents and Chemotherapy*, 45(12), 3310–3321.

Cicek, N., Yildiz, N., Kadayifci, E., Gokce, I., & Alpay, H. (2017). Invasive aspergillosis in a patient with end stage renal disease. *Medical Mycology Case Reports*, 18, 12-14.

Cornely, O. A., Alastruey-Izquierdo, A., & Arenz, D. (2019). Global guideline for the diagnosis and management of mucormycosis: an initiative of the European Confederation of Medical Mycology in cooperation with the Mycoses Study Group Education and Research Consortium. *The Lancet Infectious Diseases*, 19(12), 405-421.

Dan, S., Dutta, P., Sharma, D., Rout, A., Upadhyay, S. K., & Kumari, R. (2022). Infectivity, Morbidity, Emerged Variants of SARS-CoV-2 and Vaccination in Indian Perspectives from First Wave to Second Wave of COVID-19. *Letters in Applied NanoBioScience,* 12(3), 1-18.

Dan, S., Pant, M., & Upadhyay, S. K. (2020). The case fatality rate (CFR) in SARS-COV-2 patients with cardiovascular disease (CVD): A global health risk paradigm in COVID-19 pandemic. *Current Pharmacology Reports*, 6, 315-324.

Dan, S., Sharma, D., Mandal, M., & Sharma, D. (2020). Incidence of COVID-19 and its correlation between temperature and population density. *International Journal of Scientific Research in Biological Sciences*, 7(2), 134-140.

Dannaoui, E., Schwarz, P., & Lortholary, O. (2009). In vitro interactions between antifungals and immunosuppressive drugs against zygomycetes. *Antimicrobial Agents and Chemotherapy*, 53(8), 3549–3551.

De Locht, M., Boelaert, J. R., & Schneider, Y. J. (1994). Iron uptake from ferrioxamine and from ferrirhizoferrin by germinating spores of Rhizopus microsporus. *Biochemical Pharmacology*, 47(10), 1843–1850.

De Pauw, B., Walsh, T. J., Donnelly, J. P., Stevens, D. A., Edwards, J. E., Calandra, T., & Denning, D. W. (2008). Revised definitions of invasive fungal disease from the European organization for research and treatment of cancer/invasive fungal infections cooperative group and the national institute of allergy and infectious diseases mycoses study group (EORTC/MSG) consensus group. *Clinical infectious diseases*, 46(12), 1813-1821.

Delliere, S., Dudoignon, E., Fodil, S., Voicu, S., Collet, M., & Oillic, P. (2020). Risk factors associated with COVID-19-associated pulmonary aspergillosis in ICU patients: a French multicentric retrospective cohort. *Clinical Microbiology and Infection,* 27(5), 790-790.

Dudzinski, D. M., Hébert, P. C., Foglia, M. B., & Gallagher, T. H. (2010). The disclosure dilemma - large-scale adverse events. *New England Journal of Medicine*, 363(10), 978-986.

Elinav, H., Zimhony, O., Cohen, M. J., Marcovich, A. L., & Benenson, S. (2009). Rhinocerebral mucormycosis in patients without predisposing medical conditions: a review of the literature. *Clinical Microbiology and Infection*, 15(7), 693-697.

Falcone, M., Massetti, A., Russo, A., Vullo, V., & Venditti, M. (2011). Invasive aspergillosis in patients with liver disease. *Medical Mycology*, 49, 406-413.

Gholinejad-Ghadi, N., Shokohi, T., Seifi, Z., Aghili, S. R., Roilides, E., Nikkhah, M., Pormosa, R., Karami, H., Larjani, L. V., Ghasemi, M., & Haghani, I. (2018). Identification of Mucorales in patients with proven invasive mucormycosis by polymerase chain reaction in tissue samples. *Mycoses*, 61(12), 909-915.

Goel, S., Palaskar, S., & Shetty, V. P. (2009). Rhinomaxillary mucormycosis with cerebral extension. *Journal of Oral and Maxillofacial Pathology*, 13(1), 14-17.

Goldstein, E. J., Spellberg, B., Walsh, T. J., Kontoyiannis, D. P., Edwards, J. Jr., & Ibrahim, A. S. (2009). Recent advances in the management of mucormycosis: from bench to bedside. *Clinical Infectious Diseases*, 48(12), 1743-1751.

Greenberg, R. N., Mullane, K., & Van Burik, J. A. (2006). Posaconazole as salvage therapy for zygomycosis. *Antimicrobial Agents and Chemotherapy*, 50, 126-133.

Greene, R. E., Schlamm, H. T., & Oestmann, J. W. (2007). Imaging findings in acute invasive pulmonary aspergillosis: Clinical significance of the halo sign. *Clinical Infectious Diseases*, 44, 373-379.

Hammer, M. M., Madan, R., & Hatabu, H. (2018). Pulmonary mucormycosis: radiologic features at presentation and over time. *American Journal of Roentgenology*, 210(4), 742-747.

Hartnett, K. P., Jackson, B. R., Perkins, K. M., Glowicz, J., Kerins, J. L., Black, S. R., Lockhart, S. R., Christensen, B. E., & Beer, K. D. (2019). A guide to investigating suspected outbreaks of mucormycosis in healthcare. *Journal of Fungi*, 5(3), 69.

Hector, R. F. (1993). Compounds active against cell walls of medically important fungi. *Clinical Microbiology Reviews*, 6(1), 1–21.

Horby, P., Lim, W. S., Emberson, J. R., Mafham, M., Bell, J. L., Linsell, L., & Cao, B. (2021). Dexamethasone in hospitalized patients with COVID-19. *New England Journal of Medicine*, 384(8), 693-704.

Ibrahim, A. S., Gebremariam, T., Fu, Y., Edwards Jr, J. E., & Spellberg, B. (2008). Combination echinocandin-polyene treatment of murine mucormycosis. *Antimicrobial Agents and Chemotherapy*, 52(4), 1556-1558.

Ibrahim, A. S., Gebremariam, T., Fu, Y., Edwards Jr, J. E., & Spellberg, B. (2008). Combination echinocandin-polyene treatment of murine mucormycosis. *Antimicrobial Agents and Chemotherapy*, 52(4), 1556-1558.

Ibrahim, B., Spellberg, T., Walsh, D., & Kontoyiannis. (2012). Pathogenesis of mucormycosis. *Clinical Infectious Disease*, 54, 16-22.

Ibrahim, D., & Kontoyiannis. (2013). Update on mucormycosis pathogenesis. *Current Opinion in Infectious Disease*, 26, 508-515.

Jeong, W., Keighley, C., & Wolfe, R. (2019). The Epidemiology and Clinical Manifestations of Mucormycosis: A Systematic Review and Meta-Analysis of Case Reports. *Clinical Microbiology and Infection*, 25(1), 26-34.

Johnson, A. K., Ghazarian, Z., Cendrowski, K. D., & Persichino, J. G. (2021). Pulmonary aspergillosis and mucormycosis in a patient with COVID-19. *Medical Mycology Case Reports*, 32, 64-67.

Jung, S. H., Kim, S. W., Park, C. S., Song, C. E., Cho, J. H., & Lee, J. H. (2009). Rhinocerebral mucormycosis: Consideration of prognostic factors and treatment modality. *Auris, Nasus, Larynx*, 36(3), 274-279.

Kachalia, A., Sands, K., Niel, M. V., Dodson, S., Roche, S., Novack, V., & Mello, M. M. (2018). Effects of a communication-and-resolution program on hospitals' malpractice claims and costs. *Health Affairs,* 37(11), 1836-1844.

Khatri, A., Chang, K. M., Berlinrut, I., & Wallach, F. (2021). Mucormycosis after Coronavirus disease 2019 infection in a heart transplant recipient – Case report and review of literature. *Journal of Medical Mycology*, 31(2), 101125.

Koehler, P., Cornely, O. A., Böttiger, B. W., Dusse, F., Eichenauer, D. A., Fuchs, F., & Vehreschild, J. J. (2020). COVID-19 associated pulmonary aspergillosis. *Mycoses*, 63(6), 528-534.

Lai, W. Y. (2020). COVID-19 associated with pulmonary aspergillosis: a literature review. *Journal of Microbiology, Immunology and Infection*, 54(1), 46-53.

Lansbury, L., Lim, B., Baskaran, V., & Lim, W. S. (2020). Co-infections in people with COVID-19: a systematic review and meta-analysis. *Journal of Infection*, 81(2), 266-275.

Lanternier, F., Poiree, S., & Elie, C. (2015). Prospective pilot study of high-dose (10 mg/kg/day) liposomal amphotericin B (L-AMB) for the initial treatment of mucormycosis. *Journal of Antimicrobial Chemotherapy*, 70(11), 3116-3123.

Lass-Florl, C., Resch, G., & Nachbaur, D. (2007). The value of computed tomography-guided percutaneous lung biopsy for diagnosis of invasive fungal infection in immunocompromised patients. *Clinical Infectious Diseases*, 45, 101-104.

Legrand, M., Gits-Muselli, M., Boutin, L., Garcia-Hermoso, D., Maurel, V., Soussi, S., & Denis, B. (2016). Detection of circulating Mucorales DNA in critically ill burn patients: preliminary report of a screening strategy for early diagnosis and treatment. *Clinical Infectious Diseases*, 63(10), 1312-1317.

Lewis, R. E., Lortholary, O., Spellberg, B., Roilides, E., Kontoyiannis, D. P., & Walsh, T. J. (2012). How does antifungal pharmacology differ for mucormycosis versus aspergillosis? *Clinical Infectious Diseases*, 54, 67-72.

Li, C. S., & Pan, S. F. (2003). Analysis and causation discussion of 185 severe acute respiratory syndrome dead cases. *Zhongguo Wei Zhong Bing Ji Jiu Yi Xue*, 15(10), 582-584.

Llata, E., Blossom, D. B., Khoury, H. J., Rao, C. Y., Wannemuehler, K. A., Noble-Wang, J., & Jackson, D. R. (2011). A cluster of mucormycosis infections in hematology patients: challenges in investigation and control of invasive mold infections in high-risk patient populations. *Diagnostic Microbiology and Infectious Disease*, 71(1), 72-80.

Ma, L. J., Ibrahim, A. S., & Skory, C. (2009). Genomic analysis of the basal lineage fungus Rhizopus oryzae reveals a whole-genome duplication. *PLoS Genetics*, 5, e1000549.

Machado, M., Valerio, M., Alvarez-Uria, A., Olmedo, M., Veintimilla, C., & Padilla, B. (2021). Invasive pulmonary aspergillosis in the COVID-19 era: an expected new entity. *Mycoses*, 64, 132-143.

McCarthy, M., Rosengart, A., & Schuetz, A. N. (2014). Mold infections of the central nervous system. *New England Journal of Medicine*, 371, 150-160.

Mehta, S., & Pandey, A. (2020). Rhino-orbital mucormycosis associated with COVID-19. *Cureus*, 12(9), e10726.

Mignogna, M. D., Fortuna, G., & Leuci, S. (2011). Mucormycosis in immunocompetent patients: a case-series of patients with maxillary sinus involvement and a critical review of the literature. *International Journal of Infectious Diseases*, 15, 533-540.

Millon, L., Larosa, F., Lepiller, Q., Legrand, F., Rocchi, S., Daguindau, E., & Grenouillet, F. (2013). Quantitative polymerase chain reaction detection of circulating DNA in serum for early diagnosis of mucormycosis in immunocompromised patients. *Clinical Infectious Diseases*, 56(10), 95-101.

Mohamed, A., Rogers, T. R., & Talento, A. F. (2020). COVID-19 associated invasive pulmonary aspergillosis: Diagnostic and therapeutic challenges. *Journal of Fungi*, 6(3), 115.

Mohindra, S., Mohindra, S., & Gupta, R. (2007). Rhinocerebral mucormycosis: the disease spectrum in 27 patients. *Mycoses*, 50, 290-296.

NIH (2020). Coronavirus disease 2019 (COVID-19) treatment guidelines. *National Institutes of Health*. https://www.covid19treatmentguidelines.nih.gov [15 July 2020].

Paltauf, A. (1885). *Mycosis mucorina. Virchows Archiv fur Pathologische Anatomie und Physiologie und fur Klinische Medizin*, 102, 543-564.

Pappas, P. G., Alexander, B. D., & Andes, D. R. (2010). Invasive fungal infections among organ transplant recipients: results of the Transplant-Associated Infection Surveillance Network (TRANSNET). *Clinical Infectious Diseases*, 50(8), 1101-1111.

Pasero, Sanna, S., Liperi, C., Piredda, D., Branca, G., & Casadio, L. (2020). A challenging complication following SARS-CoV-2 infection: a case of pulmonary mucormycosis. *Infection*, 49(5), 1055-1060.

Peeri, N. C., Shrestha, N., Rahman, M. S., Zaki, R., Tan, Z., Bibi, S., & Haque, U. (2020). The SARS, MERS and novel coronavirus (COVID-19) epidemics, the newest and biggest global health threats: what lessons have we learned? *International Journal of Epidemiology*, 49(3), 717-726.

Petrikkos, G., Skiada, A., Lortholary, O., Roilides, E., Walsh, T. J., & Kontoyiannis, D. P. (2012). Epidemiology and clinical manifestations of mucormycosis. *Clinical Infectious Diseases*, 54(1), 23-34.

Placik, D. A., Wesley, T. L., & Nathan, W. M. (2020). Bronchopleural fistula development in the setting of novel therapies for acute respiratory distress syndrome in SARS-CoV-2 pneumonia. *Radiology Case Reports*, 15(11), 2378-2381.

Prabhu, S., Alqahtani, M., & Al Shehabi, M. (2018). A fatal case of rhinocerebral mucormycosis of the jaw after dental extractions and review of literature. *Journal of Infection and Public Health*, 11, 301-303.

Rammaert, B., Lanternier, F., & Zahar, J. R. (2012). Healthcare-associated mucormycosis. *Clinical Infectious Diseases*, 54(S1), 44-54.

Rawson, T. M., Moore, L. S., Zhu, N., Ranganathan, N., Skolimowska, K., Gilchrist, M., & Holmes, A. H. (2020). Bacterial and fungal coinfection in individuals with coronavirus: A rapid review to support COVID-19 antimicrobial prescribing. *Clinical Infectious Diseases*, 71(9), 2459-2468.

Reed, C., Bryant, R., & Ibrahim, A. S. (2008). Combination polyene-caspofungin treatment of rhino-orbital-cerebral mucormycosis. *Clinical Infectious Diseases*, 47(3), 364-371.

Reich, P., Shute, T., Lysen, C., Lockhart, S. R., Kelly Keating, M., Custer, P., & Orscheln, R. (2018). Saksenaea vasiformis orbital cellulitis in an immunocompetent child treated with posaconazole. *Journal of the Pediatric Infectious Diseases Society*, 7(3), 169-171.

Rochna, I. C. N., Hasan, M. M., & Goyal, S. (2021). COVID-19 and mucormycosis syndemic: Double health threat to a collapsing healthcare system in India. *Tropical Medicine and International Health*, 26(9), 1016-1018.

Roden, M. M., Zaoutis, T. E., & Buchanan, W. L. (2005). Epidemiology and outcome of zygomycosis: A review of 929 reported cases. *Clinical Infectious Diseases*, 41, 634-653.

Rodriguez, M. M., Calvo, E., Marine, M., Pastor, F. J., Fernandez-Ballart, J., & Guarro, J. (2009). Efficacy of liposomal amphotericin B combined with gamma interferon or granulocyte-macrophage colony-stimulating factor for treatment of systemic zygomycosis in mice. *Antimicrobial Agents and Chemotherapy*, 53(8), 3569-3571.

Rodriguez, M. M., Serena, C., Marine, M., Pastor, F. J., & Guarro, J. (2008). Posaconazole combined with amphotericin B, an effective therapy for a murine disseminated infection caused by Rhizopus oryzae. *Antimicrobial Agents and Chemotherapy*, 52(10), 3786-3788.

Roux, B. G., Mechinaud, F., & Gay-Andrieu, F. (2010). Successful triple combination therapy of disseminated Absidia corymbifera infection in an adolescent with osteosarcoma. *Journal of Pediatric Hematology/Oncology*, 32(2), 131-133.

Saoulidis, S., Simitsopoulou, M., & Dalakiouridou, M. (2011). Antifungal activity of posaconazole and granulocyte colony-stimulating factor in the treatment of disseminated zygomycosis (mucormycosis) in a neutropenic murine model. *Mycoses*, 54, 486-492.

Scheckenbach, K., Cornely, O., Hoffmann, T. K., Engers, R., Bier, H., & Chaker, A. (2010). Emerging therapeutic options in fulminant invasive rhinocerebral mucormycosis. *Auris, Nasus, Larynx*, 37(3), 322-328.

Shibuya, K., Ando, T., & Hasegawa, C. (2004). Pathophysiology of pulmonary aspergillosis. *Journal of Infection and Chemotherapy*, 10, 138-145.

Shpitzer, T., Keller, N., Wolf, M., Goldschmied-Reouven, A., Bahar, G., Bahar, I., & Talmi, Y. P. (2005). Seasonal variations in rhino-cerebral Mucor infection. *Annals of Otology, Rhinology and Laryngology*, 114(9), 695-698.

Sivagnanam, S., Sengupta, D. J., Hoogestraat, D., Jain, R., Stednick, Z., Fredricks, D. N., & Duchin, J. S. (2017). Seasonal clustering of sinopulmonary mucormycosis in patients with hematologic malignancies at a large comprehensive cancer center. *Antimicrobial Resistance and Infection Control*, 6(1), 1-1.

Soummer, A., Mathonnet, A., & Scatton, O. (2008). Failure of deferasirox, an iron chelator agent, combined with antifungals in a case of severe zygomycosis. *Antimicrobial Agents and Chemotherapy*, 52(4), 1585-1586.

Spellberg, B., Edwards Jr., J., & Ibrahim, A. (2005). Novel perspectives on mucormycosis: pathophysiology, presentation, and management. *Clinical Microbiology Reviews*, 18(3), 556-569.

Spellberg, B., Fu, Y., Edwards Jr, J. E., & Ibrahim, A. S. (2005). Combination therapy with amphotericin B lipid complex and caspofungin acetate of disseminated zygomycosis in diabetic ketoacidotic mice. *Antimicrobial Agents and Chemotherapy*, 49(2), 830-832.

Spellberg, B., Ibrahim, A., Roilides, E., Lewis, R. E., Lortholary, O., Petrikkos, G., Kontoyiannis, D. P., & Walsh, T. J. (2012). Combination therapy for mucormycosis: why, what, and how? *Clinical Infectious Diseases*, 54(S1), 73-78.

Talmi, Y. P., Goldschmied-Reouven, A., Bakon, M., Barshack, I., Wolf, M., Horowitz, Z., & Kronenberg, J. (2002). Rhino-orbital and rhino-orbito-cerebral mucormycosis. *Otolaryngology-Head and Neck Surgery*, 127(1), 22-31.

Thompson, G., Cornely, O., Pappas, P., Patterson, T., Hoenigl, M., & Jenks, J. (2020). Invasive aspergillosis as an under-recognized superinfection in COVID-19. *Open Forum Infectious Disease*, 7, 1-3.

Upadhyay, S. K., Dan, S., & Girdhar, M. (2021). Recent advancement in SARS-CoV-2 diagnosis, treatment, and vaccine formulation: a new paradigm of nanotechnology in strategic combating of COVID-19 pandemic. *Current Pharmacology Reports*, 7, 1-14.

Veisi, A., Bagheri, A., Eshaghi, M., Rikhtehgar, M. H., Rezaei Kanavi, M., & Farjad, R. (2021). Rhino-orbital mucormycosis during steroid therapy in COVID-19 patients: A case report. *European Journal of Ophthalmology,* 32(4), 11-16.

Viterbo, S., Fasolis, M., & Garzino-Demo, P. (2011). Management and outcomes of three cases of rhinocerebral mucormycosis. *Oral Surgery, Oral Medicine, Oral Pathology, Oral Radiology, and Endodontology*, 112, 69-74.

Wang, Y., Wang, Y., Chen, Y., & Qin, Q. (2020). Unique epidemiological and clinical features of the emerging 2019 novel coronavirus pneumonia (COVID-19) implicate special control measures. *Journal of Medical Virology*, 92(6), 568-576.

Werthman-Ehrenreich, A. (2021). Mucormycosis with orbital compartment syndrome in a patient with COVID-19. *The American Journal of Emergency Medicine*, 42, 264-264.

White, L., Dhillon, R., Cordey, A., Hughes, H., Faggian, F., Soni, S., & Borman, A. (2020). A national strategy to diagnose coronavirus disease 2019 – associated invasive fungal disease in the intensive care unit. *Clinical Infectious Diseases*, 73(7), 1634-1644.

Yang, W., Cao, Q., Qin, L., Wang, X., Cheng, Z., Pan, A., & Wang, X. (2020). Clinical characteristics and imaging manifestations of the 2019 novel coronavirus disease (COVID-19): A multi-center study in Wenzhou city, Zhejiang, China. *Journal of Infection*, 80(4), 388-393.

Yin, C. H., Wang, C., Tang, Z., Zhang, S. W., & Wang, B. S. (2004). Clinical analysis of 146 patients with critical severe acute respiratory syndrome in Beijing areas. *Clinical Journal of Emergency Medicine*, 1, 12-14.

Zhang, Y., Li, W. X., Huang, K. W., Cao, Z. X., & Hao, J. Y. (2003). Hospital acquired pneumonia occurring after acute stage of the serious SARS and its treating strategies. *Chinese Journal of Nosocomiology*, 11, 1081-1087.

Zurl, M., Hoenigl, M., Schulz, E., Hatzl, S., Gorkiewicz, G., & Krause, R. (2021). Autopsy proven pulmonary mucormycosis due to Rhizopus microsporus in a critically ill COVID-19 patient with underlying hematological malignancy. *Journal of Fungi*, 7(2), 88.

## Chapter 7

# Mucormycosis and Associated Infections in Immunocompromised COVID-19 Patients: From Pathogenesis, Advances in Diagnosis, Treatment, Pharmacology to Nanotherapy

**Siddhartha Dan[1,2]**
**Mohit Pant[3]**
**Bhawana Paliwal[4]**
**Subashani[5]**
**Samyak Nag[6]**
**Nikul B. Chavada[7]**
**and Sushil Kumar Upadhyay[8,*]**

[1]Department of Biotechnology, I. K. Gujral Punjab Technical University, Jalandhar, Punjab, India
[2]Department of Biotechnology, Dr. B. R. Ambedkar National Institute of Technology; Jalandhar, Punjab, India
[3]Department of Pharmacovigilance, Paraxel International (India) Private Limited, Chandigarh, India
[4]Department of Bioscience and Biotechnology, Banasthali Vidyapith, Banasthali (Rajasthan), India
[5]Department of Biochemistry, Institute of Biosciences and Biotechnology, Chhatrapati Shahu Ji Maharaj University, Kanpur, Uttar Pradesh, India
[6]Amity Institute of Pharmacy, Amity University, Noida, Uttar Pradesh, India
[7]OM College of Science and PG Center, Bhesan -Junagadh Road, Junagadh, Gujarat, India
[8]Department of Bio-Sciences and Technology, MMEC, Maharishi Markandeshwar (Deemed to be University), Mullana–Ambala (Haryana), India

[*] Corresponding Author's Email: upadhyay.k.sushil@gmail.com.

In: Therapeutic Advances in Human Health and Diseases
Editors: Sushil Kumar Upadhyay, Manoj Singh and Anil Kumar Sharma
ISBN: 979-8-89113-304-4

## Abstract

Invasive fungal infection (IFI), for instance, mucormycosis is usually caused by various species of saprophytic fungi. It is widespread in patients with different co–morbidities, especially diabetes and organ transplantation. The mucormycosis emerged to be a fatal fungal infection during the current COVID-19 (coronavirus disease–2019) pandemic. The present study was designed to explore the risk factors, pathogenesis, diagnosis, identification, clinical treatment, and nanotherapeutic approaches for various types of invasive fungal infections (mucormycosis) in immunocompromised persons with co-morbidities and SARS–CoV–2 (severe acute respiratory syndrome coronavirus 2) infections. Various cases of mucormycosis were recorded among those who underwent a fresh heart transplant for the management of severe cardiac failure or suffered from immunocompromised ailments. The cases of mucormycosis prevailed in COVID-19 patients and demonstrated the significantly augmented orientation among those suffering from diabetes mellitus, neutropenia, and under the improper dosage regimen of corticosteroids for managing the severe case of COVID-19. There were a number of cases of mucormycosis that have been documented among persons after three months of recovery from SARS-CoV-2. The serological, molecular, and modern diagnostic tests over conventional methods played a key role in the management of mucormycosis. The excellent treatment outcome was noticed with the combination of potent anti-IFI drugs, synergistic treatments as contemporary antifungal medicines, and magnetite surface functionalized nano–conjugated drug therapy. The immunocompromised COVID-19 patients are more prone to mucormycosis. Innovative diagnostic tests and nanotherapeutic approaches improve the efficacy of traditional antifungal medicines, helpful in targeted therapy and simultaneously reducing drug–related side effects.


**Keywords:** invasive fungal infection, mucormycosis, COVID-19, immunocompromised, nanotherapy

## 1. Introduction

The nCoV-19 (novel coronavirus 2019) was recorded in late 2019 and Wuhan, China supposed as the epicenter for the eruption of this disease called coronavirus disease-2019 (COVID-19) caused by the severe acute respiratory syndrome coronavirus 2 (SARS–CoV–2) (Ying–Hui et al., 2020; Phelan et al.,

2020; Wu et al., 2020; Zhou et al., 2020). The disease was later declared a Pandemic by the WHO (World Health Organization) and killed millions of people throughout the world and called the hardest threat to society's health, existence, and livelihood (Garg et al., 2020; Kumar et al., 2020; Jha et al., 2020; Upadhyay et al., 2020). Patients with cardiovascular illness, diabetes, organ transplant, and compromised immunity with older age were more prone to SARS–CoV–2 infection and COVID-19 (Dan et al., 2020; Sood et al., 2020; Upadhyay et al., 2020). These individuals were at a higher risk of morbidity and fatality than COVID-19 patients without the aforesaid ailments. The diseases including hypertension, atherosclerosis, and congestive heart failure are quite more linked to the RAS (renin–angiotensin system), expressed ACE2 (angiotensin-converting enzyme 2), and the response impact of hyperactivity with angiotensin–II (Upadhyay et al., 2021; Yadav et al., 2021). The fatality rate among COVID-19 patients with cardiovascular illness was around 10.5%, however, the mortality recorded was about five times higher (52%) among patients with heart failure earlier with just a 12% recovery rate (Dan et al., 2020). Patients with severe COVID-19 infection were more likely to acquire secondary fungal infection as a co-infection due to hospitalization circumstances, therapy that includes corticosteroids and antibiotics, or pre-existing comorbidities (Ibrahim et al., 2012). A superimposed *Aspergillus* infection has been observed with the COVID-19 infection from the beginning of the pandemic (Cicek et al., 2017; Mohamed et al., 2020). There were scant data records linked with mucormycosis in COVID-19 patients, but the current report has a unique instance of severe COVID-19 infection accompanied by invasive lung mucormycosis.

## 2. Mucormycosis

Mucormycosis was discovered to be a rare, dangerous fungal illness with a death rate of over 50% despite antifungal treatment and surgical epithelialization (Falcone et al., 2011; Ibrahim et al., 2012). *Rhizopus arrhizus*, which causes 70% of mucormycosis, was found to be linked with many clinical manifestations (pulmonary, cutaneous, rhino–orbital–cerebral, and stomach in the adults) (Figure 1) (Ibrahim et al., 2012). The fungal infection is renowned for its pathogenic nature, and is characterized by seizures that extend across tissue planes and rapid tissue destruction (Cicek et al., 2017). Unconstrained ketoacidosis, stem cell, and solid organ emigration are all significant danger factors for the life-threatening fungal illness known as mucormycosis. The spotting of inventive fungal structures by histological analysis of tissue prototypes from individuals with distrust signals and symptoms is used to diagnose mucormycosis (Cicek et al., 2017). Mucormycosis is often treated with advanced truculent surgical drafting of contaminating tissues, along with the administration of liposomal amphotericin B (L-AmB) or amphotericin B deoxycholate (AmB). Over 70% of all instances of meddling aspergillosis are caused by *Aspergillus fumigatus* (Cicek et al., 2017; Solano and Vazquez, 2018).

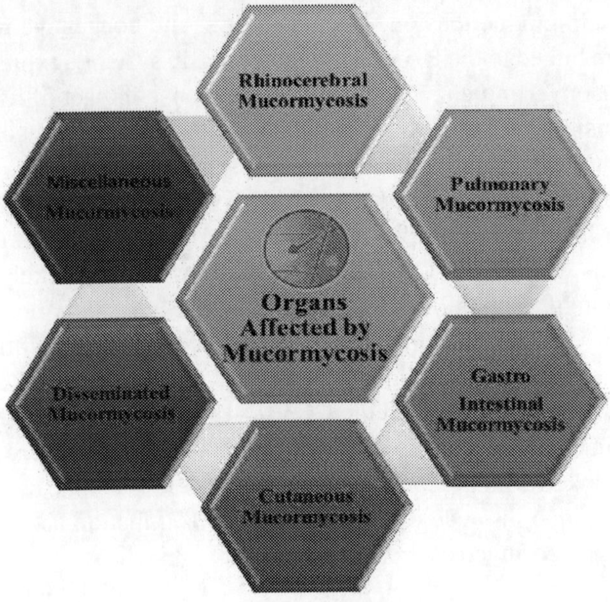


**Figure 1.** Types of mucormycosis and associated organs.

Invasive aspergillosis is more common among immunocompromised patients, such as those on long–term corticosteroid treatment or those who have long–term neutropenia due to malignancy (Falcone et al., 2011; Cicek et al., 2017; Solano and Vazquez, 2018). The combination of the host location, ventilation, light, and mycological findings over there used to identify, demonstrate, and expect the probable invasive aspergillosis (Ascioglu et al., 2002). Administration of isavuconazole or voriconazole is the best treatment for aspergillosis (Falcone et al., 2011; Cicek et al., 2017; Solano and Vazquez, 2018). The infections of both (SARS–CoV–2 and fungi) have been recognized as secondary and major obstacles to the treatment of coronavirus disease 2019 (COVID-19), particularly among patients in the intensive care unit (ICU) (Lai and Yu, 2020; Thompson et al., 2020; Machado et al., 2021). According to earlier published reports, up to 35% of these victims have interstitial pulmonary aspergillosis, which has been linked to previous corticosteroid use and is critically associated with augmented mortality (Delliere et al., 2020; Lai and Yu, 2020; Machado et al., 2021). Protruding pulmonary mucormycosis chasing COVID-19, on the other hand, is uncommon, with just two instances documented to date (Pasero et al., 2021; Zurl et al., 2021). According to the literature, this was the first instance of suspected mucormycosis coupled with likely pulmonary aspergillosis in a guy with COVID-19 admitted to the ICU (Johnson et al., 2021).

Secondary infections associated with invasive pulmonary aspergillosis are particularly common in severe cases of COVID-19 pneumonia, according to reports from several schools (Koehler et al., 2020; Mohamed et al., 2020). A research discussed the example of a 60-year-old patient who underwent diabetic therapy was carried rhino–orbital mucor infection that has been identified using a nasal biopsy culture. Later on, as the cytokine storm progressed, this patient died of shock (Mehta and Pandey, 2020). Another case recorded by Werthman–Ehrenreich in reference to a 33 years diabetic lady who was in ketoacidosis with COVID-19 pneumonia and later identified with the rhino-orbital cerebral mucormycosis by biopsy (Werthman–Ehrenreich, 2021). Because of the severe fungal involvement in her brain and the dismal prognosis, she was eventually transferred to intensive care for effective treatment (Werthman–Ehrenreich, 2021). Placik et al. (2020) also described the case of a 49-year-old COVID-19 patient who developed a bronchopleural fistula and suffered tension pneumothorax. During the treatment, a cardiothoracic surgery with a thoracotomy was done to treat the fistula, and an observation led to empyema, which developed *Rhizopus* species on culture and became lethal for the patient (Placik et al., 2020).

In the common COVID-19 infection without IFI (invasive fungal infection) or mucormycosis, the fatality rate was recorded at 40–60% among immunocompromised patients (Cornely et al., 2019). However, according to the review kinds of literature thus far, in the situations when these two illnesses (COVID-19 and IFI) were confirmed to be co-occurring, the death rate exceeds many folds up to 100% lethality. Diabetes is the most common cause of mucor infection and more likely to develop a rhino–cerebral infection, whereas other immunosuppressive patients were diagnosed with pulmonary mucormycosis (Figure 1) (Jeong et al., 2019). During the pandemic, mucormycosis arose as a crossroads of two outcomes, such as COVID-19, and comorbidities such as poorly controlled diabetes mellitus. There have been recorded examples of CAPA (COVID-19-associated pulmonary aspergillosis) and CAMCR being distinguished (COVID-19-associated mucormycosis) (Table 1). Physicians must be alert and recognize, identify, and manage CAMCR in an acutely sick patient with COVID-19 and DM (diabetes mellitus) who experiencing rhino–orbital or rhino–cerebral symptoms (Singh et al., 2021).

In individuals suffering from DM synergizing with COVID-19, cranial discomfort in the absence of swelling may manifest as neuropathic pain, and in the absence of facial asymmetry or necrosis, mucormycosis should not be suspected. The impact of preventative antifungal combination medicine, on the other hand, has yet to be scientifically demonstrated. Similarly, to other immunosuppressive diseases, such as severe viral pneumonia, which is exacerbated by additional risk factors, the patients were exposed to secondary IFIs such as mucormycosis and IAM (influenza-associated mucormycosis) (Figure 1). An extensive literature analysis was conducted and revealed that IAM was mostly caused by pulmonary mucormycosis, whereas CAM was characterized by other forms of mucormycosis, such as gastrointestinal, pulmonary, and disseminated mucormycosis (Jeong et al., 2019; Song et al., 2020; Singh et al., 2021). CAM was found to be considerably deadly even with increased medical intervention (Table 1). Extensive study is required to explore various poor prognostic factors in complementary and alternative medicine (CAM) and ways to reduce their impact on morbidity and mortality. Clinicians should be cautious when diagnosing COVID-19-infected individuals for mucormycosis. The substantial link between these two fatal diseases should be investigated through extensive and ongoing study.

## 3. Nanocomposites: Opportunity and Challenges in Treatment

The counterfeit composite polymers and polymeric particles of nanoscale size (ranging between 10 to 1000nm) are known as nanoparticles (NPs). These NPs are known for their remarkable applications in multifaceted clinical aspects. Thus the nanoparticles have been developed as a significant device in nanomedicine instead of the conventional ways of medication and techniques through a major focus on the tranquilization, carriage, and targeted drug delivery. Additionally, these carry the potency that can serve to strengthen the process of the detection along with the treatment, making use of most of the instrumentation in nanomedicine (Yadav et al., 2016; Anjali et al., 2021; Dan et al., 2021; Pant et al., 2021). Thereby, having several applications in copious fields, inclusive of branches of science and engineering, we can culminate that family of graphene along with its oxides, make silver nanoparticles efficient, and photocatalytic, metal oxides functional, coupled with multicomponent reactions which are modified with different concentrations can also inhibit growth. The NPs possess beneficial antimicrobial properties and can be applied in oral cancer, teeth infection, and gum-related diseases as well (Singh et al., 2020; Dan et al., 2021; Rashidzadeh et al., 2021; Singh et al., 2021; Tuli et al., 2021; Singh et al., 2021; Upadhyay et al., 2021). Not only this, but nanoscience has also technologically advanced in several biosensors, nano vaccines, and antiviral composites being favorably applicable for closely related viruses; thus, it serves to be a significant channel for development against SARS–CoV–2.

Henceforth, to fight against COVID-19 pandemic, nanoscience has a lot to offer, and the times coming up in the months ahead are crucially important as nanotechnological devices can be brought into relevance such as nanosized sensors, antiviral composites, and vaccination to fight against this. Presently, global health crisis on varied levels is essential to fight, mainly for avoiding the spread of infection and following the correct course of detection and treatment. In order to deal with the COVID-19 pandemic or any other similar emerging public health emergency, a comprehensive knowledge of the virulence or the transmission of the virus is essential which can further justify the understanding of the transmittance of virus from species to species. This could also lead to the discovery of the varied encoded nano–structural enzymes and proteins along with their related mechanism of action. Using surface functionalized nanoparticles, novel therapeutic targets can be identified and targeted. Along with this the comprehension of viral lifecycle and its host response can aid in generating efficient nano vaccine.

**Table 1.** Risk factors, diagnosis, identification tests, and therapeutic approaches for different invasive fungal co-infections

| Patients | Illness and Hospitalization | Risk Factors | Diagnosis and Identification Test | | | | | Therapeutic Approaches | Disease |
|---|---|---|---|---|---|---|---|---|---|
| | | | Microscopy | Culture | Serology | Molecular | Modern | | |
| COVID-19 | Severe illness accompanied by immuno-compromised state (ICU admitted, ventilation support & prolonged hospitalization | GC use, COPD, prolonged neutropenia, allo-HSCT, SOT, inherited immuno-deficiencies, CF, HM | Acute angle branching with septate hyphae observed in Calcoflour or Blankophor histopathology with special stains (e.g., PAS and GMS) | 37°C for 2-5 days to study topology | - | PCR-based assay using target genes: BenA, CAL, ITS | GM test using serum and BALF | Triazoles: Voriconazole, posaconazole, esaconazole, itraconazole<br>AmB: Its liposomes<br>Echinococcins: Micafugin, carpofenjing | Invasive aspergillosis |
| | | Parental nutrition, broad-spectrum antibacterial drugs use, invasive examination | Pseudohyphae observed in Calcoflour or Blankophor | Blood and other sterile samples turned cream-like | Mannan and antimannan IgG test, CAGTA, BDG | PCR-based assay using target genes: rDNA, ITS | $T_2$ magnetic resonance and MALDI-TOF | Echinocandin: Caspofungin, micafungin, anidulafungin<br>Triazoles: Voriconazole, fluconazole, itaconazole<br>AmB: Its liposomes | Invasive candidiasis |
| | | Trauma, diabetes mellitus, GC use, allo-HSCT, SOT, inherited immuno-deficiencies, HM | Non-septate/ pauci-septate ribbon like hyphae (6-16μm wide) observed in fluorescent brightener histopathology with special stains (e.g., PAS and GMS) | Cottony white or grayish black colony on routine media at 30°C and 37°C | - | PCR-based assay, HRM using target genes: rDNA, 18s, 28s, ITS | - | Surgical treatment: If possible<br>Primary prophylaxis: Posaconazole<br>First line treatment: AmB lipid complex, Iliposomal AmB, posaconazole oral suspension | Invasive mucormycosis |

| Patients | Illness and Hospitalization | Risk Factors | Diagnosis and Identification Test | | | | | Therapeutic Approaches | Disease |
|---|---|---|---|---|---|---|---|---|---|
| | | | Microscopy | Culture | Serology | Molecular | Modern | | |
| | | HIV infection (CD4 < 200 cells/µl), allo-HSCT, SOT | Narrow budding encapsulated yeasts observed in CSF mixed with India ink | Mucoid creamy colonies at 30°C for 7 days in aerobic condition | CrAg, LAT, EIA, LFA | Pan-fungal PCR, multiplex PCR, DNA sequencing, isothermal amplification, probe-based microarray, target genes: IGS1, CAP5, ITS | - | Induction phase: AmB deoxycholate + flucytosine followed by fluconazole; fluconazole + flucytosine; amB deoxycholate + fluconazole<br>Consolidate and maintenance phase: Fluconazole | Invasive cryptococcosis |

Despite the fact that nanotechnology provides a variety of methods for antifungal therapy, certain negative consequences of nanomaterial-based therapies have also been considered. From a clinical viewpoint, the toxicity of metallic nanoparticles, such as Ag-NPs, has been regarded as the most significant factor (Asharani et al., 2009; Panácek et al., 2009; Monteiro et al., 2013; Das et al., 2016; Niemirowicz et al., 2016). Asharani et al. (2009) conducted a series of tests and indicated that despite their effectiveness in the treatment of microbial infections, particularly those caused by *C. albicans,* Ag-NPs were characterized by significant cytotoxicity and genotoxicity. These negative consequences are related to disruption of the mitochondrial respiratory chain and increased reactive oxygen species (ROS) generation. Das et al. (2016) presented a new core-shell nanocomposite in which silver nanoparticles were enveloped with a layer of zinc oxide (Ag–ZnO), limiting the harmful effects of Ag–NPs while preserving their fungicidal activity (Das et al., 2016). Importantly, this nanocomposite was effective against *C. krusei*, which has emerged as a prominent emerging pathogen, frequently identified in patients who had previously had fluconazole or amphotericin B therapy and demonstrated resistance to routinely used antifungal medications (Orozco et al., 1998; Krcmery et al., 2002).

The application of nanoparticles in designing new antifungal treatments led to the development of mucoadhesive nanoparticle-based formulations containing fluconazole for the local treatment of oral candidiasis (Roque et al., 2018). Rencber et al. (2016) recently proposed a nanosystem that addressed a significant drawback of frequently used drug forms: the difficulty of sustaining salivary concentrations of fungicidal agents for long periods of time, which is required for full pathogen eradication. Given this limitation, developing a mucoadhesive fluconazole–loaded system for buccal delivery with fungicidal efficacy against *C. albicans* and low cytotoxicity would be a solution with a wide range of applications (Bondaryk et al., 2013; Rençber et al., 2016). In addition to the accomplishments in the creation of new nanomaterial-based fungicidal agents, it was proposed that magnetic nanoparticles with theranostic potential have a lot of promise. An increasing number of studies showed that iron oxide–based magnetic nanoparticles enable the creation of multifunctional nanosystems that are beneficial not only in the treatment of fungal infections but also have the potential to be used in diagnostic and sensitizing tools (Niemirowicz et al., 2017; Vallabani et al., 2018; Ajinkya et al., 2020; Yaqoob et al., 2020; Montiel Schneider et al., 2022).

## 4. Nanotherapeutics and Synergistic Approaches as Profound Antifungal Treatment

Despite the ongoing advancement of fungal-targeted methods, a slew of therapy-related issues, such as poor drug penetration and the emergence of drug-resistant strains, restrict the efficacy of fungal treatments. The rising body of evidence suggests that newer nanotechnology-based techniques might overcome a significant portion of these constraints. Several nanomaterials, including biodegradable polymeric and copolymeric–based structures, metallic nanoparticles, metallic nanocomposites, and lipid-based nanosystems, have been comprehensively studied and reported as novel antifungal agents (Das et al., 2016; Niemirowicz et al., 2016; Mohammadi et al., 2017). Synergistic treatments were another technique used in contemporary antifungal medicines (Cui et al., 2015; Scorzoni et al., 2017; Wambaugh et al., 2020). The use of nanostructures as agents to improve the efficacy of traditional antifungal medicines while simultaneously reducing the drug-related side effects of antifungal treatments is one innovative nanotechnology–focused antifungal approach.

The ability to provide nanomaterial–focused treatments *via* oral, nasal, parenteral, and intraocular routes, made feasible by nanoparticles' tiny size was recognized as a significant benefit (Chidambaram et al., 2011). The use of nanostructures as an agent to improve the efficacy of traditional antifungal medicines by simultaneously reducing the drug-related side effects of antifungal treatments was found to be one innovative nanotechnology–focused antifungal approach. Saldanha et al. (2016) confirmed that preparing magnetite surface functionalized nanostructures with a bilayer of lauric acid conjugated with amphotericin B suitable for the treatment of paracoccidioidomycosis caused by *Paracoccidioides brasiliens.* It resulted in a reduction in acute hepatotoxic and nephrotoxic effects of amphotericin B, as well as a reduction in the number of applications. According to Mohammadi et al. (2017), the antifungal activity of nystatin against *C. albicans* strains might be improved by employing nystatin-loaded PLGA-glucosamine nanoparticles. According to a most recent study, ketoconazole–loaded chitosan–gellan gum nanoparticles were more effective against *Aspergillus niger* than unmodified NPs or ketoconazole (Kumar et al., 2016).

Synergistic treatments are another technique used in contemporary antifungal medicines to reduce the adverse effects of drugs and improve killing capacity against drug-resistant microorganisms. Sun et al. (2016)

recently tested this method against *C. albicans*, which was resistant to fluconazole and VRC eradication. Combinatory treatment with these drugs and polyvinylpyrrolidone-coated–coated silver nanoparticles (Ag–NPs) was shown to be effective in killing all resistant cells owing to a mechanism involving disruption of cell membrane impermeability as well as impairment of ergosterol signaling and efflux pump activities (Sun et al., 2016). Pd/Ag nanosheets (palladium/silver nanosheets), a novel type of core-shell nanoparticles made by covering palladium nanosheets with silver, showed a similar behavior (Huang et al., 2011). Pd/Ag nanostructures were shown to be effective against diverse pathogen fungi including *Candida*, *Aspergillus*, *Cryptococcus*, and *Rhizopus* species, with cryptococcal and fluconazole-resistant isolates being the most susceptible. Essentially, when coupled with amphotericin B, Pd/Ag nanosheets displayed synergistic action, which was conditioned by these chemicals' membrane permeabilizing activity, disruption of intracellular protein, and energy metabolism. Surprisingly, it did not have the same impact when used with fluconazole. It's also worth noting that, even at the greatest fungicidal concentrations, Pd/Ag NPs were less hemolytic than amphotericin B (Zhang et al., 2016). The use of antifungal medicines in combination with nanoparticles may be beneficial in the treatment of *Candida*–associated denture stomatitis. Monteiro et al. investigated the antibiofilm activity of silver nanoparticles in combination with nystatin and chlorhexidine digluconate, finding that this combination therapy was effective against biofilm formed by *Candida albicans* and *C. glabrata* and has great clinical potential in the treatment of denture stomatitis (Monteiro et al., 2013). Sharma et al. (2016) discovered that ZnO nanoparticles and fluconazole/amphotericin B have additive effects against *C. neoformans* and *Trichophyton mentagrophytes*, respectively.

Surprisingly, it was discovered that unmodified nanomaterials alone might be a powerful weapon in the battle against fungal diseases. According to Panácek et al. (2009), Ag–NPs (silver nanoparticles) were effective against *C. albicans*, *C. tropicalis,* and *C. parapsilosis* strains, with profound efficacy equivalent to amphotericin B, fluconazole, and itraconazole. The employment of sodium dodecyl sulfate (SDS) as a nanoparticle stabilizer might improve the fungicidal actions; because of the high permeabilizing characteristics of SDS and result in enhanced accessibility of nanoparticles into fungal cells. Thus SDS–stabilized Ag–NPs had fungicidal activity equivalent to or better than amphotericin B, posaconazole, itraconazole, VRC and caspofungin (Panácek et al., 2009). Nanomaterials' biological potential is also included for destroying fungal cells trapped in biofilms. The ability of ZnO–NPs (zinc oxide nanoparticles) to inhibit the adherence and development of biofilm on a catheter surface by fluconazole-sensitive and fluconazole-resistant *C. tropicalis* strains had been demonstrated using XTT and ATP–based assays, highlighting the potential use of these structures in the medical field (Jothiprakasam et al., 2017). The use of ZnO to modify polymethylmethacrylate resulted in the production of an antifungal composite material for dentures. Cierech et al. (2016) recently presented that ZnO–based nanoparticles greatly improve the antibiofilm capabilities of polymethylmethacrylate due to higher induction of antioxidative stress in *C. albicans* cells. Resultantly ZnO–based NPs could be of considerable interest in the development of materials for individuals who are prone to denture stomatitis.

The ability to modify the pharmacokinetic characteristics of antifungal medicines and develop a form of drug with enhanced qualities is a huge benefit of nanotechnology-based treatments. VRC is supposed one such medication with high oral absorption, tolerable admissibility, and broad–spectrum efficacy against fungus, including drug-resistant fungi (Li et al., 2010; Arastehfar et al., 2020). However, because of its low solubility in water, it is not suitable for ocular injection as a treatment for strains that cause fungal keratitis, a fungal infection of the cornea. There have been a number of attempts to create a VRC formulation based on nanomaterials that can be used in eye drops (Pawar et al., 2013; Pahuja et al., 2014). Pahuja et al. (2014) and Pawar et al. (2013) have shown that a cyclodextrin–based eye drop solution and gel may be used to deliver ocular drugs in a stable manner. The aqueous solubility of VRC was considerably increased by adding 2–hydroxypropyl–cyclodextrin (HP–CD) to the solution. Furthermore, supplementing this formulation with gelling compounds such as pluronic F–127, F–68, and sodium alginate has a significant impact on the mucoadhesive properties and stability of the mixture, resulting in the creation of a formulation with long-lasting antifungal effects against *C. albicans* and *C. fumigatus* (Pawar et al., 2013; Pahuja et al., 2014). It was recently shown that incorporating this antifungal medication into composite polyvinyl alcohol/hydroxypropyl–cyclodextrin (HPCD) blended nanofibers might enhance VRC ocular administration and prolong its biological activity without causing ocular pain (Sun et al., 2016).

Kumar et al. (2014) suggested an oil–water microemulsion-based alternative nanoformulation of VRC. The VRC may also be integrated into liposomes made of soy phosphatidylcholine, which has a lot of application possibilities. The aforesaid nanoagent was not only easy to make, physicochemically stable, and capable of delivering medication through bovine cornea, even in laboratory conditions with simulated tear flow, but it also appeared to be safe for patients, according to the HET–CAM irritation research (De–Sá et al., 2015). According to recent research, drug-loaded niosome solutions and VRC-loaded, lipid-based nanoparticles might improve VRC bioavailability (Shukr et al., 2016; Füredi et al., 2017). The pullulan–based nanocapsule suspensions have also been shown to enhance the characteristics of tioconazole–based formulations for the treatment of *C. albicans*-caused onychomycosis (Flores et al., 2017; Dhamoon et al., 2019; Grigoras et al., 2019). Furthermore, the characteristics of these suspensions were equivalent to those of Trosid, a commercially available tioconazole formulation, and these were known for success in preventing *Trichophyton rubrum*-caused nail infections, although they had a higher irritating potential than produced nanoformulations (Flores et al., 2017; Dhamoon et al., 2019).

## 5. Theranostic Potential and Pharmacology of Magnetic Nanoparticles

Theranostics is defined as a combination of the terms therapeutics and diagnostics that is principally used to describe the blending of one efficient drug to diagnose the disease and a second drug to bring out therapy for curing life-threatening diseases including any metastatic tumors as well. Magnetic nanoparticles (MNPs) with the general formula iron oxides ($Fe_3O_4$, magnetite or $Fe_2O_3$, maghemite) were appropriate for biomedical applications due to their unique physicochemical features including magnetic behavior, external control, hyperthermal induction, and control synthesis parameters (Bozkurt–Guzel et al., 2014). The nanoparticles have a lot of potential in current medical applications because of their magnetic characteristics, such as controlled drug and gene delivery systems, magnetic resonance imaging, magnetic hyperthermia cancer treatment (MFH), and target therapy in both *in vitro* and *in vivo* contexts (Domingues et al., 2014). The chemical surface modification of nanoparticles, which led to the final stage in nanoparticle production, is known to be the most significant because it allowed medicines to be delivered to the infection site and selectively interact with pathogens (Lepock et al., 1982).

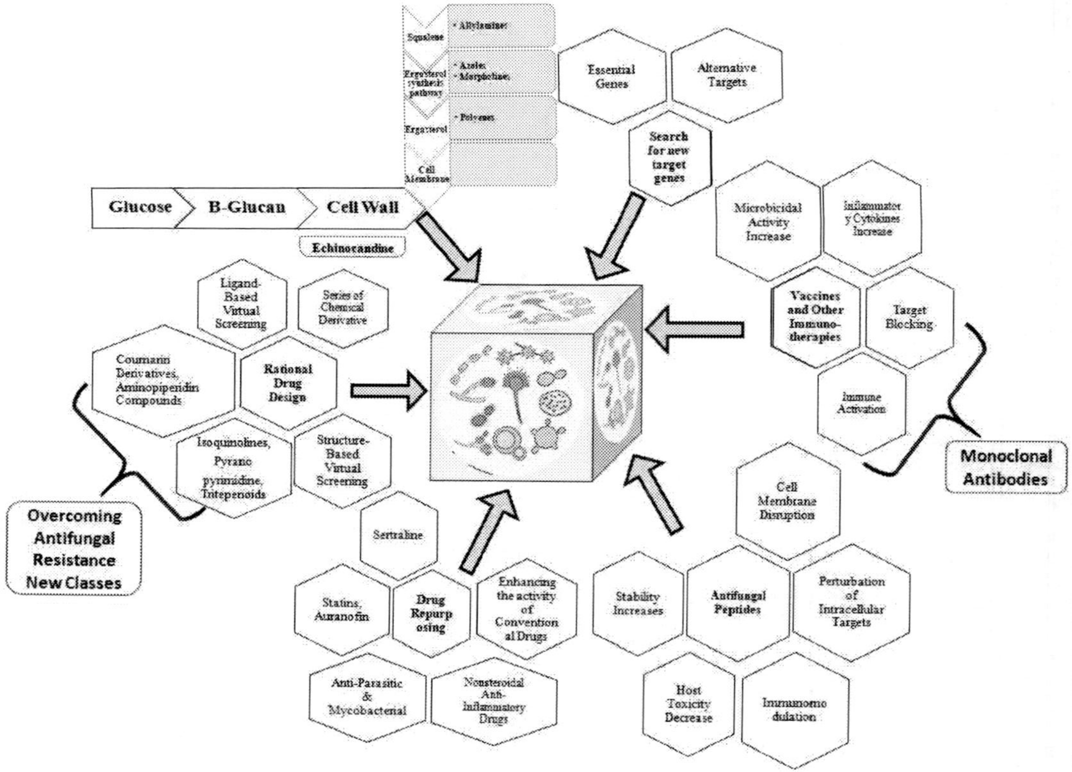


**Figure 2.** Strategies to identify efficient biopharmaceutical molecules during novel antifungal drug designing and development.

**Table 2.** The main residues of various potent antifungal drugs, mechanism of action, advantages and side effects

| Category of Drugs | Polyenes | Azoles | Echinocandins | Nucleic acid analogs (antimetabolites) |
|---|---|---|---|---|
| Main Component of Drugs | Amphotericin B (deoxycholate): Conventional formulation and its lipid formulations (lipid complex and liposomal) | Fluconazole, itraconazole, VRC, pisaconazole | Anidulafungin, caspofungin, micafungin | Flucytosine |
| Mode and Mechanism of Action | Fungicidal biding of cell membrane ergosterol and alteration of the membrane permeability | Fungistatic inhibition of the synthesis of the cell membrane ergosterol | Fungicidal and fungistatic inhibition of 1,3-βglucan synthesis, a key component of fungal cell wall | Fungicidal inhibition of pyrimidine metabolism, DNA, and RNA synthesis |
| Merits | Broad spectrum activity (Candida sp., *Aspergillus* sp., *Zygomycetes* sp., endemic fungi), fungicidal | Good penetration into CNS; VRC fungicidal against *Aspergillus fumigatus* | Good tolerance, few side effects, fungicidal against *Candida* sp., antibiofilm activity | Good penetration into most body sites |
| Demerits | Nephrotoxicity and infusion-related reactions | Low activity against *Candida glabata* and *C. crusei* (fluconazole)<br>No activity against *Aspergillus* sp. (fluconazole) and zygomyctes (posaconazole) adverse effects: hepatotoxicity, interactions with drugs that are the substrate for cytochrome P450 | No activity against Cryptococcus and Zygomycetes; tolerance against *C. parapsilosis* and *C. guillermondii* | Hepatotoxicity and bone marrow depression, only for combination therapy because of rapid resistance development |

**Table 3.** The first-line antifungal therapeutic options and suggested dosage of drugs for mucormycosis

| Drugs | Suggested Dosage | Merits and Supporting Studies | Demerits | References |
|---|---|---|---|---|
| Primary antifungal therapy | | | | |
| AmB | 1.0–1.5 mg/kg/day | Over 5 Decades of clinical experience; Inexpensive; Only licensed agents permitted to treat mucormycosis. | Poor CNS penetration; Extremely toxic. | Groll et al., 2000; Gleissner et al., 2004 |
| LAmB | 5–10 mg/kg/day | Better CNS penetration than AmB and ABLC; Less nephrotoxic than AmB; Improved outcomes in murine models and retrospective clinical review, as compared to AmB | Expensive | Groll et al., 2000, Ibrahim et al., 2003; Gleissner et al., 2004 |
| ABLC | 5–7.5 mg/kg/d | Less nephrotoxic than AmB; Retrospective clinical data and Murine models suggest the benefit of combination therapy with echinocandins | More nephrotoxic than LAmB and probably less effective than other options such as monotherapy, especially for CNS infection | Walsh et al., 1999; Wingard et al., 2000; Spellberg et al., 2005 |
| Primary combination therapy | | | | |
| Caspofungin plus lipid polyene | 70 mg IV load, then 50 mg/day for around 2 weeks; 50 mg/m$^2$ IV for children | The toxicity profile was favourable and synergistic in murine-disseminated mucormycosis; Retrospective clinical data suggested superior outcomes with a combination of caspofungin-lipid polyene therapy for rhino-orbital-cerebral mucormycosis | Clinical data for combination therapy in this case is limited. | Walsh et al., 1999; Spellberg et al., 2005; Walsh et al., 2005 |
| Micafungin or anidulafungin plus lipid polyene | 100 mg/day for ≥2 weeks; micafungin 4 mg/kg/day for children; micafungin 10 mg/kg/day for low-birth-weight infants; anidulafungin 1.5 mg/kg/day for children | The toxicity profile was favorable and synergistic with LAmB in the murine model of disseminated mucormycosis | No clinical data is available for this. | Seibel et al., 2005; Benjamin et al., 2006; Benjamin et al., 2008; Ibrahim et al., 2008 |
| Deferasirox plus lipid polyene | 20 mg/kg po qd for 2–4 weeks | Highly fungicidal for Mucorales in vitro; Synergistic with LAmB in a murine model of disseminated mucormycosis | Only available for enteral administration; No clinical data is available yet, however, a Phase 2 clinical trial is in progress. | Ibrahim et al., 2007 |

**Table 4.** Combination therapy for the treatment of mucormycosis in preclinical and clinical trials

| Combination Therapy | Description | References |
|---|---|---|
| The synergy between liposome amphotericin B (LAmB) and granulocyte-macrophage colony-stimulating factor | Its efficacy has been demonstrated in a mouse model of invasive mucormycosis. | Rodriguez et al., 2009 |
| Caspofungin and LAmB | In mice with diabetic ketoacidosis (DKA), propagated mucormycosis increased survival by a factor of two when compared to placebo. It helped patients with rhino-orbitocerebral disease live longer. | Spellberg et al., 2005; Gargouri et al., 2019 |
| LAmB and micafungin or anidulafungin | It improved survival in mice suffering from neutropenia and DKA with mucormycosis. | Ibrahim et al., 2008; Sheybani et al., 2015 |
| LAmB and deferasirox | Deferasirox has fungicidal efficacy against clinical isolates of Mucorales, according to an in vitro study. It improved the survival of DKA animals and rhinocerebral mucormycosis humans with persistent brain stem illness despite LAmB treatment. | Spellberg et al., 2012 |
| LAmB and Echinocandins | It's available as an intravenous solution. It demonstrated a substantial increase in survival in DKA animals; however, there were no clinical investigations. | Spellberg et al., 2012 |
| Posaconazole and Isavuconazole | Posaconazole and isavuconazole showed considerable efficacy against clinical isolates of Mucorales in vitro. There is no evidence of a substantial increase in survival in DKA mice, and there is no clinical evidence. Intravenous formulation is unavailable. | Rodriguez et al., 2008; Spellberg et al., 2012 |
| Triple combination of LAmB, deferasirox and caspofungin | After proving the effectiveness of dual therapy over monotherapy, triple therapy can be added. When compared to a dual medication combination and a placebo, it dramatically enhanced lifespan and reduced the load on infected tissue with mucormycosis in DKA mice. | Roux et al., 2010; Spellberg et al., 2012 |
| Echinocandins and deferasirox | Deferasirox has fungicidal efficacy against clinical isolates of Mucorales, according to an in vitro study. In DKA mice, it dramatically increased survival. It has difficulties with safety and lacks intravenous dose forms. | Soummer et al., 2008; Spellberg et al., 2012 |

Abbreviations: LAmB: Liposome amphotericin B&DKA: Diabetic ketoacidosis

The combination of homing molecules to the particle surface, such as antibodies, peptides, or tiny molecules, allowed tissue-specific interactions with cell receptors or components (Figure 2). Drugs exert their pharmacological impact on a cellular level due to the unique characteristics of nanocarriers that improved cellular absorption and resulted in an efficient therapeutic impact (De Jong et al., 2008; Wang et al., 2017; Khan et al., 2019; Vargason et al., 2021). Special systems, such as smart stimuli response shell, functionalization by fusogenic or cell penetration peptides, and coating by lipid or micelle shell, have also been proposed to avoid endosomal drug degradation. The production and assessment of nano-antimicrobial agents have grown in the recent decade (Bucki et al., 2008). Therefore, the majority of these agents were metal-based nanoparticles that employed noble metals like gold, silver, and copper, as well as iron and other elements supposed to be employed for the treatment of several life-threatening diseases, mucormycosis, associated fungal infection in the immunocompromise COVID-19 patients.

## 6. Efficacy and Pharmacodynamics of Antifungal Agents in Mucormycosis

### 6.1. Polyenes

For the treatment of mucormycosis, the only licensed antifungal agent is Amphotericin B deoxycholate (AmB) known so far (Table 2). Being less nephrotoxic and safe for administration even at higher doses and could be given for longer durations, the formulations related to the lipid of Amphotericin B (LFABs) were chosen over normal AmB (Reed et al., 2008; Nicola et al., 2019; Walsh et al., 1999). According to research, the salvage therapy of mucormycosis showed a 71% success rate when treated with amphotericin B lipid complex (ABLC) (Walsh et al., 1998). Moreover, about a 67% survival rate was observed while treated with LAmB in comparison to a 39% survival rate when treated with AmB amid cancer patients who encountered mucormycosis (Gleissner et al., 2004). Hence, these observations made clear that for the treatment of mucormycosis LFAmBs were safe and efficient substitutions to AmB (Table 3).

The primary therapy for mucormycosis generally included polyene (Figure 2, Table 2). Patients refusing to take polyene–based regimens were given non-polyene–based regimens. Nonpolyene-based regimens were also appropriate for patients with mild disease in relatively immunocompetent hosts that can be surgically eradicated (e.g., isolated suprafacial cutaneous infection). In the future, randomized trials would be really necessary to understand and confirm the efficacy of combination therapy in animal and small human studies of mucormycosis (Figure 2, Table 4). Also, increasing the dosage of any of the echinocandin was not recommended based on the paradoxical loss of benefit of combination therapy at echinocandin dosages of ≥3 mg/kg/d (Table 2).

## 6.2. Azoles

Fluconazole and voriconazole have no reliable activity against the pathogen of mucormycosis, and the activity of itraconazole was mainly limited to the *Absidia* species (Van Cutsem et al., 1989; Rickerts et al., 2002; Sun et al., 2002; Dannaoui et al., 2003; Ide et al., 2004; Imhof et al., 2004; Kauffman et al., 2004; Marty et al., 2004; Vigouroux et al., 2005; Trifilio et al., 2007). In contrast, the *in vitro* activity against the Mucorales was increased by posaconazole with reported 90% minimum inhibitory concentrations ($MIC_{90}$) of 1 to ≥ 4 μg/mL (Pfaller et al., 2000; Sun et al., 2002; Ullmann et al., 2006; Almyroudis et al., 2007; Arikan et al., 2008; Lass-Florl et al., 2008). However, in febrile patients with neutropenia or invasive fungal infection, posaconazole was administered orally at a dose of 400 mg twice a day, resulting in a serum level of <1 μg/mL, which had an equivalent large variability (Krishna et al., 2007; Walsh et al., 2007). Although such levels might produce favorable results in the treatment of invasive aspergillosis with MIC of *Aspergillus fumigatus* usually ≤0.5 μg/mL (Pfaller et al., 2003; Andes et al., 2008). Therefore, compared with aspergillosis pharmacokinetics and pharmacodynamics, the data raised concerns about the reliability of oral posaconazole at sufficient levels in the body to treat mucormycosis (Table 2). Hence, during the treatment of mucormycosis with posaconazole, it might be necessary to monitor the treatment, especially in patients with a high risk of malabsorption (e.g., patients with mucositis and gastrointestinal graft *vs.* host disease) (Andes et al., 2004).

Additionally, the data from mouse models of mucormycosis (including serum posaconazole levels >5 μg/mL) further raised concerns about the efficacy of posaconazole in the treatment of mucormycosis (Figure 2) (Andes et al., 2004). The neutropenic *Mucor* species was found to be infectious for the mice model. Sun et al. found that posaconazole was statistically significantly lower than AmB (Sun et al., 2002). Similarly, Dannaoui et al. (2003) found that posaconazole was less effective than AmB in treating mice infected with *Rhizopus microsporus* or *Absidia* species. Furthermore, reported that posaconazole was not better than a placebo in treating *Rhizopus oryzae* which caused more than 70% of clinical mucormycosis cases (Reed et al., 2008). A recent study also showed posaconazole monotherapy was not better than placebo in the treatment of *R. oryzae* infection in neutropenia or DKA mice model (Rodriguez et al., 2008; Ibrahim et al., 2009). Thus, data from aforesaid four groups of researchers showed that posaconazole was not as effective as AmB in the treatment of mucormycosis in mice model; however, the three groups found that it was not better than placebo in treating mice infected with *R. oryzae* (Table 2). Based on the available animal data and lack of clinical data, posaconazole monotherapy could not be recommended as the main treatment for mucormycosis (Figure 2). On the contrary, the existing clinical data from open-label therapy studies indicated that posaconazole was a reasonable choice for patients with mucormycosis who were found to be refractory or intolerant to polyenes (Greenberg et al., 2006; Van Burik et al., 2006).

## 7. Combination Therapy in Mucormycosis

Mucormycosis, also known as zygomycosis or phycomycosis, was originally described in 1885 by Paltauf as an unusual and severe fungal infection that affects patients by altering their immune and rhinocerebral system (Paltauf, 1885; Arnáiz–García et al., 2009). However, it has a low incidence rate of up to 1.7 per million people, and numerous instances have been reported, leading to a significant increase in incidence in the current context of the exceptional COVID-19 pandemic (Awal et al., 2021). Many accidental exploratory case reports have been documented previously, however, there was no solid link between COVID-19 and increased fungal infections. Mehta and Pandey described a case of rhino–orbital mucormycosis in one patient who was accompanied by COVID-19 in September 2020 (White et al., 2020). In another study Werthman–Ehrenreich published a comparable instance in the same month (Awal et al., 2021; Werthman–Ehrenreich et al., 2021).

Clinical analysis of antifungal intervention for mucormycosis treatment is essential. Studies including Caillot et al. (1997) and Greene et al. (2007) revealed that the treatment applied in the course of the initial stage suggested radiographic investigations of the invasive pulmonary aspergillosis. Perhaps, the halo sign was associated with a better approach of effective treatment with a significant response and chances of survival, as compared to the patients who have been intervened with antifungal medication prescribed *via* the CT imaging results lasting for 7–10 days in general. Delays in the treatment allowed the clear spread of Angio–invasive fungal including thrombotic necrosis of neighboring tissue that limits lifesaving drug delivery to the infection areas (Berenguer et al., 1995; Shibuya et al., 2004; Ben–Ami et al., 2009). Combination therapy was found to be profoundly effective for the treatment of mucormycosis which has been studied in both preclinical and clinical settings (Figure 2, Table 4).

## Conclusion

As the rate of fungal infections emerged and escalated, novel methods of drug designing and therapeutic models have come into effect to proliferate resistance to the current models or designs of therapeutics. A constructive substitution to antifungal agents' progression needs to establish the notion wherein the resemblance in fungal and neoplastic cells is to be used for treatment through targeted nanotherapeutics. Yet there have been several outcomes of the novel strategies, still a varied number of factors limit the designing of NP–based antifungal drugs. Reviews have intimated that these strategies for drug designing, and development should gain surplus efforts so that the multifunctional nanoparticles can be used for the utmost benefit. The novel approaches for the treatment via antifungal agents can involve a combination of hyperthermia/photodynamic therapy along with real-time imaging of targeted treatment, and drug delivery which can offer the greatest possibilities in advancement. The obstacle in antifungal nano-systems was its biocompatibility resolved through various research in the field of nanotoxicology, analysis of pharmacokinetic and pharmacodynamic properties of the nano-systems *in vitro* followed by *in vivo* models as well. Further, to obtain the desired results herein, a higher stable nano-carrier system having appropriate solubility in physiological fluids must be developed which also possesses the potential to release the active compound *via* the newly made nano-formulations. The innovative diagnostic tests and nanotherapeutic approaches improved the efficacy of traditional antifungal medicines, helpful in targeted therapy and simultaneously reducing drug-related side effects during the treatment of immunocompromised COVID-19 patients with mucormycosis. In accordance with the available data through the review, it can be assumed that further research on nanotechnology-based approaches can generate desired outcomes for the improvisation in the biodistribution of the antifungal drugs even after oral administration, inadequacy relating to the injection–associated adverse effects and significant decline in the drug-related toxicity.

## References


Ajinkya, N., Yu, X., Kaithal, P., Luo, H., Somani, P., & Ramakrishna, S. (2020). Magnetic iron oxide nanoparticle (IONP) synthesis to applications: present and future. *Materials*, 13(20), 4644.

Almyroudis, N. G., Sutton, D. A., Fothergill, A. W., Rinaldi, M. G., & Kusne, S. (2007). In vitro susceptibilities of 217 clinical isolates of zygomycetes to conventional and new antifungal agents. *Antimicrobial Agents and Chemotherapy*, 51(7), 2587-2590.

Andes, D., Marchillo, K., Conklin, R., Krishna, G., Ezzet, F., Cacciapuoti, A., & Loebenberg, D. (2004). Pharmacodynamics of a new triazole, posaconazole, in a murine model of disseminated candidiasis. *Antimicrobial Agents and Chemotherapy*, 48(1), 137-142.

Andes, D., Pascual, A., & Marchetti, O. (2009). Antifungal therapeutic drug monitoring: established and emerging indications. *Antimicrobial Agents and Chemotherapy*, *53*(1), 24-34.

Arastehfar, A., Gabaldón, T., Garcia–Rubio, R., Jenks, J. D., Hoenigl, M., Salzer, H. J. F., Ilkit, M., Lass–Flörl, C., & Perlin, D. S. (2020). Drug–resistant fungi: An emerging challenge threatening our limited antifungal armamentarium. *Antibiotics*, 9(12), 877.

Arikan, S., Sancak, B., Alp, S., Hascelik, G., & Mcnicholas, P. (2008). Comparative *in vitro* activities of posaconazole, voriconazole, itraconazole, and amphotericin B against *Aspergillus* and *Rhizopus*, and synergy testing for *Rhizopus*. *Sabouraudia*, 46(6), 567-573.

Arnáiz-García, M. E., Alonso-Peña, D., del Carmen González-Vela, M., García-Palomo, J. D., Sanz-Giménez-Rico, J. R., & Arnáiz-García, A. M. (2009). Cutaneous mucormycosis: Report of five cases and review of the literature. *Journal of Plastic, Reconstructive and Aesthetic Surgery*, 62(11), e434-e441.

Ascioglu, S., Rex, J. H., De Pauw, B., Bennett, J. E., Bille, J., Crokaert, F., & Stevens, D. A. (2003). Defining opportunistic invasive fungal infections in immunocompromised patients with cancer and hematopoietic stem cell transplants: an international consensus. *Проблемы Медицинской Микологии*, 5(1), 10-16.

AshaRani, P. V., Low Kah Mun, G., Hande, M. P., & Valiyaveettil, S. (2009). Cytotoxicity and genotoxicity of silver nanoparticles in human cells. *ACS Nano*, 3(2), 279-290.

Awal, S. S., Biswas, S. S., & Awal, S. K. (2021). Rhino-orbital mucormycosis in COVID-19 patients—a new threat? *Egyptian Journal of Radiology and Nuclear Medicine*, 52, 1-6.

Ben-Ami, R., Luna, M., Lewis, R. E., Walsh, T. J., & Kontoyiannis, D. P. (2009). A clinicopathological study of pulmonary mucormycosis in cancer patients: extensive angioinvasion but limited inflammatory response. *Journal of Infection*, 59(2), 134-138.

Berenguer, J., Allende, M. C., Lee, J. W., Garrett, K., Lyman, C., Ali, N. M., & Walsh, T. J. (1995). Pathogenesis of pulmonary aspergillosis. Granulocytopenia versus cyclosporine and methylprednisolone-induced immunosuppression. *American Journal of Respiratory and Critical Care Medicine*, 152(3), 1079-1086.

Bondaryk, M., Kurzątkowski, W., & Staniszewska, M. (2013). Antifungal agents commonly used in the superficial and mucosal candidiasis treatment: mode of action and resistance development. *Advances in Dermatology and Allergology/Postępy Dermatologii I. Alergologii*, 30(5), 293-301.

Bozkurt-Guzel, C., Savage, P. B., Akcali, A., & Ozbek-Celik, B. (2014). Potential synergy activity of the novel ceragenin, CSA-13, against carbapenem-resistant Acinetobacter baumannii strains isolated from bacteremia patients. *BioMed Research International,* 710273, 1–5.

Bucki, R., Byfield, F. J., Kulakowska, A., McCormick, M. E., Drozdowski, W., Namiot, Z., Hartung, T., & Janmey, P. A. (2008). Extracellular gelsolin binds lipoteichoic acid and modulates cellular response to proinflammatory bacterial wall components. *Journal of Immunology,* 181(7), 4936–4944.

Caillot, D., Casasnovas, O., Bernard, A., Couaillier, J. F., Durand, C., Cuisenier, B., & Guy, H. (1997). Improved management of invasive pulmonary aspergillosis in neutropenic patients using early thoracic computed tomographic scan and surgery. *Journal of Clinical Oncology*, 15(1), 139-147.

Chidambaram, M., Manavalan, R., & Kathiresan, K. (2011). Nanotherapeutics to overcome conventional cancer chemotherapy limitations. *Journal of Pharmacy and Pharmaceutical Sciences*, 14(1), 67-77.

Cicek, N., Yildiz, N., Kadayifci, E. K., Gokce, I., & Alpay, H. (2017). Invasive aspergillosis in a patient with end stage renal disease. *Medical Mycology Case Reports*, 18, 12-14.

Cierech, M., Kolenda, A., Grudniak, A. M., Wojnarowicz, J., Woźniak, B., Gołaś, M., & Mierzwińska-Nastalska, E. (2016). Significance of polymethylmethacrylate (PMMA) modification by zinc oxide nanoparticles for fungal biofilm formation. *International Journal of Pharmaceutics*, 510(1), 323-335.

Cornely, O. A., Alastruey-Izquierdo, A., Arenz, D., Chen, S. C., Dannaoui, E., Hochhegger, B. & Chakrabarti, A. (2019). Global guideline for the diagnosis and management of mucormycosis: an initiative of the European Confederation of Medical Mycology in cooperation with the Mycoses Study Group Education and Research Consortium. *The Lancet Infectious Diseases*, 19(12), e405-e421.

Cui, J., Ren, B., Tong, Y., Dai, H., & Zhang, L. (2015). Synergistic combinations of antifungals and anti-virulence agents to fight against *Candida albicans*. *Virulence*, 6(4), 362-371.

Dan, S., Pant, M., & Upadhyay, S. K. (2020). The case fatality rate in COVID-19 patients with cardiovascular disease: Global health challenge and paradigm in the current pandemic. *Current Pharmacology Reports*, 6, 315-324.

Dan, S., Sharma, D., Rastogi, K., Shaloo, Ojha, H., Pathak, M., & Singhal, R. (2021). Therapeutic and diagnostic applications of nanocomposites in the treatment Alzheimer's disease studies. *Biointerface Research in Applied Chemistry*, 12(1), 940-960.

Dan, S., Upadhyay, S. K., Girdhar, M., Mandal, M., & Sakshi. (2021). Oral carcinoma and therapeutic approaches of nanotechnology: from fundamental concept, incidence, molecular mechanism to emerging treatment techniques. *Biointerface Research in Applied Chemistry,* 12(3), 3900–37.

Dan, S., Upadhyay, S. K., Pant, M. & Shaloo. (2021). Synergistic approach of graphene oxide–silver–titanium nanocomposite film in oral and dental studies: A new paradigm of infection control in dentistry. *Biointerface Research in Applied Chemistry,* 11(2), 9680–9703.

Dannaoui, E., Meis, J. F., Loebenberg, D., & Verweij, P. E. (2003). Activity of posaconazole in treatment of experimental disseminated zygomycosis. *Antimicrobial Agents and Chemotherapy*, 47(11), 3647-3650.

Dannaoui, E., Meletiadis, J., Mouton, J. W., Meis, J. F., & Verweij, P. E. (2003). *In vitro* susceptibilities of zygomycetes to conventional and new antifungals. *Antimicrobial Agents and Chemotherapy*, 51(1), 45-52.

Das, B., Khan, M. I., Jayabalan, R., Behera, S. K., Yun, S. I., Tripathy, S. K., & Mishra, A. (2016). Understanding the antifungal mechanism of Ag/ ZnO core-shell nanocomposites against *Candida krusei*. *Scientific Reports*, 6(1), 36403.

De Jong, W. H., & Borm, P. J. (2008). Drug delivery and nanoparticles: Applications and hazards. *International Journal of Nanomedicine*, *3*(2), 133-149.

De Sá, F. A. P., Taveira, S. F., Gelfuso, G. M., Lima, E. M., & Gratieri, T. (2015). Liposomal voriconazole (VOR) formulation for improved ocular delivery. *Colloids and Surfaces B: Biointerfaces*, 133, 331-338.

Dellière, S., Dudoignon, E., Fodil, S., Voicu, S., Collet, M., Oillic, P. A., Salmona, M., Dépret, F., Ghelfenstein-Ferreira, T., Plaud, B., Chousterman, B., Bretagne, S., Azoulay, E., Mebazaa, A., Megarbane, B., & Alanio, A. (2020). Risk factors associated with COVID-19-associated pulmonary aspergillosis in ICU patients: a French multicentric retrospective cohort. *Clinical Microbiology and Infection*, 27(5), e7901–e7905.

Dhamoon, R. K., Popli, H., & Gupta, M. (2019). Novel drug delivery strategies for the treatment of onychomycosis. *Pharmaceutical Nanotechnology*, 7(1), 24–38.

Domingues, M. M., Silva, P. M., Franquelim, H. G., Carvalho, F. A., Castanho, M. A., & Santos, N. C. (2014). Antimicrobial protein rBPI21-induced surface changes on Gram-negative and Gram-positive bacteria. *Nanomedicine: Nanotechnology, Biology and Medicine*, 10(3), 543-551.

Falcone, M., Massetti, A. P., Russo, A., Vullo, V., & Venditti, M. (2011). Invasive aspergillosis in patients with liver disease. *Medical Mycology*, 49(4), 406–413.

Flores, F. C., Rosso, R. S., Cruz, L., Beck, R. C., & Silva, C. B. (2017). An innovative polysaccharide nanobased nail formulation for improvement of onychomycosis treatment. *European Journal of Pharmaceutical Sciences*, 100, 56-63.

Füredi, P., Pápay, Z. E., Kovács, K., Kiss, B. D., Ludányi, K., Antal, I., & Klebovich, I. (2017). Development and characterization of the voriconazole loaded lipid-based nanoparticles. *Journal of Pharmaceutical and Biomedical Analysis*, 132, 184-189.

Garg, S., Aggarwal, D., Upadhyay, S. K., Kumar, G., & Singh, G. (2020). Effect of COVID-19 on school education system: Challenges and opportunities to adopt online teaching and learning. *Humanities and Social Sciences Reviews*, 8(6), 10-17.

Gleissner, B., Schilling, A., Anagnostopolous, I., Siehl, I., & Thiel, E. (2004). Improved outcome of zygomycosis in patients with hematological diseases? *Leukemia and Lymphoma*, 45(7), 1351-1360.

Greenberg, R. N., Mullane, K., Van Burik, J. A., Raad, I., Abzug, M. J., Anstead, G., & Hare, R. (2006). Posaconazole as salvage therapy for zygomycosis. *Antimicrobial Agents and Chemotherapy*, 50(1), 126-133.

Greene, R. E., Schlamm, H. T., Oestmann, J. W., Stark, P., Durand, C., Lortholary, O., & Rubin, R. H. (2007). Imaging findings in acute invasive pulmonary aspergillosis: Clinical significance of the halo sign. *Clinical Infectious Diseases*, 44(3), 373-379.

Grigoras, A. G. (2019). Drug delivery systems based on pullulan polysaccharides and their derivatives. In: *Pharmaceuticals from Microbes: The Bioengineering Perspective*, pp. 99-141.

Huang, X., Tang, S., Liu, B., Ren, B., & Zheng, N. (2011). Enhancing the photothermal stability of plasmonic metal nanoplates by a core-shell architecture. *Advanced Materials*, 23(30), 3420-3425.

Ibrahim, A. S., Gebremariam, T., Schwartz, J. A., Edwards Jr, J. E., & Spellberg, B. (2009). Posaconazole mono-or combination therapy for treatment of murine zygomycosis. *Antimicrobial Agents and Chemotherapy*, 53(2), 772-775.

Ibrahim, A. S., Spellberg, B., Walsh, T. J., & Kontoyiannis, D. P. (2012). Pathogenesis of mucormycosis. *Clinical Infectious Diseases*, 54, S16-S22.

Ide, L., Buysschaert, I., Demuynck, H., De Man, R., Verlinde, A., De Laere, E., & Surmont, I. (2004). Zygomycosis in neutropenic patients with past Aspergillus infection: a role for posaconazole? *Clinical Microbiology and Infection*, 10(9), 862-863.

Imhof, A., Balajee, S. A., Fredricks, D. N., Englund, J. A., & Marr, K. A. (2004). Breakthrough fungal infections in stem cell transplant recipients receiving voriconazole. *Clinical Infectious Diseases*, 39(5), 743-746.

Jeong, W., Keighley, C., Wolfe, R., Lee, W. L., Slavin, M. A., Kong, D. C. M., & Chen, S. A. (2019). The epidemiology and clinical manifestations of mucormycosis: A systematic review and meta-analysis of case reports. *Clinical Microbiology and Infection*, 25(1), 26-34.

Jha, D., Sharma, V., Sharma, J. K., Kumar, S., Sharma, V., Kamboj, P., Upadhyay, S. K. and & Sharma, A. K. (2020). Plausible state-specific plans and recommendations to avert COVID-19 community transmission. *Bulletin of Pure and Applied Sciences (Zoology)*, 39A(2), 447-454.

Jin, Y. H., Cai, L., Cheng, Z. S., Cheng, H., Deng, T., Fan, Y. P., Fang, C., Huang, D., Huang, L. Q., Huang, Q., Han, Y., Hu, B., Hu, F., Li, B. H., Li, Y. R., Liang, K., Lin, L. K., Luo, L. S., Ma, J., Ma, L. L., Peng, Z. Y., Pan, Y. B., Pan, Z. Y., Ren, X. Q., Sun, H. M., Wang, Y., Wang, Y. Y., Weng, H., Wei, C. J., Wu, D. F., Xia, J., Xiong, Y., Xu, H. B., Yao, X. M., Yuan, Y. F., Ye, T. S., Zhang, X. C., Zhang, Y. W., Zhang,

Y. G., Zhang, H. M., Zhao, Y., Zhao, M. J., Zi, H., Zeng, X. T., Wang, Y. Y. & Wang, X. H. (2020). A rapid advice guideline for the diagnosis and treatment of 2019 novel coronavirus (2019-nCoV) infected pneumonia (standard version). *Military Medical Research*, 7(1), 4.

Johnson, A. K., Ghazarian, Z., Cendrowski, K. D., & Persichino, J. G. (2021). Pulmonary aspergillosis and mucormycosis in a patient with COVID-19. *Medical Mycology Case Reports*, 32, 64-67.

Jothiprakasam, V., Sambantham, M., Chinnathambi, S., & Vijayaboopathi, S. (2017). *Candida tropicalis* biofilm inhibition by ZnO nanoparticles and EDTA. *Archives of Oral Biology*, 73, 21-24.

Kauffman, C. A. (2004). Zygomycosis: Reemergence of an old pathogen. *Clinical Infectious Diseases*, 39(4), 588-590.

Khan, I., Saeed, K. & Khan, I. (2019). Nanoparticles: Properties, applications and toxicities. *Arabian Journal of Chemistry*, 12(7), 908–931.

Koehler, P., Cornely, O. A., Böttiger, B. W., Dusse, F., Eichenauer, D. A., Fuchs, F., Hallek, M., Jung, N., Klein, F., Persigehl, T., Rybniker, J., Kochanek, M., Böll, B., & Shimabukuro-Vornhagen, A. (2020). COVID-19 associated pulmonary aspergillosis. *Mycoses*, 63(6), 528–534.

Krcmery, V., & Barnes, A. J. (2002). Non-albicans *Candida* spp. causing fungaemia: Pathogenicity and antifungal resistance. *Journal of Hospital Infection*, 50(4), 243-260.

Krishna, G., Martinho, M., Chandrasekar, P., Ullmann, A. J., & Patino, H. (2007). Pharmacokinetics of oral posaconazole in allogeneic hematopoietic stem cell transplant recipients with graft-versus-host disease. *Pharmacotherapy*, 27(12), 1627-1636.

Krishna, G., Sansone-Parsons, A., Martinho, M., Kantesaria, B., & Pedicone, L. (2007). Posaconazole plasma concentrations in juvenile patients with invasive fungal infection. *Antimicrobial Agents and Chemotherapy*, 51(3), 812-818.

Kumar, G., Singh, G., Bhatnagar, V., Gupta, R., & Upadhyay, S. K. (2020). Outcome of online teaching-learning over traditional education during COVID-19 pandemic. *International Journal*, 9(5), 77014-7711.

Kumar, R., & Sinha, V. R. (2014). Preparation and optimization of voriconazole microemulsion for ocular delivery. *Colloids and Surfaces B: Biointerfaces*, 117, 82-88.

Kumar, S., Kaur, P., Bernela, M., Rani, R., & Thakur, R. (2016). Ketoconazole encapsulated in chitosan-gellan gum nanocomplexes exhibits prolonged antifungal activity. *International Journal of Biological Macromolecules*, 93, 988-994.

Lai, C. C., & Yu, W. L. (2021). COVID-19 associated with pulmonary aspergillosis: A literature review. *Journal of Microbiology, Immunology and Infection*, 54(1), 46-53.

Lass-Flörl, C., Mayr, A., Perkhofer, S., Hinterberger, G., Hausdorfer, J., Speth, C., & Fille, M. (2008). Activities of antifungal agents against yeasts and filamentous fungi: assessment according to the methodology of the European Committee on Antimicrobial Susceptibility Testing. *Antimicrobial Agents and Chemotherapy*, 52(10), 3637-3641.

Lepock, J. R. (1982). Involvement of membranes in cellular responses to hyperthermia. *Radiation Research*, 92(3), 433-438.

Li, Y., Theuretzbacher, U., Clancy, C. J., Nguyen, M. H., & Derendorf, H. (2010). Pharmacokinetic/pharmacodynamic profile of posaconazole. *Clinical Pharmacokinetics*, 49, 379-396.

Machado, M., Valerio, M., Álvarez-Uría, A., Olmedo, M., Veintimilla, C., Padilla, B., & Vicente, T. (2021). Invasive pulmonary aspergillosis in the COVID-19 era: An expected new entity. *Mycoses*, 64(2), 132-143.

Marty, F. M., Cosimi, L. A., & Baden, L. R. (2004). Breakthrough zygomycosis after voriconazole treatment in recipients of hematopoietic stem-cell transplants. *New England Journal of Medicine*, 350(9), 950-952.

Mehta, S., & Pandey, A. (2020). Rhino-orbital mucormycosis associated with COVID-19. *Cureus*, 12(9), e10726.

Mohamed, A., Rogers, T. R., & Talento, A. F. (2020). COVID-19 associated invasive pulmonary aspergillosis: Diagnostic and therapeutic challenges. *Journal of Fungi*, 6(3), 115.

Mohammadi, G., Shakeri, A., Fattahi, A., Mohammadi, P., Mikaeili, A., Aliabadi, A., & Adibkia, K. (2017). Preparation, physicochemical characterization and anti-fungal evaluation of nystatin-loaded PLGA-glucosamine nanoparticles. *Pharmaceutical Research*, 34, 301-309.

Monteiro, D. R., Silva, S., Negri, M., Gorup, L. F., de Camargo, E. R., Oliveira, R., & Henriques, M. (2013). Antifungal activity of silver nanoparticles in combination with nystatin and chlorhexidine digluconate against *C. andida, C. albicans* and *C. glabrata* biofilms. *Mycoses*, 56(6), 672-680.

Montiel Schneider, M. G., Martín, M. J., Otarola, J., Vakarelska, E., Simeonov, V., Lassalle, V., & Nedyalkova, M. (2022). Biomedical applications of iron oxide nanoparticles: Current insights progress and perspectives. *Pharmaceutics*, 14(1), 204.

Nicola, A. M., Albuquerque, P., Paes, H. C., Fernandes, L., Costa, F. F., Kioshima, E. S., Abadio, A. K. R., Bocca, A. L., & Felipe, M. S. (2019). Antifungal drugs: New insights in research and development. *Pharmacology and Therapeutics*, 195, 21–38.

Niemirowicz, K., Durnaś, B., Piktel, E., & Bucki, R. (2017). Development of antifungal therapies using nanomaterials. *Nanomedicine*, 12(15), 1891-1905.

Niemirowicz, K., Durnaś, B., Tokajuk, G., Głuszek, K., Wilczewska, A. Z., Misztalewska, I. & Bucki, R. (2016). Magnetic nanoparticles as a drug delivery system that enhance fungicidal activity of polyene antibiotics. *Nanomedicine: Nanotechnology, Biology and Medicine*, 12(8), 2395-2400.

Niemirowicz, K., Durnaś, B., Tokajuk, G., Piktel, E., Michalak, G., Gu, X., & Bucki, R. (2017). Formulation and candidacidal activity of magnetic nanoparticles coated with cathelicidin LL-37 and ceragenin CSA-13. *Scientific Reports*, 7(1), 4610.

Orozco, A. S., Higginbotham, L. M., Hitchcock, C. A., Parkinson, T., Falconer, D., Ibrahim, A. S., & Filler, S. G. (1998). Mechanism of fluconazole resistance in *Candida krusei*. *Antimicrobial Agents and Chemotherapy*, 42(10), 2645-2649.

Pahuja, P., Kashyap, H., & Pawar, P. (2014). Design and evaluation of HP-β-CD based voriconazole formulations for ocular drug delivery. *Current Drug Delivery*, 11(2), 223-232.

Paltauf, A. (1885). Mycosis mucorina. *Virchows Archiv für pathologische Anatomie und Physiologie und für klinische Medizin,* 102, 543–64.

Panácek, A., Kolár, M., Vecerová, R., Prucek, R., Soukupová, J., Krystof, V., Hamal, P., Zboril, R., & Kvítek, L. (2009). Antifungal activity of silver nanoparticles against *Candida* spp. *Biomaterials*, 30(31), 6333–6340.

Pant, M., Dan, S., Pant, S., Raj, A., & Upadhyay, S. K. (2021). Progression in Alzheimer's disease correlates with epigenetics and cerebral formaldehyde: from potential hereditary mechanism and environmental factors to therapeutic measures. *Current Pharmacology Reports*, 7(5), 187-205.

Pasero, D., Sanna, S., Liperi, C., Piredda, D., Branca, G. P., Casadio, L., & Terragni, P. (2021). A challenging complication following SARS-CoV-2 infection: A case of pulmonary mucormycosis. *Infection*, 49, 1055-1060.

Pawar, P., Kashyap, H., Malhotra, S., & Sindhu, R. (2013). Hp-CD-voriconazole in situ gelling system for ocular drug delivery: *in vitro*, stability, and antifungal activities assessment. *BioMed Research International*, 1–9.

Pfaller, M. A., Messer, S. A., Boyken, L., Hollis, R. J., & Diekema, D. J. (2003). In vitro susceptibility testing of filamentous fungi: Comparison of Etest and reference M38-A microdilution methods for determining posaconazole MICs. *Diagnostic Microbiology and Infectious Disease*, 45(4), 241-244.

Pfaller, M. A., Messer, S. A., Hollis, R. J., & Jones, R. N. (2002). Antifungal activities of posaconazole, ravuconazole, and voriconazole compared to those of itraconazole and amphotericin B against 239 clinical isolates of *Aspergillus* spp. and other filamentous fungi: Report from SENTRY Antimicrobial Surveillance Program, 2000. *Antimicrobial Agents and Chemotherapy*, 46(4), 1032-1037.

Phelan, A. L., Katz, R., & Gostin, L. O. (2020). The novel coronavirus originating in Wuhan, China: Challenges for global health governance. *Journal of American Medical Association*, 323(8), 709-710.

Placik, D. A., Taylor, W. L., & Wnuk, N. M. (2020). Bronchopleural fistula development in the setting of novel therapies for acute respiratory distress syndrome in SARS-CoV-2 pneumonia. *Radiology Case Reports*, 15(11), 2378-2381.

Rashidzadeh, H., Danafar, H., Rahimi, H., Mozafari, F., Salehiabar, M., Rahmati, M. A., Rahamooz–Haghighi, S., Mousazadeh, M., Mohammadi, A., Ertas, Y. N., Ramazani, A., Huseynova, I., Khalilov, R., Davaran, S., Webster, T. J., Kavetskyy, T., Eftekhari, A., Nosrati, H., & Mirsaeidi, M. (2021). Nanotechnology against the novel coronavirus (Severe Acute Respiratory Syndrome Coronavirus 2): Diagnosis, treatment, therapy and future perspectives. *Nanomedicine*, 16(6), 497-516.

Reed, C., Bryant, R., Ibrahim, A. S., Edwards Jr, J., Filler, S. G., Goldberg, R., & Spellberg, B. (2008). Combination polyene-caspofungin treatment of rhino-orbital-cerebral mucormycosis. *Clinical Infectious Diseases*, 47(3), 364-371.

Rencber, S., Karavana, S. Y., Yılmaz, F. F., Eraç, B., Nenni, M., Özbal, S., & Ertan, G. (2016). Development, characterization, and *in vivo* assessment of mucoadhesive nanoparticles containing fluconazole for the local treatment of oral candidiasis. *International Journal of Nanomedicine*, 11, 2641- 53.

Rickerts, V., Böhme, A., & Just-Nübling, G. (2002). Risk factor for invasive zygomycosis in patients with hematologic malignancies. *Mycoses*, 45, 27-30.

Rodríguez, M. M., Serena, C., Mariné, M., Pastor, F. J., & Guarro, J. (2008). Posaconazole combined with amphotericin B, an effective therapy for a murine disseminated infection caused by *Rhizopus oryzae*. *Antimicrobial Agents and Chemotherapy*, 52(10), 3786-3788.

Roque, L., Alopaeus, J., Reis, C., Rijo, P., Molpeceres, J., Hagesaether, E., & Reis, C. (2018). Mucoadhesive assessment of different antifungal nanoformulations. *Bioinspiration and Biomimetics*, 13(5), 055001.

Saldanha, C. A., Garcia, M. P., Iocca, D. C., Rebelo, L. G., Souza, A. C. O., Bocca, A. L., & Azevedo, R. B. (2016). Antifungal activity of amphotericin B conjugated to nanosized magnetite in the treatment of paracoccidioidomycosis. *PLoS Neglected Tropical Diseases*, 10(6), e0004754.

Scorzoni, L., de Paula e Silva, A. C., Marcos, C. M., Assato, P. A., de Melo, W. C., de Oliveira, H. C., & Fusco-Almeida, A. M. (2017). Antifungal therapy: new advances in the understanding and treatment of mycosis. *Frontiers in Microbiology*, 8, 36.

Sharma, N., Jandaik, S., & Kumar, S. (2016). Synergistic activity of doped zinc oxide nanoparticles with antibiotics: ciprofloxacin, ampicillin, fluconazole and amphotericin B against pathogenic microorganisms. *Anais da Academia Brasileira de Ciências*, *88*, 1689-1698.

Shibuya, K., Hasegawa, C., Hamatani, S., Hatori, T., Nagayama, T., Nonaka, H., & Wakayama, M. (2004). Pathophysiology of pulmonary aspergillosis. *Journal of Infection and Chemotherapy*, 10(3), 138-145.

Shukr, M. H. (2016). Novel in situ gelling ocular inserts for voriconazole-loaded niosomes: design, *in vitro* characterisation and in vivo evaluation of the ocular irritation and drug pharmacokinetics. *Journal of Microencapsulation*, *33*(1), 71-79.

Singh, H., Dua, S., Goel, A., Dhar, A., Bhadauria, V., Garg, A., Katyar, V., Sharma, S & Shukla, A. (2021). Rhino-orbital-cerebral mucormycosis in times of COVID-19: A neurosurgical experience. *Surgical Neurology International*, *12*.

Singh, M., Kamboj, S., Kumari, S., Kamboj, V., & Upadhyay, S. K. (2020). One pot synthesis of physico–chemically stabilized ZnO nanoparticles *via* biological method and its potential application as antimicrobial agent. *Bulletin* of *Pure* and *Applied Sciences- Zoology,* 39A(1), 116–29.

Singh, M., Kumar, V., Sehrawat, N., Yadav, M., Chaudhary, M., Upadhyay, S. K., Kumar, S., Sharma, V., Kumar, S., Dilbaghi, N. & Sharma, A. K. (2021). Current paradigms in epigenetic anticancer therapeutics and future challenges. *Seminars in Cancer Biology*, 83, 422-440.

Singh, M., Renu Kumar, V., Upadhyay, S. K., Singh, R., Yadav, M., Seema Kumari, S., Sharma, A. K. & Manikandan, S. (2021). Biomimetic synthesis of silver nanoparticle from aqueous extract of *Saraca indica* and its profound antibacterial activity. *Biointerface Research in Applied Chemistry,* 11(1), 8110–20.

Singh, R., Sharma, I., Sharma, P., Gupta, M., Singhal, P., Goyal, S., Yadav, M. & Upadhyay, S. K. (2021). Nanoparticles and Nanotechnology: From source, properties, types, synthesis to multifaceted functional potential in agriculture. *BioScience Research Bulletin,* 37(1), 23–34.

Solano, C., & Vazquez, L. (2018). Invasive aspergillosis in the patient with oncohematologic disease. *Revista Iberoamericana de Micologia*, 35(4), 198-205.

Song, G., Liang, G., & Liu, W. (2020). Fungal co-infections associated with global COVID-19 pandemic: A clinical and diagnostic perspective from China. *Mycopathologia*, 185(4), 599-606.

Sood, S., Aggarwal, V., Aggarwal, D., Upadhyay, S. K., Sak, K., Tuli, H. S., & Talwar, S. (2020). COVID-19 pandemic: from molecular biology, pathogenesis, detection, and treatment to global societal impact. *Current Pharmacology Reports*, 6, 212-227.

Sun, L., Liao, K., Li, Y., Zhao, L., Liang, S., Guo, D., & Wang, D. (2016). Synergy between polyvinylpyrrolidone-coated silver nanoparticles and azole antifungal against drug-resistant *Candida albicans*. *Journal of Nanoscience and Nanotechnology*, 16(3), 2325-2335.

Sun, Q. N., Fothergill, A. W., McCarthy, D. I., Rinaldi, M. G., & Graybill, J. R. (2002). In vitro activities of posaconazole, itraconazole, voriconazole, amphotericin B, and fluconazole against 37 clinical isolates of zygomycetes. *Antimicrobial Agents and Chemotherapy*, 46(5), 1581-1582.

Sun, Q. N., Najvar, L. K., Bocanegra, R., Loebenberg, D., & Graybill, J. R. (2002). *In vivo* activity of posaconazole against *Mucor* spp. in an immunosuppressed-mouse model. *Antimicrobial Agents and Chemotherapy*, 46(7), 2310-2312.

Sun, X., Yu, Z., Cai, Z., Yu, L., & Lv, Y. (2016). Voriconazole composited polyvinyl alcohol/hydroxypropyl-β-cyclodextrin nanofibers for ophthalmic delivery. *PloS one*, 11(12), e0167961.

Thompson Iii, G. R., Cornely, O. A., Pappas, P. G., Patterson, T. F., Hoenigl, M., Jenks, J. D., & Nguyen, M. H. (2020). Invasive aspergillosis as an under-recognized superinfection in COVID-19. *Open Forum Infectious Diseases,* 7(7), 242.

Trifilio, S. M., Bennett, C. L., Yarnold, P. R., McKoy, J. M., Parada, J., Mehta, J., & Kontoyiannis, D. P. (2007). Breakthrough zygomycosis after voriconazole administration among patients with hematologic malignancies who receive hematopoietic stem-cell transplants or intensive chemotherapy. *Bone Marrow Transplantation*, 39(7), 425-429.

Tuli, H. S., Mittal, S., Aggarwal, D., Parashar, G., Parashar, N. C., Upadhyay, S. K., Barwal, T. S., Jain, A., Kaur, G., Salva, R., Sak, K., Kumar, M., Varol, M., Iqubal, A. & Sharma, A. K. (2021). Path of silibinin from diet to medicine: A dietary polyphenolic flavonoid having potential anti–cancer therapeutic significance. *Seminars in Cancer Biology*, 73, 196–218.

Tuli, H. S., Sak, K., Aggarwal, P., Iqubl, A., Upadhyay, S. K., Kaur, J., Kaur, G., & Aggarwal D. (2021). Molecular evolution of SARS–CoV–2 virus: Hazardous and more hazardous strains behind the COVID-19 pandemic. *Frontiers in Cellular and Infection Microbiology,* 11, 763687.

Ullmann, A. J., Cornely, O. A., Burchardt, A., Hachem, R., Kontoyiannis, D. P., Topelt, K., & Raad, I. (2006). Pharmacokinetics, safety, and efficacy of posaconazole in patients with persistent febrile neutropenia or refractory invasive fungal infection. *Antimicrobial Agents and Chemotherapy*, 50(2), 658-666.

Upadhyay, S. K., Dan, S., Girdhar, M., & Rastogi, K. (2021). Recent advancement in SARS-CoV-2 diagnosis, treatment, and vaccine formulation: A new paradigm of nanotechnology in strategic combating of COVID-19 pandemic. *Current Pharmacology Reports*, 7, 1-14.

Upadhyay, S. K., Singh, R., Babita, K. G. & Singh, G. (2020). The outbreak and challenges of novel coronavirus (COVID–19): The global pandemic emergency of early 2K20 and Indian scenario. *International Journal of Biology, Pharmacy and Allied Sciences*, 9(5):1173–99.

Upadhyay, S. K., Singh, R., Singh, M., Kumar, V., Yadav, M., Aggarwal, D., & Sehrawat, N. (2020). COVID-19 in republic of India: A report on situation and precautionary strategies to global pandemic. *Bulletin of Environment Pharmacology and Life Sciences*, 9(6), 39-48.

Upadhyay, S. K., Prakash, S., Singh, M., Upadhyay, K., Rani, K. & Singh, R. (2022). Ayurvedic approach of some indigenous flora in curbing SARS–CoV–2 infection: I. Traditional spices as immunity booster for COVID-19 patients. *International Journal of Botany Studies*, 7(1), 655–61.

Upadhyay, S. K., Yadav, D., Singh, M., Yadav, M., Upadhyay, K. & Singh, R. (2022). Ayurvedic approach of some indigenous flora in curbing SARS–CoV–2 infection: II. Traditional medicinal plants for strengthening of immune system and treatment of COVID–19. *International Journal of Botany Studies*, 7(3), 72–8.

Vallabani, N. S., & Singh, S. (2018). Recent advances and future prospects of iron oxide nanoparticles in biomedicine and diagnostics. *3 Biotech*, 8(6), 279.

van Burik, J. A. H., Hare, R. S., Solomon, H. F., Corrado, M. L., & Kontoyiannis, D. P. (2006). Posaconazole is effective as salvage therapy in zygomycosis: A retrospective summary of 91 cases. *Clinical Infectious Diseases*, 42(7), e61-e65.

Van Cutsem, J., Van Gerven, F., Fransen, J., & Janssen, P. A. J. (1989). Treatment of experimental zygomycosis in guinea pigs with azoles and with amphotericin B. *Chemotherapy*, 35(4), 267-272.

Vargason, A. M., Anselmo, A. C., & Mitragotri, S. (2021). The evolution of commercial drug delivery technologies. *Nature Biomedical Engineering*, 5(9), 951-967.

Vigouroux, S., Morin, O., Moreau, P., Méchinaud, F., Morineau, N., Mahé, B., & Milpied, N. (2005). Zygomycosis after prolonged use of voriconazole in immunocompromised patients with hematologic disease: Attention required. *Clinical Infectious Diseases*, 40(4), e35-e37.

Walsh, T. J., Finberg, R. W., Arndt, C., Hiemenz, J., Schwartz, C., Bodensteiner, D., Pappas, P., Seibel, N., Greenberg, R. N., Dummer, S., Schuster, M., & Holcenberg, J. S. (1999). Liposomal amphotericin B for empirical therapy in patients with persistent fever and neutropenia. National Institute of Allergy and Infectious Diseases Mycoses Study Group. *The New England Journal of Medicine*, 340(10), 764–771.

Walsh, T. J., Hiemenz, J. W., Seibel, N. L., Perfect, J. R., Horwith, G., Lee, L., & Anaissie, E. J. (1998). Amphotericin B lipid complex for invasive fungal infections: Analysis of safety and efficacy in 556 cases. *Clinical Infectious Diseases*, 26(6), 1383-1396.

Walsh, T. J., Raad, I., Patterson, T. F., Chandrasekar, P., Donowitz, G. R., Graybill, R., & Perfect, J. R. (2007). Treatment of invasive aspergillosis with posaconazole in patients who are refractory to or intolerant of conventional therapy: An externally controlled trial. *Clinical Infectious Diseases*, 44(1), 2-12.

Wambaugh, M. A., Denham, S. T., Ayala, M., Brammer, B., Stonhill, M. A., & Brown, J. C. (2020). Synergistic and antagonistic drug interactions in the treatment of systemic fungal infections. *Elife*, 9, e54160.

Wang, L., Hu, C., & Shao, L. (2017). The antimicrobial activity of nanoparticles: Present situation and prospects for the future. *International Journal of Nanomedicine*, 12, 1227–1249.

Werthman-Ehrenreich, A. (2021). Mucormycosis with orbital compartment syndrome in a patient with COVID-19. *The American Journal of Emergency Medicine*, 42, e264-e265.

White, P. L., Dhillon, R., Cordey, A., Hughes, H., Faggian, F., Soni, S., & Backx, M. (2021). A national strategy to diagnose coronavirus disease 2019–associated invasive fungal disease in the intensive care unit. *Clinical Infectious Diseases*, 73(7), e1634-e1644.

Wu, F., Zhao, S., Yu, B., Chen, Y. M., Wang, W., Song, Z. G., Hu, Y., Tao, Z. W., Tian, J. H., Pei, Y. Y., Yuan, M. L., Zhang, Y. Z., Dai, F. H., Liu, Y., Wang, Q. M., Zheng, J. J., Xu, L., Holmes, E. C. & Zhang, Y. Z. (2020). A new coronavirus associated with human respiratory disease in China. *Nature*, 579(7798), 265-269.

Yadav, D., Upadhyay, S. K., Anwar, M. F., & Unnithan, J. S. (2016). A review on the patents of various metal nanoparticles: Preparations and formulations. *World Journal of Pharmacy and Pharmaceutical Sciences*, 5(2), 1309-1317.

Yadav, R., Dhiman, U., Parihar, R. D., & Upadhyay, S. K. (2021). Virtual screening of potential drug molecules against Covid-19 targets: A drug repurposing approach. *Letters in Appllied NanoBioScience*, 11(1), 2965-2980.

Yadav, R., Parihar, R. D., Dhiman, U., Dhamija, P., Upadhyay, S. K., Imran, M. & Prasad, T. K. (2020). Docking of FDA approved drugs targeting nsp-16, n-protein and main protease of SARS-CoV-2 as dual inhibitors. *Biointerface Research in Applied Chemistry,* 11(3), 9848-9861.

Yaqoob, A. A., Ahmad, H., Parveen, T., Ahmad, A., Oves, M., Ismail, I. M., & Mohamad Ibrahim, M. N. (2020). Recent advances in metal decorated nanomaterials and their various biological applications: A review. *Frontiers in Chemistry*, 8, 341.

Zhang, C., Chen, M., Wang, G., Fang, W., Ye, C., Hu, H., & Liao, W. Q. (2016). Pd/ Ag nanosheets in combination with Amphotericin B exert a potent anti-cryptococcal fungicidal effect. *PLoS One*, 11(6), e0157000.

Zhou, P., Yang, X. L., Wang, X. G., Hu, B., Zhang, L., Zhang, W., Si, H. R., Zhu, Y., Li, B., Huang, C. L., Chen, H. D., Chen, J., Luo, Y., Guo, H., Jiang, R. D., Liu, M. Q., Chen, Y., Shen, X. R., Wang, Zheng, X. S. & Shi, Z. L. (2020). A pneumonia outbreak associated with a new coronavirus of probable bat origin. *Nature*, 579(7798), 270-273.

Zurl, C., Hoenigl, M., Schulz, E., Hatzl, S., Gorkiewicz, G., Krause, R., & Prattes, J. (2021). Autopsy proven pulmonary mucormycosis due to *Rhizopus microsporus* in a critically ill COVID-19 patient with underlying hematological malignancy. *Journal of Fungi*, 7(2), 88.

## Chapter 8

# Advancements in the Testing Methods of SARS-CoV-2: From Conventional Clinical Diagnostic, Serological, Rapid-Biomolecular Tests to Nanobased Biosensors

**Siddhartha Dan[1,2]**
**Pritika Dutta[3]**
**Pallavi Dutta[4]**
**Deeksha Sharma[5]**
**Sakshi Tyagi[6]**
**Sushil Kumar Upadhyay[7,*]**
**and Anil K. Sharma[8]**

[1]Department of Biotechnology, I. K. Gujral Punjab Technical University, Jalandhar, Punjab, India
[2]Department of Biotechnology; Dr. B. R. Ambedkar National Institute of Technology, Jalandhar, Punjab, India
[3]Department of Physiology, All India Institute of Medical Sciences, New Delhi, India
[4]Department of Biotechnology, Jawaharlal Nehru University, New Delhi, India
[5]Faculty of Applied Sciences and Biotechnology, Shoolini University, Solan, Himachal Pradesh, India
[6]Department of Biotechnology, Jaypee Institute of Information Technology, Noida, Uttar Pradesh, India
[7]Department of Bio-Sciences and Technology, M.M.E.C., Maharishi Markandeshwar (Deemed to be University), Mullana-Ambala (Haryana), India
[8]Department of Biotechnology, Amity University, Mohali, Punjab, India

---

[*] Corresponding Author's Email: upadhyay.k.sushil@gmail.com.

In: Therapeutic Advances in Human Health and Diseases
Editors: Sushil Kumar Upadhyay, Manoj Singh and Anil Kumar Sharma
ISBN: 979-8-89113-304-4

## Abstract

The novel Coronavirus Disease 2019 (COVID-19) which is primarily caused by severe acute respiratory syndrome coronavirus 2 (SARS-CoV-2) has created a major impact on the lives of people worldwide. After the severe global outbreak of the Middle East Respiratory Syndrome-CoV (MERS-CoV) in 2002 and Severe Acute Respiratory Syndrome-CoV (SARS-CoV) in 2012, SARS-CoV-2 emerged as the third pandemic related to coronavirus and successfully caught the attention of all clinicians thereby becoming the reason of paramount concern. After its origin in Wuhan and quick escalation throughout the world, WHO announced it as an immediate international emergency to public health that needs to be attended to and managed promptly to control any further catastrophic health hazards in the near or far future. Tremendous efforts have been put forth and several research-based, technical tests have been introduced after the approval from the food and drug administration sector of respective countries. Clinical diagnostic and molecular-level biochemical tests have been introduced for quick diagnosis of this viral disease. Some of the accessible methods of testing include real-time polymerase chain reaction, quantitative reverse transcription-polymerase chain reaction, real-time isothermal loop-mediated amplification, rapid serological test, antigen-based test, electrochemical biosensors and enzyme-linked immunosorbent assay and nano-biotechnology. This review therefore primarily aims to provide the detailed features and exact shortcomings of the available testing techniques to furnish timely detection of COVID-19 thereby aiming for proper clinical assistance. Undoubtedly, RT-PCR is the most recommended test for the detection of viral load, yet for quick results, rapid immunological testing is considered to be more valuable.

**Keywords:** SARS-CoV-2, COVID-19, rapid antigen tests, real-time PCR, nano-based biosensor

## Introduction

A novel coronavirus termed by the World Health Organization as Severe Acute Respiratory Syndrome Coronavirus 2 (SARS-CoV-2) was detected in Wuhan, the capital of Central China's Hubei Province around December 2019 (Mohamadian et al., 2021). Due to its likeness of the structure to severe acute respiratory syndrome-related coronaviruses, this novel coronavirus was termed SARS-CoV-2 (Dan et al., 2020). Soon after its detection, it promptly spread across China and in several other countries throughout the world, raising major global concerns (Caruana et al., 2020; Wang et al., 2020; WHO, 2020; Awadasseid et al., 2021). In general, Coronaviruses are considered a species of viruses that belong to the family Coronaviridae and are capable of generating diseases in humans as well as in animal species. The said coronavirus family is further classified into four subfamilies namely, Alphacoronavirus, Betacoronavirus, Gammacoronavirus, and Deltacoronavirus (Hossain et al., 2021).

Coronaviruses are a family of viruses that are naturally hosted and evolutionarily designed by bats (Cui et al., 2019; Li et al., 2020). Certainly, it has been claimed that most of the coronaviruses in human beings are derived from the bat reservoir (Li et al., 2005; Dominguez et al., 2007). Currently, numerous teams have established the genetic resemblance between SARS-CoV-2 and a bat betacoronavirus of the sub-genus *Sarbecovirus* (Benvenuto et al., 2020; Chan et al., 2020; Wei et al., 2020; Wu et al., 2020; Xu et al., 2020; Zhou et al., 2020). The complete genome sequence of this novel virus, SARS-CoV-2 has 96.2% similarity to that of a bat SARS-related coronavirus (SARSr-CoV; RaTG13) collected in Yunnan province, China (Paraskevis et al., 2020; Zhou et al., 2020a) nonetheless has little similarity to that of SARS-CoV (about 79%) or MERS-CoV (about 50%) (Gralinski and Menachery, 2020; Lu et al., 2020). It is to be noted that in total, about seven coronaviruses in humans have been established till now such as Human Coronavirus (HCo) 229E, OC43, NL63, HKU1, SARS-COV and SARS-COV-2 and MERS-COV (Chia et al., 2020; Mohamadian et al., 2021) the most advanced coronavirus that is linked with humans is none other than COVID19 that is typically caused by the SARS-COV-2, a single-strand RNA virus responsible for acute respiratory syndrome in the human population (Hui et al., 2020; Wu et al., 2020; Hossain et al., 2021; Yesudhas et al., 2021). Even though the available genome sequence related to the virus provides a close association between SARS-COV-1 and SARS-COV-2, the latter is tremendously transferable as and when compared to the former (Zhong et al., 2003; Hossain et al., 2021).

Studies have reported angiotensin-converting enzyme-2 (ACE2) as a recognized receptor for the binding of the SARS-CoV-2 virus to cells (Kuba et al., 2005; Campbell et al., 2021). The fact that this receptor is specifically expressed in the nasopharyngeal and alveolar epithelial cells of the airway furnishes a reasonable explanation of respiratory distress in patients suffering from COVID-19 (Manne et al., 2020; Xu et al., 2020). Multiple independent studies have been carried out over the past few years wherein it has been established that platelets tend to be hyperactive in COVID-19 cases which may further give rise to vascular inflammatory responses thereby serving as a molecular reservoir for the disease to spread rapidly (Abdelrahman et al., 2020; Elrashdy et al., 2020; Manne et al., 2020; Zaid et al., 2020). Several transcriptomic analyses and proteomics assays have been performed but the precise route of transmission from natural reservoirs to humans remains vague (Li et al., 2020; Wei et al., 2020).

Regardless of these latest discoveries, quite a few fundamental and major issues associated with the evolutionary patterns and driving forces behind this deadly outbreak of SARS-CoV-2 remain to be fully characterized (Yang, 2007; Hanson and Coller, 2018; Wu and Poo, 2020). Eminent researchers have studied the degree of molecular divergence between SARS-CoV-2 and other correlated coronaviruses and also carried out population genetic analyses of 103 sequenced genomes of SARS-CoV-2 thereby providing new comprehensions about the evolution of SARS-CoV-2 along with insights about its pattern of spread through the human population (Tang et al., 2020).

Since its detection, this virus has been spreading at alarming rates and has become a foremost public health concern across the globe. As with any other health issue, early diagnosis plays an important role as it is critical for better patient management and outbreak control. Maximum diagnosis tests which are being currently used for the detection of SARS-CoV-2 depend on viral RNA amplification by using real-time PCR (RT-PCR) and need some hours before the result is released. On that account, exceptionally sensitive immunological-related diagnostics techniques that could detect the viral antigens in the samples would prove to be highly effective for fast and correct diagnosis of COVID-19 (Tang et al., 2020). Molecular detection of the causative pathogen, SARS-CoV-2 is the diagnostic reference standard for coronavirus disease 2019 (COVID-19) (CDC, 2020; Corman et al., 2020; Hong et al., 2020). However, it takes around three to four hours to identify the nucleic acid and necessitates dedicated instruments, knowledge, and skilled laboratory workforces who are acquainted with molecular techniques (Mak et al., 2020).

Moreover, several countries have faced a scarcity of test kits (Albert et al., 2021). To tackle this problem, many rapid antigen tests (RATs) were made for the prompt and low-cost detection of SARS-CoV-2 which can be used at the point of care (POC). It has been seen that most of the RATs generate test outcomes in less than 1.5 hours as it primarily involve immune-chromatographic assays from nasopharyngeal specimens (CDC, 2020; Cerutti et al., 2020). Even though in NP specimens their diagnostic sensitivity for SARS-CoV-2 detection is subordinate to that of molecular tests (CDC, 2020), undoubtedly the development of a new test system that is more cost-effective, high-throughput along with a rapid turnaround time would be significant for inhibiting viral spread.

Additionally, SARS-CoV-2 antigen kinetics was scrutinized based on the number of days post-symptom onset (PSO) (Kweon et al., 2021). Approaches to control the SARS-CoV-2 pandemic majorly depend on readily accessible and dependable diagnostic assays to detect the virus in respiratory material. Various RT-PCR assays were introduced just after the first full-length SARS-CoV-2 genome sequence was made available to the public (CDC, 2020; Corman et al., 2020; Konrad et al., 2020; Muenchhoff et al., 2020; van Kasteren et al., 2020; WHO, 2021). Though the inclusive performance of these assays is variable (Muenchhoff et al., 2020), the quantifiable and sensitive detection of the SARS-CoV-2 genome by laboratory-based RT-PCR assays has undeniably simplified clinical management, surveillance, contact management, and disease control. On the other hand, the shortage of skilled laboratory staff to function complex PCR platforms, scarcities in equipment and reagents as well as the extensive turn-around times until test results are available, clarify glitches in a "PCR-only"-based testing strategy (Osterman et al., 2021). Possibilities for additional, non-PCR-based point-of-care testing (POCT) are receiving great consideration and are being widely applied in national test strategies. In principle, such assays are thought to provide rapid and reliable statistics on the SARS-CoV-2 infection status, for instance, in emergency departments or other healthcare facility settings. Initial published reports have indicated sensitivities of SARS-CoV-2 antigen tests of 75.6% to 87.5% (Young et al., 2020; Diao et al., 2021).

## 1. Methods of Testing

Similar to other viral infections, SARS-CoV-2 infection diagnosis is also grounded on the direct identification of viral RNA or antigens or the indirect identification of particular antibody responses. For an active infection, a direct diagnosis is a benchmark, while the detection of specific anti-SARS-CoV-2 antibodies is the foundation stone for the identification of earlier interaction with the virus, both for diagnostic and epidemiological aims (WHO, 2020).

### 1.1. Respiratory Isolates

The SARS-CoV-2 culture isolate (strain hCoV-19/Hong Kong/ VM20001097/2020, the first COVID-19 case detected in Hong Kong) was used to achieve a serial tenfold dilution to find out the limit of detection (LOD) between diverse assays (Mak et al., 2020). A total of thirteen non-SARS-CoV-2 respiratory virus isolates were tested to assess the cross-reactivity of the RAD test. They were influenza A(H3), influenza B, influenza A (H1pdm09), adenovirus, coronavirus type 229E, coronavirus type OC43, parainfluenza virus type 1, parainfluenza virus type 2, parainfluenza virus type 3, parainfluenza virus type 4, rhinovirus, respiratory syncytial virus, and enterovirus(Mak et al., 2020).

### 1.2. Respiratory Samples

For this evaluation, respiratory samples from patients confirmed with SARS-CoV-2 infection by RT-PCR pointing to the SARS-CoV-2 virus-specific RdRp gene were regained, dated from February 1, 2020, to April 21, 2020. All these collected samples were carefully placed in viral transport media (VTM) or Phosphate-Buffered Saline (PBS) for RNA extraction. The residual part of the suspension was put in safekeeping at −70 °C until use in this study. Virus concentrations in samples were projected from the cycle threshold (Ct) value (Mak et al., 2020).

Since April 2020, the Public Health Laboratory Services Branch (PHLSB) in Hong Kong has been entitled to a COVID-19 reference laboratory, and all confirmed cases in Hong Kong were either diagnosed or confirmed by PHLSB (WHO, 2020). Recently, a study was conducted to diagnose coronavirus infection among symptomatic patients by taking respiratory samples based on the nucleic acid amplification model and to evaluate the accuracy of nucleic acid amplification tests among these patients. As and when compared, among all the PCR tests, RT-PCR proved to have higher sensitivity, thereby proving to be an effective method for testing (Hellou et al., 2021).

### 1.3. RAD Kits for SARS−CoV−2 Detection

With the help of two rapid antigen detection (RAD) kits available in the market in Egypt: BIOCREDIT COVID-19 Ag (RapiGENInc., Korea) and Standard Q COVID-19 Ag (SD Biosensor, Korea), all samples were tested for SARS-CoV-2 antigens that were provided to the CPHL to assess the performance of these tests afore introduction to routine(Khairat et al., 2020). COVID-19 RAD kits are quick and qualitative tests that permit identifying SARS-CoV-2 antigen in nasopharyngeal specimens. The RAD kits are designed to employ a format that can easily detect the viral antigen with the help of the SARS-COV-2 antibody present. To target the SARS-CoV-2 antigen, these tests exploit monoclonal antibodies conjugated to colloidal gold nanoparticles. These antibodies are secured onto the nitrocellulose membrane.

Antigen detection was lead following the manufacturers' instructions by mixing 100 µL of nasopharyngeal secretions with four drops of dilution buffer in a tube, which is then added to the strip, where solubilized conjugate together with the sample flows with passive diffusion and reacts with SARS-CoV-2 antibodies, which are fixed onto the nitrocellulose membrane. To safeguard the right flow of the sample, the strip contains a control line. The results were inferred visually after 15 minutes (Khairat et al., 2020; Mertens et al., 2020). During the evaluation of the performance of both kits, sensitivity, specificity, and accuracy were considered, in comparison with the benchmark viral nucleic acid detection using RT-PCR (Khairat et al., 2020). A study performed by Mak et al. (2020) has concluded that the limit of detection of the reference kit was $10^5$ less sensitive compared to the RT-PCR kit with respect to BIOCREDIT COVID-19 Ag thereby can be considered safe to use for the detection of the novel virus. These findings were per the results of studies done previously (West et al., 2021).

### 1.4. Biocredit COVID-19 Ag

The proposed use for the BIOCREDIT COVID-19 Ag kit is for nasopharyngeal swab samples. As nasopharyngeal swab and throat swab (NPS TS), nasopharyngeal swab and throat swab (NPS TS), sputum and throat saliva had either been eluted in VTM or suspended in PBS, the test was carried out with reformed sample processing methods (Mak et al., 2020).

**Table 1.** Comparing PCR Kits for 2019-nCoV Detection: Exploring Kit Names and PCR equipment with targeted genes

| Kit name, Manufacturer | PCR equipment | Target genes/ No. Tubes | Internal Control | Volume of RNA elutes per test (μl) | No. of amplifications | Running Time of PCR | Cut Off Ct |
|---|---|---|---|---|---|---|---|
| Allplex 2019-nCoV seegene | CFX96 | E, RdRd, N/one | Bacteriophage M52 spiked into the sample | 8 | 45 | 110 min. | <40 |
| Power check 2019-nCoV Real-time PCR, Kogene Biotech | CFX96, ABI7500, Gentier 96 | E, RdRd/two | Recombinant DNA Plasmid spiked into PCR mixture | 5 | 40 | 120 min. | ≤35 |
| Real-Q 2019-nCoV Detection, Biosewoon | CFX96, ABI7500 | E, RdRd/one | Human RNase P, Intrinsic | 5 | 40 | 110 min. | Target genes:<38 Internal Control:≤35 |
| Standard Mn CoV Real-time Detection, SD Biosensor | CFX96, ABI7500, LC480 | E, RdRd/one | Pseudovirus particle Spiking of 5μl into the sample or 0.5μl into the PCR mixture | 10 | 45, including 5 pre-amplifications | 90 min. | Target genes:≤36* Internal Control:≤32* |

SARS-CoV-2, Severe acute respiratory syndrome corona virus 2; Ct, cycle threshold.
*Pre-amplification was not counted for Ct.

## 1.5. Sample Processing by Biocredit COVID-19 Ag

The sample volume recommended by the BIOCREDIT COVID-19 Ag kit was 90–150 μL. To unify the sample volume, 100 μL sample volume was used. We assessed two sample processing methods based on the nature of the samples (Mak et al., 2020).

### *1.5.1. For Less Viscous Samples*

Preparation was not needed for these samples, 100 μL sample was added straight into a sample well of the device (Mak et al., 2020).

### *1.5.2. For Viscous Samples*

For collecting samples, the swab which was provided by the kit was used and the swab was immersed in the provided assay diluent tube. The succeeding processes were carried out as per the manufacturer's instructions. For effectively comparing the performance of these two sample processing methods (i.e., methods for handling less viscous and viscous samples), LOD was determined using a serial tenfold dilution of the virus. After that, the results were compared with viral culture and RT-PCR (Mak et al., 2020). Table 1 shows the comparison of PCR Kits for 2019-nCoV Detection: Exploring Kit Names and PCR equipment with targeted genes (Hur et al., 2020).

## 1.6. Viral Culture for SARS-CoV-2 Virus

The viral culture was conducted by inoculating samples onto Vero E6 cells. When the virus-induced cytopathic effect was scrutinized, the identification of the SARS-CoV-2 virus in culture fluid was established by the RT-PCR (Mak et al., 2020).

## 1.7. Virus Culture

By standard methodology, the virus culture can be done as defined by Kim et al. (2020). Concisely the Vero cells which were cultured 1 × Dulbecco's modified Eagle's medium (DMEM) supplemented with 2% fetal bovine serum at 37°C with 5% $CO_2$; used for the inoculation of nasopharyngeal and oropharyngeal samples (Kim et al., 2020). Three days afterwards of inoculation the particular cytopathic effects were detected. Later on, by using real-time RT PCR they are also deep-rooted. Investigators from Wuhan, China have completed virus isolation on human airway epithelial cells and Vero E6 and Huh-7 cell lines by inoculation of bronchoalveolar-lavage samples, and the isolated virus was titled 2019-nCoV (Zhu et al., 2020). Using the human airway epithelial cell cultures for virus isolation is a skillful labor concentrated chore, nonetheless, these were found very promising for the investigation of respiratory pathogens in humans (Jonsdottir and Dijkman, 2016).

An Indian study recently reported the First isolation of SARS-CoV-2 by using Vero CCL-81 cells (Sarkale et al., 2020). The inoculated cells with upper respiratory samples were then fastened, dried out, and carefully cut into sections using the standard methodology described by Kim et al., (2020). Kim et al., (2020) stated that they have witnessed Coronavirus-specific morphology and found the virus particle size ranged from 70 to 90 nm. They also found that the virus is observed in a wide variety of intracellular organelles particularly in vesicles (Kim et al., 2020). These kinds of sensitive cultures need to be conducted in a bio-safety Level-3 facility. The cell culture is very beneficial for the isolation and characterization of viruses; however, ultimately the cell culture for virus isolation is not suggested for diagnostic purposes (Mathuria and Yadav, 2020).

## 2. Indirect Diagnosis of SARS-CoV-2 Infection

The indirect diagnosis of SARS-CoV-2 infection is grounded on the finding of particular Immunoglobulin G (IgG) and/or Immunoglobulin M (IgM) antibodies. Even though nucleic acid testing is the common standard technique to measure the viral load in an individual, its low positivity rate has necessitated the need to develop other indirect possibilities with higher diagnostic accuracy. Prominently, the World Health Organization (WHO) highlights a strong requirement for serological IgM and IgG testing and a quick design of easy and economical point-of-care (POC) tests (Cheng et al., 2020; Gomes, 2020; Yang et al., 2020). Many authors have studied the dynamics of antibody responses.

The prime viral load and antibody expression on deep-throat saliva specimens (posterior nasopharyngeal samples) were evaluated by To et al., (2020) signifying that serological testing might be harmonizing with RT-PCR testing; the authors observed that typically within 10 days after symptom onset and positively correlated with neutralizing antibody titers, IgG and IgM responses against the internal viral NP and the S protein receptor-binding domain (RBD) occurred; antibodies against RBD displayed an earlier upsurge when matched to those against NP, and an increase of IgG former to IgM was perceived. Furthermore, they exhibited a more extended RT-PCR positivity in patients who formed antibodies in the initial stages with a poor prognosis (Zhang et al., 2006; Liu et al., 2019) Examining 173 patients with SARS-CoV-2 infection, seroconversion was observed in less than 40% of the patients by Zhao et al. (2020) within 1-week from the onset of symptoms and in all patients (94.3% for IgM and 79.8% for IgG) within day 15 after clinical presentation.

In April 2020, antibody dynamics were evaluated by Lee et al., (2020) in a Chinese cohort of 285 COVID-19 patients, using a magnetic chemiluminescence immunoassay (MCLIA). All individuals had virus-specific IgG nearly at day 17–19 after the onset of symptoms, while 94.1% had virus-specific IgM at day 20–22. Besides, greater IgG titers were witnessed in patients with a severe course of sickness compared to those without ($P = 0.001$) (Lee et al., 2020). Xie et al., (2020) developed an IgM-IgG combined assay to check the sensitivity among suspected COVID-19 patients. They concluded that IgM-IgG tests prove to be an accurate method as patients with severe illness tend to get exposed to the virus for a prolonged time duration thereby developing serious inflammatory responses. However, it is to be noted that for future aspects, a combination of both, nucleic acid testing as well as immunoglobulin markers might validate to be more successful for early detection and treatment of this novel virus (Xie et al., 2020). More than a few serological immunoassays have been developed for the correct detection of SARS-CoV-2 viral proteins and antibodies in human serum or plasma samples. The most extensively used commercial tests are established on rapid lateral flow immunoassay (LFIA), automated chemiluminescence immunoassay (CLIA), and enzyme-linked immunosorbent assay (ELISA) (Vashist, 2020). Table 2 shows the characteristics of different indirect tests for SARS-CoV-2 (Vashist, 2020).

### 2.1. Enzyme-Linked Immunosorbent Assay (ELISA)

ELISA is a scientific technique to detect anti-SARS-CoV-2 IgG and IgM responses by recognizing antibodies against the NP and spike proteins; however, the absenteeism of well-defined standards symbolizes a drawback.

**Table 2.** Characteristics of Different Indirect Test for SARS-CoV-2

| SARS-CoV-2 Test | Type | Specimen | Specific Infrastructural requirement | Optimal Timing for testing | Turnaround Time (days) | Se (%) | Sp (%) |
|---|---|---|---|---|---|---|---|
| ELISA | IgG and IgM | Human serum, Plasma, whole blood | Yes | After 17-19 days from infection | 240 | ≈82* | ≈97* |
| CLIA | IgM and IgG | Human serum, Plasma, whole blood | Yes | After 17-19 days from infection | 30 | ≈79.9§ | ≈100§ |
| Rapid Detection test | IgG and IgM | Finger prick samples | No | After 17-19 days from infection | 10-30 | ≈88§ | ≈90.63§ |

Abbreviations: ELISA, enzyme-linked immunosorbent assay; CLIA, chemiluminescence immunoassay; Se, sensitivity; Sp, specificity.
*Data from meta-analysis: §Data from small cohort.

In the latest meta-analysis whose objective was to scrutinize the precision of available tests to detect SARS-CoV-2 infection in Brazil, the pooled diagnostic measures of ELISA tests had a sensitivity ratio of 82% and a specificity ratio of 97% for IgM antibodies, and 97% sensitivity ratio and 98% specificity ratio for IgG antibodies respectively (Castro et al., 2020). As ELISA is a time-consuming procedure, companies prepare automated methods for quick detection of the antibodies in the samples provided. However, when it comes to COVID-19, several other facts come into consideration as well as the seroconversion is highly based on the onset of symptoms thereby the day on which the test is being performed is considered highly important (Ejazi et al., 2021). Lie et al. (2020) have established that the sensitivity of the ELISA test to detect IgM/IgG antibodies is at its peak when performed five days before the onset of symptoms or ten days after (Liu et al., 2020). Similar results have been concurred by Adam et al. (2020).

## 2.2. Chemiluminescent Immunoassay (CLIA)

CLIA offers noteworthy benefits over outdated assay detection methods, specifically in the quantification of antibodies. Light-producing chemical reactions (a substrate reacts with the Avidin-Horseradish Peroxidase resulting in light development) permitted approximating the titers of IgG and IgM by the total of the emitted luminous signal. Apart from this, Padoan et al. (2020), analyzed the kinetics of anti-SARS-CoV-2 IgG and IgM antibodies by CLIA, presenting a prompt upsurge in IgM and IgG after 6–7 days from symptom onset. Precisely from day 1 to day 5 after symptom onset, no patient had measurable IgM and IgG; between days 6-7, about 50% were positive for IgM and 66.6% for IgG antibodies, and between days 12-13 the positivity ratio has increased to 77.8% for IgM and 100% for IgG respectively (Russo et al., 2020).

With the occurrence of the pandemic, numerous researchers have scrutinized the response of antibodies through CLIA immunoassay (Ejazi et al., 2021). On one hand, a retrospective study has shown that the positivity rate of IgM antibodies increases only during the initial stage followed by a continuous rapid drop whereas the positivity rate of IgG antibodies reaches as far as a hundred percent (Jin et al., 2020). On the other hand, another study performed retrospectively communicated that the rate of detection was maximum during 16-18 days in the case of IgM and 19-21 with respect to IgM (Hu et al., 2020). Various other serological studies performed across the globe have exhibited a high rate of sensitivity for IgG as and when compared with IgM when performed with the commercial CLIA test (Bryan et al., 2020; Padoan et al., 2020; Zhong et al., 2020). Incidentally, Zeng et al. (2020) have claimed higher IgG antibodies among the female population when compared with the males specifically during the early stage of the viral infection (Zeng et al., 2020).

## 2.3. Rapid Serological Tests

Many companies have developed several rapid IgM/IgG tests, chiefly based on immunoassay technology (Li et al., 2020) providing results in less time than 10–15 minutes. These test devices encompass not only the colloidal gold-labeled recombinant protein but also are surrounded by the murine anti-human IgG and murine anti-human IgM antibodies immobilized in the G and M area (Russo et al., 2020). However, before the authorization of rapid tests for mass screening of COVID-19, their clinical accuracy needs to be rigorously estimated. The manufacturers proclaim a relative specificity of 100% and a sensitivity of 81% in cases wherein observations have taken place between day 4 and day 10 post the onset of symptoms and a relative sensitivity of 97% between days 11 and 24. Cassaniti et al. (2020) did a comparison of the results of rapid serological tests with those of nasopharyngeal swabs in 30 healthy individuals who tested positive for SARS-CoV-2 and 50 individuals who were admitted with fever and respiratory troubles.

The result of the IgM/IgG testing claimed all the healthy individuals to be negative for the viral infection whereas the patients admitted to the emergency department with respiratory syndrome expressed positive for both IgG as well as IgM antibodies, however, the percentage of positivity differed among the cases. Remarkably, out of the 50 patients, thirty-eight were tested positive with RT-PCR and only seven with the rapid testing method. Based on current data, WHO does not acclaim the use of antibody-detecting rapid diagnostic tests for patient care and management, nevertheless, their committee members keep encouraging the continuation of hard work in disease surveillance and epidemiological research (WHO, 2021).

## 2.4. Direct Diagnosis of SARS-CoV-2 Infection

The direct diagnosis of SARS-CoV-2 infection is fundamentally grounded on the recognition of SARS-CoV-2 RNA on nasopharyngeal swabs or lower respiratory tract samples (WHO, 2020). The former is most extensively used in clinical practice, even though tests on lower respiratory tract specimens are performed in certain defined cases (WHO, 2020). In patients with good results, the RNA virus can be detected for as long as twenty days or even more after the onset of customary symptoms. Also, it has been noted that even after the viral load becomes undetectable with a polymerase chain reaction, a rebound of the viral load is possible (To et al., 2020).

Additionally, as accounted earlier, the RT-PCR positivity rate for SARS-CoV-2 RNA peaks around 7-10 days in the upper respiratory tracts of humans after the initial onset of the infection-related symptoms followed by a gradual drop; on the contrary, RT-PCR RNA detection in lower respiratory tract specimens remains unchanged for three weeks after symptom onset/clinical presentation (To et al., 2020). The features for ideal testing for a direct diagnosis of SARS-CoV-2 infection comprise short turnaround time, high throughput, least batching, low infrastructural necessities, raised precision, low price to allow access to testing, also bearing in mind testing primacies to diagnose susceptible populations, and to lessen viral spread, specifically in nosocomial, family, and closed community settings (Russo et al., 2020; Wang et al., 2020).

Nucleic acid testing (real-time RT-qPCR) on respiratory tract samples has many of these mentioned features, hence demonstrating the current benchmark in the diagnosis of SARS-CoV-2 infection (WHO, 2021). But, several factors, either procedural or virus-related, may weaken its dependability, (Lippi et al., 2020) for instance a single-time point (Lee et al., 2020) and an unmet need for procedural standardization (Liu et al., 2020) (from sample collection, as well as swab types, to processing) remains complex by lacks of workforces and resources (Cheng et al., 2020; Osterman et al., 2021). For these explanations, innovative rapid tests (either based on antigens or antibodies), point-of-care (POC) assays, and digital technologies would support infection detection and containment, also in low- and middle-income settings, but need cautious estimation (Cheng et al., 2020; Edward, 2020; Mahmood et al., 2020; Yang et al., 2020).

### *2.4.1. Reverse-Transcription-PCR for SARS-CoV-2 Virus*

Among all the nucleic acid-based testing methodologies, RT-PCR stands out to be the most widely used among scientists and clinicians because of certain desirable features like quick detection and high sensitivity. Several diagnostic companies and scientific teams have come together over the past couple of months to detect the viral infection with improved efficacy. A one-step method was introduced that can effectively produce ten copies but its limitations to generate false-positive made it undesirable, thereby giving rise to a novel RNA-dependant RNA polymerase assay (Li and Ren, 2020). For the detection of SARS-CoV-2 virus nucleic acid presence in provided samples, in-house developed RT-PCR was used. It was conducted using Master Mix (Roche Diagnostics GmbH, Germany) and NxtScript Enzyme. The reaction mixture constituted of 5 μL RNA samples, 0.06 μL Adpta Taq DNA polymerase, 0.05 μL NxtScript RT Enzyme, and 0.9 μL volume of working primer/probe mix. The mixture was brought to the final volume of 10 μL with the addition of nuclease-free water. The working primer/probe mix was prepared by mixing an equal volume of the forward primer. RT-PCR was then performed in the LC 480 system at the given standard temperature and duration (Mak et al., 2020).

### *2.4.2. The Quantitative Reverse-Transcription Polymerase Chain Reaction (RT-PCR)*

In January 2020, from Wuhan's patients providing information on viral genetic sequencing, the novel coronavirus was isolated, accessible at the Global Initiative on Sharing All Influenza Data (GISAID), sanctioning the development of the particular diagnostic methods for COVID-19 through RT-PCR system, i.e, quantitative Real-Time amplifications headed by RNA extraction from the nasopharyngeal and oropharyngeal secretions, followed by a reverse transcription step to transform RNA into complementary DNA (cDNA) that will undergo amplification. The RT-PCRs that have been applied to COVID-19 diagnosis comprise fluorescent probes that will identify and hybridize to sections of the amplification products, raising the specificity of the assays (Corman et al., 2020; Singh et al., 2020; Tan et al., 2020). The RT-PCR is the touchstone for the confirmation of COVID-19 infection in upper respiratory samples (nasopharyngeal and oropharyngeal secretion). Numerous RT-PCR protocols were published by WHO to provide an appropriate diagnosis, aid testing populations, and contribute to controlling the further spread of the disease (Table 3) (Singh et al., 2020; Wang et al., 2020).

**Table 3.** Description of the most used RT-PCR for diagnosing SARS-Cov-2

| Institution/country | Primer ID | Method | Findings | References |
|---|---|---|---|---|
| China's CDC – China | ORF1ab, E, and N | Three singleplex RT-PCR using fluorescent-labeled probes | The lowest detection limit of ORF1ab was 203 copies/mL<br>The lowest detection limit of the E gene was 664 copies/mL<br>The lowest detection limit of the N gene was 667 copies/mL | Castro et al., 2020; Vashist, 2020 |
| Institut Pasteur – France | RdRp gene/nCoV_IP2<br>RdRp gene/nCoV_IP4 | Two singleplex RT-PCR or one multiplex RT-PCR with fluorescent-labeled probes | 95% assertiveness in samples containing ~100 viral copies<br>The multiplex RT-PCR detects 10 viral copies<br>No cross-reactivity with other viruses | Vashist, 2020 |
| CDC – USA | 2019-nCoV_N1<br>2019-nCoV_N2<br>2019-nCoV_N3 | Three singleplex RT-PCR using fluorescent-labeled probes | 95% assertiveness in samples containing 100,5 RNA copies/µL using automatic RNA extraction and 100<br>RNA copies/µL using manual RNA extraction | Vashist, 2020; Ejazi et al., 2021 |
| Charité – Germany | RdRP_SARSr<br>E_Sarbeco | Two singleplex RT-PCR, the screening made by the E gene amplification confirmed by RdRP | The lowest detection limit of RdRp and E_Sarbeco 3.8 and 5.2 copies/reaction, respectively | Liu et al., 2020; Vashist, 2020 |
| HKU - Hong Kong | ORF1b-nsp14<br>N | Two RT-PCR, firstly the N gene amplification with fluorescent-labeled probe followed by confirmation by amplifying the ORF1b-nsp14 with the fluorescent-labeled probe | N gene Ct values up to 35.43 were positive corresponding to 15 copies/reaction<br>ORF1b Ct values up to 38.97 were positive corresponding to 1.5 copies/reaction | Adams et al., 2020; Vashist, 2020 |
| National Institute of Health – Thailand | N | Singleplex RT-PCR with the fluorescent-labeled probe | N gene Ct values were positive up to 38.12, corresponding to 15 copies/reaction | Adams et al., 2020; Vashist, 2020 |

CDC = Center for Disease Control and Prevention; HKU = Hong Kong University.

Institut Pasteur (France) has designed the protocol for RT-PCR which exhibited brilliant results in comparison with the protocol from Charité (Germany), considered the reference RT-PCR, getting close 95% assertiveness in samples encompassing about 100 copies of the SARS-CoV-2 genome. In this protocol, two targets from the RNA-dependent RNA Polymerase (RdRP) gene of SARS-CoV-2 were assessed distinctly, and then the primers were joined in multiplex RT-PCR assays bring about the detection of samples comprising 10 copies of the virus genome (Habibzadeh et al., 2021). Evaluation of the specificity was done using samples containing some other respiratory viruses (H1N1, H3N2, B-Victoria, B-Yamagata, influenza C, RSV A and B, hBoV, hPIV, hMPV, HRV/enterovirus, adenovirus, HKU1, OC43, 229E and NL63) and no one of them was detected with the RdRp gene/nCoV-IP2 and 429 (Oliveira et al., 2020).

With the unprecedented rise in the current pandemic, healthcare facilities have brought forward diagnostic tools to detect the presence of SARS-CoV-2 either with the help of RT-qPCR alone or in a pool of different sizes, varying from 2- to 64-sample pools. Application of such a grouping system, when implemented with standard protocols and associated reagents for the identification of COVID-19, has proven to be of adequate predictive value not only in close-knit groups like hospital or army units but also in the community in general (Yelin et al., 2020). Hirotsu et al. (2020) have validated the accomplishment of a new antigen test that has been developed based on the chemiluminescence enzyme immunoassay henceforth confirming the so-called LUMIULSE antigen test to be one of the most effective tests that can rapidly identify symptomatic individuals carrying moderate to severe viral load (Hirotsu et al., 2020).

Even though RT-PCR has been labeled as the gold standard for diagnosing COVID-19, there are quite a few problems involving its use (Li and Ren, 2020; Singh et al., 2020; Wang et al., 2020; Zhang et al., 2020). The RT-PCR kit which was distributed by China's CDC was aimed to detect the nucleocapsid (N) and the Open Reading Frame ORF1ab of the SARS-CoV-2 genome, and the infection is confirmed when both the markers are amplified. But, it is not uncommon that the results are varying owing to the amplification of only one of the targets (Li et al., 2020; Wang et al., 2020). One of the setbacks associated with RT-PCR for the diagnosis of COVID-19 is the inappropriate collection and processing of samples. As per some studies, samples that are obtained from the upper respiratory tract (bottom of the nostrils and the oropharynx) (Singh et al., 2020; Wang et al., 2020; Xiang et al., 2020) are optimum clinical samples due to the high viral copy amount in the respiratory tract. Apart from oral and nasal swabs, viral load levels can also be detected in the gastrointestinal tract and ultimately in blood samples, but in lesser amounts (Corman et al., 2020; Sridhar et al., 2020; Wang et al., 2020).

Yang et al. (2020) performed a study, using unalike samples (throat swabs, nasal swabs, sputum, and bronchoalveolar lavage fluid – BALF) collected in different time periods (0 to 7, 8 to 14, and more than 15 days after the onset of disease) demonstrated that excluding BALF, sputum samples conferred the highest rate of positivity followed by nasal swabs in patients from severe to mild symptoms in the initial 14 days after the onset of the infectious disease. It has been noted that the positivity rate subsequently reduced after the $15^{th}$ day of the disease (Tahamtan and Ardebili, 2020; Yang et al., 2020). BALF was considered significant for observing and diagnosing severe cases, whereas throat swabs presented the lowest positivity among the samples (CDC, 2020; Tahamtan and Ardebili, 2020).

Different viral load kinetics were found in a report of two Korean patients signifying distinctions among infected people. In the first patient between two and three days after the onset of symptoms in both, the lower and the upper respiratory tract, the virus was detected. However, viral load levels reduced on the $7^{th}$ day, continuing to be positive until the $13^{th}$ day. On the other hand, in the second patient, the virus was detected on the $14^{th}$ day of symptoms in the lower and the upper respiratory tract, becoming untraceable from the $18^{th}$ to $20^{th}$ day, but then coming back positive on the $25^{th}$ day (Tahamtan and Ardebili, 2020). To guarantee the paramount performance of the technique and to evade RNA degradation, following the swab collection, the samples are submerged in a transport medium/lysis buffer or a sterile saline solution1, (CDC, 2020; Sridhar et al., 2020; Habibzadeh et al., 2021). Specimens must be kept at 2-8°C for up to 72 hours after sampling. When the test will not be done in a short period, the samples should be kept at even much lower temperatures, as a minimum of -70°C (CDC, 2020; Habibzadeh et al., 2021).

An additional struggle in carrying out RT-PCR is the postponement of releasing results during the pandemic (Singh et al., 2020; Wang et al., 2020). The RNA extraction step, part of the diagnostic protocol, takes a lot of time, particularly if there is no computerized platform to execute this process (Arumugam and Wong, 2020; Grant et al., 2020), opening ambiguities for the happening of cross-contamination between samples and of biological hazards to the handler, if the laboratory worker is not using appropriate personal protection equipment when manipulating high viral load respiratory secretions (Aslanzadeh, 2004; Schmid-Burgk et al., 2020; Wang et al., 2020). Certain studies have been carried out to reduce the diagnostic period using RT-PCR, and the outcomes have shown that the RNA extraction step can be side-stepped in the diagnosis of COVID-19 (Grant et al., 2020; Merindol et al., 2020). Grant et al., (2020) designed an RT-PCR for COVID-19 that does not go through a preceding RNA extraction step, and this system was compared with a high-yield automated platform (Panther Fusion Hologic) that reached 98% sensitivity and 100% specificity. The authors established that the RT-PCR with no previous RNA extraction step has improved the performance of the technique. To strengthen this idea, Arumugam and Wong (2020), dealing with samples from influenza-suspected cases, confirmed that the RNA extraction step is not essential, provided that the patient's nasal swab is submerged in a viral transport medium. These results were validated in samples from COVID-19 patients (Beltrán-Pavez et al., 2020; Bruce et al., 2020).

Besides the formerly stated difficulties related to RT-PCR, precise information and expert technical training are required to perform these amplifications, apart from the high expenditures of reagents and thermocyclers. The occurrence of RT-PCR false-positive results is related to handling inaccuracies and cross-contamination of samples, whereas false-negative results are related to inappropriate sample collection, storage, and processing (Singh et al., 2020; Wang et al., 2020).

### *2.4.3. Real-Time PCR Tests*

With the ongoing pandemic, sensitive and specific testing has become an important criterion for the clinical management of COVID-19. Primers were typically designed keeping the ongoing scenario and LOD in mind. Employing 96 SARS-CoV-2 AND 104 non-SARS-CoV-2 specific virus genomes, the GolayMEtaMiner genome subtraction was locally identified which showed complete concordance with the pre-developed reference assay (Yip et al., 2020). So far, Real-time RT-PCR is the utmost choice for SARS-CoV-2 RNA detection technology (CDC, 2020). In many real-time PCR tests, the primers were designed such that they stand against the envelope (E) and RNA-dependent RNA polymerase (RdRp) regions (Corman et al., 2020) for first-line screening the E-region was used, whereas for confirmatory testing the RdRp section was engaged. The open reading frame (ORF) 1b and N regions of SARS-CoV-2 were used for screening and as confirmatory tests simultaneously. Apart from this, other investigators developed one-step RT-PCR assays (Chu et al., 2020). The precise primers could also bind other coronaviruses and closely related viruses since ORF1b and N regions are highly preserved in *Sarbecoviruses*. As regards the RT-PCR performances, a current meta-analysis by Kim et al., (2020) considering 19 studies acknowledged a pooled sensitivity of 89% (95% CI = 81–94%; I2 = 90%), but the positive predictive value (PPV) stretched from 47.3–98.3% and the negative predictive value (NPV) stretched from 93.4–99.9%. Indeed, false-negative results might not only originate from poor sensitivity, but they can also be due to little amount of sample, insufficient conservation, or the existence of amplification inhibitors or mutations in the target regions of the particular primer used (Kim et al., 2020; Wang et al., 2020; Xiao et al., 2020). For instance, it was observed that, of the 610 patients registered, 63% had negative specimens at baseline, 12% turned out to be positive at the second swab whereas only 3% showed positive results at the third (Li et al., 2020). Comparable results were reported by Xiao et al., (2020) as well. Therefore, a negative result does not eliminate SARS-CoV-2 infection and should not be used unaccompanied for clinical management (Russo et al., 2020).

To identify an optimal sample type, the nasopharyngeal swab remains the benchmark for SARS-CoV-2 RNA detection. The probability of performing RT-PCR on saliva samples was highlighted by Azzi et al., (2020) whereof all the patients included in the study resulted in coronavirus-positive with RT-PCR employing nasopharyngeal swabs of significance, the collection of a single lower respiratory specimen or sequential upper respiratory specimens may be indispensable to detect the virus in subjects exhibiting symptoms with early negative RT-PCR testing. In reality, Guo et al., (2020) displayed that RT-PCR executed on throat washing samples was more correct for COVID-19 diagnosis than nasopharyngeal swab samples *($P < 0.031$).*

### 2.4.4. Reverse-Transcription-Loop-Mediated Isothermal Amplification (RT-LAMP)

Over the past few years, for the prompt detection of virus-specific genes, with a specificity and sensitivity comparable to that stated for RT-PCR assays, the loop-mediated isothermal amplification (LAMP) method, which consists of exponential amplification of particular nucleic acid sequences at a constant temperature, has been commonly used. The Loop-mediated isothermal amplification (LAMP) is a new-age nucleic acid amplification method that has the highest potency. Due to its effective augmented feature, it is considered to be most efficient in amplifying RNA and DNA strands. Not only the technique is rapid but also the reagents involved in it are cost-effective. Multiple strategies have been formulated to detect the novel coronavirus through this assay (Enosawa et al., 2003; Mohamadian et al., 2021). Some studies have highlighted the feasibility of the LAMP assay testing in the detection of the viral load, whereas others have proven the close connection of the level of accuracy of LAMP with that of conventional PCR testing (Poon et al., 2004; Pyrc et al., 2011). Recently, Okamaoto et al., (2020) have developed an advantageous RT-LAMP assay for subsequent monitoring of human MERS-CoV, which proved to be of great value without any cross-reaction with other categories of viruses. A grouping of LAMP with reverse transcription (rt-LAMP) allows the direct finding of RNA, together with SARS-CoV-2 RNA. It is regarded as a rapid, single-step methodology that is reliable enough to be used as screening for COVID-19 (Jiang et al., 2020; Kashir and Yaqinuddin, 2020). In a minor study, Huang et al., (2020); confirmed the RT-LAMP method by employing 16 clinical samples, eight positive and eight negatives for SARS-CoV-2 by rt-PCR: the testing outcomes were constant with the conventional rt-PCR. The LAMP technique evades a few PCR limitations, for example, the requirement for high-purity samples, trained personnel, and costly laboratory instruments (Baek et al., 2020).

### *2.4.5. Antigen-Based Tests*

Direct methods for the diagnosis of COVID-19 incorporate a double-antibody sandwich enzyme-linked immunoassay as well as recognizing the SARS-CoV-2 nucleoprotein (NP) by a microplate pre-coated with particular antibodies against SARS-CoV-2 NP and the use of horseradish peroxidase (HRP)-labeled secondary antibody against the same protein. This direct method is simple, quick, and does not need skilled workers and costly laboratory instruments. Nonetheless, Castro et al., (2020) did a meta-analysis in which the sensitivity of this test fluctuated from 70–86%, while the specificity fluctuated from 95–97%, and therefore a single negative test result cannot exclude SARS-CoV-2 infection (Khandker et al., 2021).

### *2.4.6. Electrochemical Biosensors*

They are the combination of the enantioselectivity of the electrochemical signal accelerometers and the precision of the bio-molecular recognition approach. Even though they have been extensively studied in various fields of diagnostics, their usage has not been broadly commercialized till now. With the onset of the pandemic scenario, electrochemical objectives have shown tremendous potency in addressing the limitations and setbacks of the otherwise traditional platforms thereby making the electrochemical biological sensors a strong indicator for the detection of SARS-CoV-2 viral infection (Mahshid et al., 2021).

## Conclusion

The outburst of COVID-19 occurred at the end of December 2019 and straight away surged like wildfire. It massively succeeded in challenging the worldwide health resources on one hand whereas questioning the status of general public health on the other. An early and timely diagnosis of the disease would therefore play a pivotal role as it not only helps in the early identification of the infectious cases and their clinical management but also prevents further community transmission. Currently, numerous technologies are available in the commercialized field of work for providing better diagnostic services to people in this outbreak. For proper diagnosis, it is essential to collect the right specimen at the right time. As the virus is highly infectious, one of the key challenges is to keep healthcare professionals safe by having proper PPE kits and avoiding any possibilities of infectious contact. For etiologic diagnosis of the COVID-19 cases, real-time RT-PCR assay remains the gold-standard molecular test of choice; whereas antibody-based immunological tests are used as supplementary tools for screening the mass population and sanctioning with the molecular assay. Real-time RT-PCR, as well as immunological assay, helps us to tackle this major outbreak of COVID-19 which has created havoc in peoples' lives as well as in the global economy. Additionally, rapid test kits are in great demand for providing quick diagnostic services at the patient's bedside in cases of emergencies. Selecting the suitable choice of testing technique to recognize the severity of the viral load in a particular individual based on the patients' current health condition and market-based technical availabilities plays a key role in bringing a pandemic situation under control globally. As a result, the prompt diagnosis of the novel coronavirus using the right and reliable testing method is advantageous for both patient management as well as community management.

## References

Abdelrahman, Z., Li, M., & Wang, X. (2020). Comparative review of SARS-CoV-2, SARS-CoV, MERS-CoV, and influenza a respiratory viruses. *Frontiers in Immunology*, 2, 309.

Adams, E. R., Ainsworth, M., Anand, R., Andersson, M. I., Auckland, K., Baillie, J. K., & Whitehouse, J. (2020). Evaluation of antibody testing for SARS-Cov-2 using ELISA and lateral flow immunoassays. *MedRxiv*.

Albert, E., Torres, I., Bueno, F., Huntley, D., Molla, E., Fernández-Fuentes, M. Á., & Navarro, D. (2021). Field evaluation of a rapid antigen test (Panbio™ COVID-19 Ag Rapid Test Device) for COVID-19 diagnosis in primary healthcare centers. *Clinical Microbiology and Infection*, 27(3), 472--e7.

Ao, C., Li, A., Elzaawely, A. A., Xuan, T. D., & Tawata, S. (2008). Evaluation of antioxidant and antibacterial activities of Ficus microcarpa L. fil. extract. *Food Control*, 19(10), 940–948.

Arumugam, A., & Wong, S. L. (2020). The potential use of unprocessed sample for RT-qPCR detection of COVID-19 without an RNA extraction step. *BioRxiv*.

Aslanzadeh, J. (2004). Preventing PCR amplification carryover contamination in a clinical laboratory. *Annals of Clinical \& Laboratory Science*, 34(4), 389–396.

Awadasseid, A., Wu, Y., Tanaka, Y., & Zhang, W. (2021). SARS-CoV-2 variants evolved during the early stage of the pandemic and effects of mutations on adaptation in Wuhan populations. *International Journal of Biological Sciences*, 17(1), 97.

Azzi, L., Carcano, G., Gianfagna, F., Grossi, P., Dalla Gasperina, D., Genoni, A., & Baj, A. (2020). Saliva is a reliable tool to detect SARS-CoV-2. *Journal of Infection*, 81(1), e45--e50.

Baek, Y. H., Um, J., Antigua, K. J. C., Park, J. H., Kim, Y., Oh, S., & Song, M. S. (2020). Development of a reverse transcription-loop-mediated isothermal amplification as a rapid early-detection method for novel SARS-CoV-2. *Emerging Microbes and Infections*, 9(1), 998–1007.

Beltrán-Pavez, C., Márquez, C. L., Muñoz, G., Valiente-Echeverría, F., Gaggero, A., Soto-Rifo, R., & Barriga, G. P. (2020). SARS-CoV-2 detection from nasopharyngeal swab samples without RNA extraction. *BioRxiv*.

Benvenuto, D., Giovanetti, M., Ciccozzi, A., Spoto, S., Angeletti, S., & Ciccozzi, M. (2020). The 2019-new coronavirus epidemic: evidence for virus evolution. *Journal of Medical Virology*, 92(4), 455–459.

Bruce, E. A., Huang, M. L., Perchetti, G. A., Tighe, S., Laaguiby, P., Hoffman, J. J., & Botten, J. W. (2020). Direct RT-qPCR detection of SARS-CoV-2 RNA from patient nasopharyngeal swabs without an RNA extraction step. *PLoS Biology*, *18*(10), e3000896.

Bryan, A., Pepper, G., Wener, M. H., Fink, S. L., Morishima, C., Chaudhary, A., & Greninger, A. L. (2020). Performance characteristics of the Abbott Architect SARS-CoV-2 IgG assay and seroprevalence in Boise, Idaho. *Journal of Clinical Microbiology*, 58(8), e00941-e00960.

Campbell, R. A., Boilard, E., & Rondina, M. T. (2021). Is there a role for the ACE2 receptor in SARS-CoV-2 interactions with platelets? *Journal of Thrombosis and Haemostasis*, 19(1), 46–50.

Caruana, G., Croxatto, A., Coste, A. T., Opota, O., Lamoth, F., Jaton, K., & Greub, G. (2020). Diagnostic strategies for SARS-CoV-2 infection and interpretation of microbiological results. *Clinical Microbiology and Infection*, 26(9), 1178–1182.

Cassaniti, I., Novazzi, F., Giardina, F., Salinaro, F., Sachs, M., Perlini, S., & Baldanti, F. (2020). Performance of VivaDiag COVID-19 IgM/IgG Rapid Test is inadequate for diagnosis of COVID-19 in acute patients referring to emergency room department. *Journal of Medical Virology*, 92(10):1724-1727.

Castro, R., Luz, P. M., Wakimoto, M. D., Veloso, V. G., Grinsztejn, B., & Perazzo, H. (2020). COVID-19: a meta-analysis of diagnostic test accuracy of commercial assays registered in Brazil. *Brazilian Journal of Implantology and Health Sciences*, 24, 180–187.

CDC (2020). Interim guidelines for collecting, handling, and testing clinical specimens from persons under investigation (PUIs) for coronavirus disease 2019 (COVID-19)-Overview of testing for SARS-CoV-2 (COVID-19). Centers for Disease Control and Prevention.

Cerutti, F., Burdino, E., Milia, M. G., Allice, T., Gregori, G., Bruzzone, B., & Ghisetti, V. (2020). Urgent need of rapid tests for SARS CoV-2 antigen detection: Evaluation of the SD-Biosensor antigen test for SARS-CoV-2. *Journal of Clinical Virology*, 132, 104654.

Chan, J. F. W., Kok, K. H., Zhu, Z., Chu, H., To, K. K. W., Yuan, S., & Yuen, K. Y. (2020). Genomic characterization of the 2019 novel human-pathogenic coronavirus isolated from a patient with atypical pneumonia after visiting Wuhan. *Emerging Microbes and Infections*, 9(1), 221–236.

Cheng, M. P., Papenburg, J., Desjardins, M., Kanjilal, S., Quach, C., Libman, M., & Yansouni, C. P. (2020). Diagnostic testing for severe acute respiratory syndrome--related coronavirus 2: a narrative review. *Annals of Internal Medicine*, 172(11), 726–734.

Chia, W. N., Tan, C. W., Foo, R., Kang, A. E. Z., Peng, Y., Sivalingam, V., Tiu, C., Ong, X. M., Zhu, F., & Young, B. E. (2020). Serological differentiation between COVID-19 and SARS infections. *Emerging Microbes and Infections*, 9(1), 1497–1505.

Chu, D. K., Pan, Y., Cheng, S. M., Hui, K. P., Krishnan, P., Liu, Y., & Poon, L. L. M. (2020). Molecular diagnosis of a novel coronavirus (2019-nCoV) causing an outbreak of pneumonia. *Clinical Chemistry*, 66(4), 549–555.

Corman, V. M., Landt, O., Kaiser, M., Molenkamp, R., Meijer, A., Chu, D. K. W., & Drosten, C. (2020). Detection of 2019 novel coronavirus (2019-nCoV) by real-time RT-PCR. *Eurosurveillance*, 25(3), 2000045.

Cui, J., Li, F., & Shi, Z. L. (2019). Origin and evolution of pathogenic coronaviruses. *Nature Reviews Microbiology*, 17(3), 181–192.

Dan, S., Pant, M., & Upadhyay, S. K. (2020). The case fatality rate in COVID-19 patients with cardiovascular disease: global health challenge and paradigm in the current pandemic. *Current Pharmacology Reports*, 6, 315–324.

Diao, B., Wen, K., Zhang, J., Chen, J., Han, C., Chen, Y., & Wu, Y. (2021). Accuracy of a nucleocapsid protein antigen rapid test in the diagnosis of SARS-CoV-2 infection. *Clinical Microbiology and Infection*, 27(2), 289--e1.

Dominguez, S. R., O'Shea, T. J., Oko, L. M., & Holmes, K. V. (2007). Detection of group 1 coronaviruses in bats in North America. *Emerging Infectious Diseases*, 13(9), 1295.

Edward, R. (2020). *An overview of the rapid test situation for COVID-19 diagnosis in the EU/EEA*. European Centre for Disease Prevention and Control: An agency of the European Union. https://www.ecdc.europa.eu/en/publications-data/overview-rapid-test-situation-covid-19-diagnosis-eueea.

Ejazi, S. A., Ghosh, S., & Ali, N. (2021). Antibody detection assays for COVID-19 diagnosis: an early overview. *Immunology and Cell Biology*, 99(1), 21–33.

Elrashdy, F., Redwan, E. M., & Uversky, V. N. (2020). Why COVID-19 transmission is more efficient and aggressive than viral transmission in previous coronavirus epidemics? *Biomolecules*, 10(9), 1312.

Enosawa, M., Kageyama, S., Sawai, K., Watanabe, K., Notomi, T., Onoe, S., & Yokomizo, Y. (2003). Use of loop-mediated isothermal amplification of the IS 900 sequence for rapid detection of cultured Mycobacterium avium subsp. paratuberculosis. *Journal of Clinical Microbiology*, 41(9), 4359–4365.

Gomes, C. (2020). Report of the WHO-China joint mission on coronavirus disease 2019 (COVID-19). *Brazilian Journal of Implantology and Health Sciences*, 2(3).

Gralinski, L. E., & Menachery, V. D. (2020). Return of the Coronavirus: 2019-nCoV. *Viruses*, 12(2), 135.

Grant, P. R., Turner, M. A., Shin, G. Y., Nastouli, E., & Levett, L. J. (2020). Extraction-free COVID-19 (SARS-CoV-2) diagnosis by RT-PCR to increase capacity for national testing programmes during a pandemic. *BioRxiv*.

Guo, W. L., Jiang, Q., Ye, F., Li, S. Q., Hong, C., Chen, L. Y., & Li, S. Y. (2020). Effect of throat washings on detection of 2019 novel coronavirus. *Clinical Infectious Diseases*, 71(8), 1980–1981.

Habibzadeh, P., Mofatteh, M., Silawi, M., Ghavami, S., & Faghihi, M. A. (2021). Molecular diagnostic assays for COVID-19: an overview. *Critical Reviews in Clinical Laboratory Sciences*, 58(6), 385–398.

Hanson, G., & Coller, J. (2018). Codon optimality, bias and usage in translation and mRNA decay. *Nature Reviews Molecular Cell Biology*, 19(1), 20–30.

Hellou, M. M., Górska, A., Mazzaferri, F., Cremonini, E., Gentilotti, E., De Nardo, P., & Paul, M. (2021). Nucleic acid amplification tests on respiratory samples for the diagnosis of coronavirus infections: a systematic review and meta-analysis. *Clinical Microbiology and Infection*, 27(3), 341–351.

Hirotsu, Y., Maejima, M., Shibusawa, M., Nagakubo, Y., Hosaka, K., Amemiya, K., & Omata, M. (2020). Comparison of automated SARS-CoV-2 antigen test for COVID-19 infection with quantitative RT-PCR using 313 nasopharyngeal swabs, including from seven serially followed patients. *International Journal of Infectious Diseases*, 99, 397–402.

Hong, K. H., Lee, S. W., Kim, T. S., Huh, H. J., Lee, J., Kim, S. Y., & Yoo, C. K. (2020). Guidelines for laboratory diagnosis of coronavirus disease 2019 (COVID-19) in Korea. *Annals of Laboratory Medicine*, 40(5), 351–360.

Hossain, M. G., Javed, A., Akter, S., & Saha, S. (2021). SARS-CoV-2 host diversity: An update of natural infections and experimental evidence. *Journal of Microbiology, Immunology and Infection*, 54(2), 175–181.

Hu, Q., Cui, X., Liu, X., Peng, B., Jiang, J., & Wang, X. (2020). The production of antibodies for SARS-CoV-2 and its clinical implication. *MedRxiv*.

Huang, W. E., Lim, B., Hsu, C.-C., Xiong, D., Wu, W., Yu, Y., & Cui, Z. (2020). RT-LAMP for rapid diagnosis of coronavirus SARS-CoV-2. *Microbial Biotechnology*, 13(4), 950–961.

Hui, D. S., Azhar, E. I., Madani, T. A., Ntoumi, F., Kock, R., Dar, O., Ippolito, G., Mchugh, T. D., Memish, Z. A., & Drosten, C. (2020). The continuing 2019-nCoV epidemic threat of novel coronaviruses to global health—The latest 2019 novel coronavirus outbreak in Wuhan, China. *International Journal of Infectious Diseases*, 91, 264–266.

Hur, K. H., Park, K., Lim, Y., Jeong, Y.-S., Sung, H., & Kim, M.-N. (2020). Evaluation of four commercial kits for SARS-CoV-2 real-time reverse-transcription polymerase chain reaction approved by emergency-use-authorization in Korea. *Frontiers in Medicine*, 5, 521.

Jiang, M., Pan, W., Arasthfer, A., Fang, W., Ling, L., Fang, H., & Lass-Flörl, C. (2020). Development and validation of a rapid, single-step reverse transcriptase loop-mediated isothermal amplification (RT-LAMP) system potentially to be used for reliable and high-throughput screening of COVID-19. *Frontiers in Cellular and Infection Microbiology*, 10, 331.

Jin, Y., Wang, M., Zuo, Z., Fan, C., Ye, F., Cai, Z., & Xu, A. (2020). Diagnostic value and dynamic variance of serum antibody in coronavirus disease 2019. *International Journal of Infectious Diseases*, 94, 49–52.

Jonsdottir, H. R., & Dijkman, R. (2016). Coronaviruses and the human airway: a universal system for virus-host interaction studies. *Virology Journal*, 13(1), 1–9.

Kashir, J., & Yaqinuddin, A. (2020). Loop mediated isothermal amplification (LAMP) assays as a rapid diagnostic for COVID-19. *Medical Hypotheses*, 141, 109786.

Khairat, S. M., Guindy, N. E., Motaleb, M. S. E. A., & Soliman, N. S. (2020). Evaluation of two rapid antigen tests for detection of SARS-CoV-2 virus. *Journal of Microbiology and Biotechnology*, 5(3), 131–134.

Khandker, S. S., Nik Hashim, N. N., Deris, Z. Z., Shueb, R. H., & Islam, M. A. (2021). Diagnostic accuracy of rapid antigen test kits for detecting SARS-CoV-2: A systematic review and meta-analysis of 17,171 suspected COVID-19 Patients. *Journal of Clinical Medicine*, 10(16), 3493.

Kim, H., Hong, H., & Yoon, S. H. (2020). Diagnostic performance of CT and reverse transcriptase polymerase chain reaction for coronavirus disease 2019: a meta-analysis. *Radiology*, 296(3), E145--E155.

Kim, J. M., Chung, Y. S., Jo, H. G., Lee, N. J., Kim, M. S., Woo, S. H., & Han, M. G. (2020). Identification of coronavirus isolated from a patient in Korea with COVID-19. *Osong Public Health and Research Perspectives*, 11(1), 3–7.

Konrad, R., Eberle, U., Dangel, A., Treis, B., Berger, A., Bengs, K., & Sing, A. (2020). Rapid establishment of laboratory diagnostics for the novel coronavirus SARS-CoV-2 in Bavaria, Germany, February 2020. *Eurosurveillance*, 25(9), 2000173.

Kuba, K., Imai, Y., Rao, S., Gao, H., Guo, F., Guan, B., & Penninger, J. M. (2005). A crucial role of angiotensin converting enzyme 2 (ACE2) in SARS coronavirus--induced lung injury. *Nature Medicine*, 11(8), 875–879.

Kweon, O. J., Lim, Y. K., Kim, H. R., Choi, Y., Kim, M. C., Choi, S. H., Chung, J. W., & Lee, M. K. (2021). Evaluation of rapid SARS-CoV-2 antigen tests, AFIAS COVID-19 Ag and ichroma COVID-19 Ag, with serial nasopharyngeal specimens from COVID-19 patients. *PloS One*, 16(4), e0249972.

Lee, Y. H., Hong, C. M., Kim, D. H., Lee, T. H., & Lee, J. (2020). Clinical course of asymptomatic and mildly symptomatic patients with coronavirus disease admitted to community treatment centers, South Korea. *Emerging Infectious Diseases*, 26(10), 2346.

Li, C., & Ren, L. (2020). Recent progress on the diagnosis of 2019 Novel Coronavirus. *Transboundary and Emerging Diseases*, 67(4), 1485–1491.

Li, W., Shi, Z., Yu, M., Ren, W., Smith, C., Epstein, J. H., Wang, H., Crameri, G., Hu, Z., & Zhang, H. (2005). Bats are natural reservoirs of SARS-like coronaviruses. *Science*, 310(5748), 676–679.

Li, X., Geng, M., Peng, Y., Meng, L., & Lu, S. (2020). Molecular immune pathogenesis and diagnosis of COVID-19. *Journal of Pharmaceutical Analysis*, 10(2), 102–108.

Li, X., Song, Y., Wong, G., & Cui, J. (2020). Bat origin of a new human coronavirus: there and back again. *Science China Life Sciences*, 63(3), 461–462.

Li, Y., Yao, L., Li, J., Chen, L., Song, Y., Cai, Z., & Yang, C. (2020). Stability issues of RT-PCR testing of SARS-CoV-2 for hospitalized patients clinically diagnosed with COVID-19. *Journal of Medical Virology*, 92(7), 903–908.

Li, Z., Yi, Y., Luo, X., Xiong, N., Liu, Y., Li, S., & Ye, F. (2020). Development and clinical application of a rapid IgM-IgG combined antibody test for SARS-CoV-2 infection diagnosis. *Journal of Medical Virology*, 92(9), 1518–1524.

Lippi, G., Simundic, A. M., & Plebani, M. (2020). Potential preanalytical and analytical vulnerabilities in the laboratory diagnosis of coronavirus disease 2019 (COVID-19). *Clinical Chemistry and Laboratory Medicine*, 58(7), 1070–1076.

Liu, L., Liu, W., Zheng, Y., Jiang, X., Kou, G., Ding, J., & Zheng, S. (2020). A preliminary study on serological assay for severe acute respiratory syndrome coronavirus 2 (SARS-CoV-2) in 238 admitted hospital patients. *Microbes and Infection*, 22(4–5), 206–211.

Liu, L., Wei, Q., Lin, Q., Fang, J., Wang, H., Kwok, H., & Chen, Z. (2019). Anti--spike IgG causes severe acute lung injury by skewing macrophage responses during acute SARS-CoV infection. *Journal of Clinical Investigation Insight*, 4(4).

Liu, Y., Yan, L. M., Wan, L., Xiang, T. X., Le, A., Liu, J. M., & Zhang, W. (2020). Viral dynamics in mild and severe cases of COVID-19. *The Lancet Infectious Diseases*, 20(6), 656–657.

Lu, R., Zhao, X., Li, J., Niu, P., Yang, B., Wu, H., Wang, W., Song, H., Huang, B., & Zhu, N. (2020). Genomic characterisation and epidemiology of 2019 novel coronavirus: implications for virus origins and receptor binding. *The Lancet*, *395*(10224), 565–574.

Mahmood, S., Hasan, K., Carras, M. C., & Labrique, A. (2020). Global preparedness against COVID-19: we must leverage the power of digital health. *Journal of Medical Internet Research*, 6(2), e18980.

Mahshid, S. S., Flynn, S. E., & Mahshid, S. (2021). The potential application of electrochemical biosensors in the COVID-19 pandemic: A perspective on the rapid diagnostics of SARS-CoV-2. *Biosensors and Bioelectronics*, 176, 112905.

Mak, G. C., Cheng, P. K., Lau, S. S., Wong, K. K., Lau, C. S., Lam, E. T., & Tsang, D. N. (2020). Evaluation of rapid antigen test for detection of SARS-CoV-2 virus. *Journal of Clinical Virology*, 129, 104500.

Mak, G. C., Lau, S. S., Wong, K. K., Chow, N. L., Lau, C. S., Lam, E. T., & Tsang, D. N. (2020). Analytical sensitivity and clinical sensitivity of the three rapid antigen detection kits for detection of SARS-CoV-2 virus. *Journal of Clinical Virology*, 133, 104684.

Manne, B. K., Denorme, F., Middleton, E. A., Portier, I., Rowley, J. W., Stubben, C., & Campbell, R. A. (2020). Platelet gene expression and function in patients with COVID-19. *Blood*, 136(11), 1317–1329.

Mathuria, J. P., & Yadav, R. (2020). Laboratory diagnosis of SARS-CoV-2-A review of current methods. *Journal of Infection and Public Health*, 13(7), 901–905.

Merindol, N., Pépin, G., Marchand, C., Rheault, M., Peterson, C., Poirier, A., & Danylo, A. (2020). Optimization of SARS-CoV-2 detection by RT-QPCR without RNA extraction. *BioRxiv*.

Mertens, P., De Vos, N., Martiny, D., Jassoy, C., Mirazimi, A., Cuypers, L., & Vanderlinden, J. (2020). Development and potential usefulness of the COVID-19 Ag Respi-Strip diagnostic assay in a pandemic context. *Frontiers in Medicine*, 7, 225.

Mohamadian, M., Chiti, H., Shoghli, A., Biglari, S., Parsamanesh, N., & Esmaeilzadeh, A. (2021). COVID-19: Virology, biology and novel laboratory diagnosis. *The Journal of Gene Medicine*, 23(2), e3303.

Muenchhoff, M., Mairhofer, H., Nitschko, H., Grzimek-Koschewa, N., Hoffmann, D., Berger, A., Rabenau, H., Widera, M., Ackermann, N., & Konrad, R. (2020). Multicentre comparison of quantitative PCR-based assays to detect SARS-CoV-2, Germany, March 2020. *Eurosurveillance*, 25(24), 2001057.

Okamaoto, K., Shirato, K., Nao, N., Saito, S., Kageyama, T., Hasegawa, H., & Takeda, M. (2020). An assessment of real-time RT-PCR kits for SARS-CoV-2 detection. *Japanese Journal of Infectious Diseases, JJID-2020.*

Oliveira, B. A., Oliveira, L. C. de, Sabino, E. C., & Okay, T. S. (2020). SARS-CoV-2 and the COVID-19 disease: a mini review on diagnostic methods. *Revista Do Instituto de Medicina Tropical de São Paulo*, 62.

WHO (2020). Laboratory testing for coronavirus disease 2019 (COVID-19) in suspected human cases: interim guidance, 2 March 2020 (No. WHO/COVID-19laboratory/ 2020.4).

Osterman, A., Baldauf, H. M., Eletreby, M., Wettengel, J. M., Afridi, S. Q., Fuchs, T., & Keppler, O. T. (2021). Evaluation of two rapid antigen tests to detect SARS-CoV-2 in a hospital setting. *Medical Microbiology and Immunology*, 210(1), 65–72.

Padoan, A., Cosma, C., Sciacovelli, L., Faggian, D., & Plebani, M. (2020). Analytical performances of a chemiluminescence immunoassay for SARS-CoV-2 IgM/IgG and antibody kinetics. *Clinical Chemistry and Laboratory Medicine*, 58(7), 1081–1088.

Paraskevis, D., Kostaki, E. G., Magiorkinis, G., Panayiotakopoulos, G., Sourvinos, G., & Tsiodras, S. (2020). Full-genome evolutionary analysis of the novel corona virus (2019-nCoV) rejects the hypothesis of emergence as a result of a recent recombination event. *Infection, Genetics and Evolution*, 79, 104212.

Poon, L. L. M., Leung, C. S. K., Tashiro, M., Chan, K.-H., Wong, B. W. H., Yuen, K.-Y., & Peiris, J. S. M. (2004). Rapid detection of the severe acute respiratory syndrome (SARS) coronavirus by a loop-mediated isothermal amplification assay. *Clinical Chemistry*, 50(6), 1050–1052.

Pyrc, K., Milewska, A., & Potempa, J. (2011). Development of loop-mediated isothermal amplification assay for detection of human coronavirus-NL63. *The Journal of Virological Methods*, 175(1), 133–136.

Russo, A., Minichini, C., Starace, M., Astorri, R., Calò, F., & Coppola, N. (2020). Current status of laboratory diagnosis for COVID-19: a narrative review. *Infection and Drug Resistance*, 13, 2657–2665.

Sarkale, P., Patil, S., Yadav, P. D., Nyayanit, D. A., Sapkal, G., Baradkar, S., & Abraham, P. (2020). First isolation of SARS-CoV-2 from clinical samples in India. *Indian Journal of Medical Research*, 151(2–3), 244.

Schmid-Burgk, J. L., Schmithausen, R. M., Li, D., Hollstein, R., Ben-Shmuel, A., Israeli, O., & Zhang, F. (2020). LAMP-Seq: population-scale COVID-19 diagnostics using combinatorial barcoding. *BioRxiv*.

Singh, A., Shaikh, A., Singh, R., & Singh, A. K. (2020). COVID-19: From bench to bedside. *Diabetology \& Metabolic Syndrome*, 14(4), 277–281.

Sridhar, S., Forrest, S., Kean, I., Young, J., Scott, J. Ben, Maes, M., & Baker, S. (2020). A blueprint for the implementation of a validated approach for the detection of SARS-Cov2 in clinical samples in academic facilities. *Wellcome Open Research*, 5.

Tahamtan, A., & Ardebili, A. (2020). Real-time RT-PCR in COVID-19 detection: issues affecting the results. *Expert Review of Molecular Diagnostics*, 20(5), 453–454.

Tan, C., Huang, Y., Shi, F., Tan, K., Ma, Q., Chen, Y., & Li, X. (2020). C-reactive protein correlates with computed tomographic findings and predicts severe COVID-19 early. *Journal of Medical Virology*, *92*(7), 856–862.

Tang, X., Wu, C., Li, X., Song, Y., Yao, X., Wu, X., & Lu, J. (2020). On the origin and continuing evolution of SARS-CoV-2. *National Science Review*, 7(6), 1012–1023.

To, K. K. W., Tsang, O. T. Y., Leung, W. S., Tam, A. R. M., Wu, T. C., Lung, D. C., & Yuen, K. Y. (2020). Temporal profiles of viral load in posterior oropharyngeal saliva samples and serum antibody responses during infection by SARS-CoV-2: an observational cohort study. *The Lancet Infectious Diseases*, 20(5), 565–574.

van Kasteren, P. B., van Der Veer, B., van den Brink, S., Wijsman, L., de Jonge, J., van den Brandt, A., & Meijer, A. (2020). Comparison of seven commercial RT-PCR diagnostic kits for COVID-19. *Journal of Clinical Virology*, 128, 104412.

Vashist, S. K. (2020). *In vitro* diagnostic assays for COVID-19: recent advances and emerging trends. *Diagnostics*, 10(4), 202.

Wang, D., Hu, B., Hu, C., Zhu, F., Liu, X., Zhang, J., & Peng, Z. (2020). Clinical characteristics of 138 hospitalized patients with 2019 novel coronavirus--infected pneumonia in Wuhan, China. *Journal of Americam Medical Association*, 323(11), 1061–1069.

Wang, M., Wu, Q., Xu, W., Qiao, B., Wang, J., Zheng, H., & Li, Y. (2020). Clinical diagnosis of 8274 samples with 2019-novel coronavirus in Wuhan. *MedRxiv*.

Wang, X., Yao, H., Xu, X., Zhang, P., Zhang, M., Shao, J., & Wang, H. (2020). Limits of detection of 6 approved RT--PCR kits for the novel SARS-Coronavirus-2 (SARS-CoV-2). *Clinical Chemistry*, 66(7), 977–979.

Wang, Y., Wang, Y., Chen, Y., & Qin, Q. (2020). Unique epidemiological and clinical features of the emerging 2019 novel coronavirus pneumonia (COVID-19) implicate special control measures. *Journal of Medical Virology*, 92(6), 568–576.

Wei, X., Li, X., & Cui, J. (2020). Evolutionary perspectives on novel coronaviruses identified in pneumonia cases in China. *National Science Review*, 7(2), 239–242.

West, R., Kobokovich, A., Connell, N., & Gronvall, G. K. (2021). COVID-19 antibody tests: a valuable public health tool with limited relevance to individuals. *Trends in Microbiology*, 29(3), 214–223.

WHO (2021). *Coronavirus disease (COVID-19) technical guidance: 251 laboratory testing for 2019-nCoV in humans*. World Health Oorganization (WHO) Reference Laboratories of Confirmatory Testing for COVID-19.

Wu, A., Peng, Y., Huang, B., Ding, X., Wang, X., Niu, P., Meng, J., Zhu, Z., Zhang, Z., Wang, J., & others. (2020). Genome composition and divergence of the novel coronavirus (2019-nCoV) originating in China. *Cell Host and Microbe*, 27(3), 325–328.

Wu, C. I., & Poo, M. M. (2020). Moral imperative for immediate release of 2019-nCoV sequence data. *National Science Review*, 7(4), 719–720.

Wu, Y., Ho, W., Huang, Y., Jin, D.-Y., Li, S., Liu, S.-L., Liu, X., Qiu, J., Sang, Y., & Wang, Q. (2020). SARS-CoV-2 is an appropriate name for the new coronavirus. *The Lancet*, 395(10228), 949–950.

Xiang, J., Yan, M., Li, H., Liu, T., Lin, C., Huang, S., & Shen, C. (2020). Evaluation of enzyme-linked immunoassay and colloidal gold-immunochromatographic assay kit for detection of novel coronavirus (SARS-Cov-2) causing an outbreak of pneumonia (COVID-19). *MedRxiv*.

Xiao, A. T., Tong, Y. X., & Zhang, S. (2020). False-negative of RT-PCR and prolonged nucleic acid conversion in COVID-19: rather than recurrence. *Journal of Medical Virology*, 92(10):1755-1756.

Xie, J., Ding, C., Li, J., Wang, Y., Guo, H., Lu, Z., & He, H. (2020). Characteristics of patients with coronavirus disease (COVID-19) confirmed using an IgM-IgG antibody test. *Journal of Medical Virology*, 92(10), 2004–2010.

Xu, H., Zhong, L., Deng, J., Peng, J., Dan, H., Zeng, X., & Chen, Q. (2020). High expression of ACE2 receptor of 2019-nCoV on the epithelial cells of oral mucosa. *International Journal of Oral Science*, 12(1), 1–5.

Xu, X., Chen, P., Wang, J., Feng, J., Zhou, H., Li, X., Zhong, W., & Hao, P. (2020). Evolution of the novel coronavirus from the ongoing Wuhan outbreak and modeling of its spike protein for risk of human transmission. *Science China Life Sciences*, 63, 457–460.

Yang, T., Wang, Y. C., Shen, C. F., & Cheng, C. M. (2020). Point-of-care RNA-based diagnostic device for COVID-19. *Diagnostics*, 10(3), 165.

Yang, Y., Yang, M., Shen, C., Wang, F., Yuan, J., Li, J., & Liu, Y. (2020). Evaluating the accuracy of different respiratory specimens in the laboratory diagnosis and monitoring the viral shedding of 2019-nCoV infections. *MedRxiv*.

Yang, Z. (2007). PAML 4: phylogenetic analysis by maximum likelihood. *Molecular Biology and Evolution*, 24(8), 1586–1591.

Yelin, I., Aharony, N., & Tamar, E. S. (2020). Evaluation of COVID-19 RT-qPCR test in multi-sample pools. *Clinical Infectious Diseases*, 71(16), 2073-2078.

Yesudhas, D., Srivastava, A., & Gromiha, M. M. (2021). COVID-19 outbreak: history, mechanism, transmission, structural studies and therapeutics. *Infection*, 49(2), 199–213.

Yip, C. C. Y., Ho, C. C., Chan, J. F. W., To, K. K. W., Chan, H. S. Y., Wong, S. C. Y., & Yuen, K. Y. (2020). Development of a novel, genome subtraction-derived, SARS-CoV-2-specific COVID-19-nsp2 real-time RT-PCR assay and its evaluation using clinical specimens. *International Journal of Molecular Sciences*, 21(7), 2574.

Young, S., Taylor, S. N., Cammarata, C. L., Varnado, K. G., Roger-Dalbert, C., Montano, A., & Cooper, C. K. (2020). Clinical evaluation of BD Veritor SARS-CoV-2 point-of-care test performance compared to PCR-based testing and versus the Sofia 2 SARS Antigen point-of-care test. *Journal of Clinical Microbiology*, 59(1), e02338-20.

Zaid, Y., Puhm, F., Allaeys, I., Naya, A., Oudghiri, M., Khalki, L., & Boilard, E. (2020). Platelets can associate with SARS-Cov-2 RNA and are hyperactivated in COVID-19. *Circulation Research*, 127(11), 1404–1418.

Zeng, F., Dai, C., Cai, P., Wang, J., Xu, L., Li, J., & Wang, L. (2020). A comparison study of SARS-CoV-2 IgG antibody between male and female COVID-19 patients: a possible reason underlying different outcome between sex. *Journal of Medical Virology*, 92(10), 2050–2054.

Zhang, L., Zhang, F., Yu, W., He, T., Yu, J., Yi, C. E., & Ho, D. (2006). Antibody responses against SARS coronavirus are correlated with disease outcome of infected individuals. *Journal of Medical Virology*, 78(1), 1–8.

Zhang, Y., Odiwuor, N., Xiong, J., Sun, L., Nyaruaba, R. O., Wei, H., & Tanner, N. A. (2020). Rapid molecular detection of SARS-CoV-2 (COVID-19) virus RNA using colorimetric LAMP. *MedRxiv*.

Zhao, J., Yuan, Q., Wang, H., Liu, W., Liao, X., Su, Y., & Zhang, Z. (2020). Antibody responses to SARS-CoV-2 in patients with novel coronavirus disease 2019. *Clinical Infectious Diseases*, 71(16), 2027–2034.

Zhong, L., Chuan, J., Gong, B. O., Shuai, P., Zhou, Y., Zhang, Y., & Yang, Z. (2020). Detection of serum IgM and IgG for COVID-19 diagnosis. *Science China Life Sciences*, 63(5), 777–780.

Zhong, N., Zheng, B. J., Li, Y. M., Poon, L. L. M., Xie, Z. H., Chan, K. H., & Guan, Y. (2003). Epidemiology and cause of severe acute respiratory syndrome (SARS) in Guangdong, People's Republic of China, in February, 2003. *The Lancet*, 362(9393), 1353–1358.

Zhou, P., Yang, X. L., Wang, X. G., Hu, B., Zhang, L., Zhang, W., Si, H. R., Zhu, Y., Li, B., & Huang, C. L. (2020a). A pneumonia outbreak associated with a new coronavirus of probable bat origin. *Nature*, 579(7798), 270–273.

Zhou, P., Yang, X. L., Wang, X. G., Hu, B., Zhang, L., Zhang, W., Si, H. R., Zhu, Y., Li, B., & Huang, C. L. (2020b). Discovery of a novel coronavirus associated with the recent pneumonia outbreak in humans and its potential bat origin. *BioRxiv*, 2001–2020.

Zhu, N., Zhang, D., Wang, W., Li, X., Yang, B., Song, J., & Tan, W. (2020). A novel coronavirus from patients with pneumonia in China, 2019. *The New England Journal of Medicine*, 382(8), 727–733.

Chapter 9

# Multifaceted Therapeutics Advances in Life-Threatening Human Diseases: From Traditional, Complementary and Integrative Medicine to Nano-Based Targeted Drug Delivery

**Siddhartha Dan**[1]
**Deeksha Sharma**[2]
**and Sushil Kumar Upadhyay**[3,*]

[1]Department of Biotechnology, Dr. B. R. Ambedkar, National Institute of Technology, Jalandhar (Punjab), India
[2]Faculty of Applied Sciences and Biotechnology, Shoolini University, Solan, Himachal Pradesh, India
[3]Department of Bio-Sciences and Technology, M. M. E. C., Maharishi Markandeshwar (Deemed to be University), Mullana-Ambala (Haryana), India

## Abstract

Human diseases are largely influenced by microorganisms, and recent developments in diverse therapies have completely changed the landscape of available treatments. The integration of conventional, alternative, and integrative medicine as well as the development of nano-based targeted drug delivery systems are the main topics of this abstract, which also examines the microbiological viewpoint on the advancements made in treating life-threatening human diseases. Recent developments in nanotechnology have opened up exciting new avenues for the

* Corresponding Author's Email: upadhyay.k.sushil@gmail.com.

In: Therapeutic Advances in Human Health and Diseases
Editors: Sushil Kumar Upadhyay, Manoj Singh and Anil Kumar Sharma
ISBN: 979-8-89113-304-4

development of targeted pharmaceutical delivery techniques, with the potential to greatly enhance therapeutic efficacy while decreasing adverse effects. Therapeutics can be delivered directly to the site of an infection or cancer by engineering nano-based drug carriers such as liposomes, nanoparticles, and viral vectors. Since microorganisms have developed sophisticated mechanisms for effective targeting and delivery of biomolecules, they can provide insights into the creation and application of these nanocarriers. Understanding disease-causing bacteria from a microbiological perspective has proven crucial in the creation of efficient treatments. Antibiotics and probiotics are examples of microbial compounds that traditional medicine has used to treat infectious disorders. In order to maintain health and treat disorders, complementary and integrative medicine has made use of the symbiotic interaction between humans and microorganisms. Additionally, the development of nano-based tailored drug delivery systems offers great hope for the treatment of fatal diseases. The design and improvement of these delivery systems can be influenced by the valuable insights that microorganisms offer into the mechanisms of infection and cellular connections. In order to improve the effectiveness of medicine delivery, they have also served as inspiration for the creation of novel biomimetic techniques. In conclusion, this abstract illustrates the numerous therapeutic developments in serious human diseases, including nanobased targeted drug delivery as well as conventional, alternative, and integrative medicine. Understanding the complex interactions between bacteria and their hosts has molded these developments from a microbiological perspective, opening new possibilities for successful treatment methods. Future advances in illness management can be facilitated by closing the information gap between treatment approaches and microorganisms.

**Keywords**: human diseases, nanocarriers, multifaceted therapy, complementary medicine, targeted drug delivery

## 1. Introduction

As animal-transmitted pathogens account for more than 60% of infectious diseases in humans, diseases that humans and animals share are as old as humanity itself (Pikaard, 2000). Zoonoses are complex diseases that arise and spread as a result of pathogen and host interactions, evolution, variability, and selection. The ecology and distribution of vectors also have an impact on the development and transmission of vector-borne zoonoses. Additionally, because vectors are frequently not dependent on a single host species, vector-borne zoonoses frequently have numerous reservoirs or hosts or species. It makes their dynamics more difficult to anticipate and their eradication more difficult (Egger et al., 2004). Environmental factors have a big impact on host, pathogen, and vector properties. The One Health Trial asserts a connection and interaction between the health of people, animals, and the environment (Reik et al., 2003).

Human activities and climatic changes cause changes in the environment, which in turn affect the transmission and spread of zoonoses. Arthropod vectors are frequently the primary factor influencing the spread of disease and are typically highly sensitive to environmental changes. Since vectors are ectotherms, changes in the environment's temperature patterns have a significant impact on them (Portela and Esteller, 2010; Sharma et al., 2010). Higher temperatures encourage the growth, survival, and area-wide proliferation of ticks and mosquitoes as well as their rising population (Lund and van Lohuizen, 2004; Fraga et al., 2005; Hewagama and Richardson, 2009; Fedoriw et al., 2012). Additionally, higher temperatures enhance the spread of disease by accelerating the replication of pathogens (Keating et al., 2016). These findings are related to the rise in vector-borne zoonosis incidence that has recently been observed and that certain climatic models have also indicated will occur more frequently in the near future (Lund and van Lohuizen, 2004; Fraga et al., 2005; Ballestar et al., 2006; Hewagama and Richardson, 2009). Additionally, other environmental elements, particularly extreme weather conditions like floods and storms, frequently have a supportive impact on the vector density (Fedoriw et al., 2012). Extensive farming and manufacturing, too much grazing, the draining of wetlands, and cutting down of trees all contribute to altered landscapes. Alterations in vegetation cover and water management may alter local climate by influencing the amount and timing of precipitation and temperature. This has an impact on the dispersal of disease-carrying vectors and plant and animal ecosystems (Bhavsar et al., 2008; Ho, 2010).

On a local level, several human activities have a direct impact on pathogen spread. Pathogen, vector, and human contact rates are influenced by local lifestyles, human demographics, and how the landscape is used, and they are rising as a result of global changes (Urdinguio et al., 2009; Hewagama and Richardson, 2009; Hansen et al., 2010; Park et al., 2014). Global trade and accessible travel make it possible for diseases to spread across great distances by transporting diseased persons, animals, or vectors along with agricultural products (Sadri-Vakili and Cha, 2006).

Environmental factors as well as the socioeconomic circumstances in the area have a major bearing on the prevalence and incidence of vector-borne diseases worldwide. Malaria and dengue fever are two of the most devastating vector-borne diseases, and many of the world's poorest countries are located in tropical or subtropical regions. The rising number of people in the world means that more and more close together and frequently near both domestic and wild animals. The likelihood of contracting an infection may rise if your health is compromised due to your living situation (Adcock et al., 2005; Guo et al., 2012). The healthcare system in these areas is inadequate, and a sizeable portion of the population cannot access preventative and vaccination programs. Programs to prevent the density of mosquitoes and sandflies have very little impact (Gray and De Meyts, 2005). These elements encourage the quick and vigorous transmission of zoonotic illnesses and the typically rising frequency of outbreaks (Baylin, 2005; Robertson, 2005).

The geographic distribution of zoonotic illnesses transmitted by vectors and the spread of those infections' vectors are strongly related. In tropical regions, mosquitoes, and sandflies are the most prevalent vectors, whereas in milder regions of Europe, they only occasionally operate as zoonotic carriers (Ehrlich, 2009). However, lately, emerging tropical diseases have also been found in Europe as a result of climate change and the ensuing spread of mosquitoes to the north (Varier and Timmers, 2011). Additionally, excessive human and animal migration and the ensuing infection of pre-existing vectors were to blame for infrequent outbreaks of non-autochthonous zoonoses, such as the malaria outbreak that occurred in Greece from 2009 to 2012 (Glozak and Seto, 2007; Berdasco et al., 2009).

The most significant zoonoses in Europe are those transmitted by ticks, and over the past ten years, their prevalence has increased (Quintero-Ronderos et al., 2012). Ticks are becoming more prevalent in higher latitudes and altitudes as a result of climate change, human activity, and landscape management (Jones and Takai, 2001; Quintero-Ronderos et al., 2012; Zeng et al., 2014; Zhang and Zhang, 2015). The reduction of game, invasive, and pest species populations is one strategy for regulating tick density, as their high concentrations encourage tick populations and the transmission of diseases carried by ticks (Quintero-Ronderos et al., 2012). In Europe, there is an increase in the popularity of outdoor leisure activities, cultural practices (such as hunting and gathering berries and mushrooms), and human-tick contact rates, which increases the risk of infection (Esteller, 2011).

Pathogen spread to new locations frequently has a significant effect on host populations. The infection can be very difficult and may turn into an epidemic, which could have a major influence on the host population's health if the host population and the pathogen have no shared evolutionary history and the host population's immune system is undeveloped and unprepared (Doi et al., 2009; Jin et al., 2011), similar to the 1999 West Nile virus epidemic that swept the East Coast of the United States (Kanwal andGupta, 2012). When viruses infect people, they swiftly develop new mutations that make them more powerful and make gullible host populations even more vulnerable (Gopalakrishnan et al., 2008). The most significant and dangerous vector-borne zoonotic illnesses that are now emerging and/or spreading quickly throughout Europe and/or the world are listed below, along with variables affecting their distribution and severity.

## 2. Conventional or Traditional Medicine System

Parasitic infections affect millions of people globally and considerably raise morbidity and mortality rates. Both modern medicine and traditional medicine have made great strides in treating parasite infestations. While Western medicine relies on synthetic drugs and modern technology, traditional medicinal systems use herbal remedies and local expertise (Serban, 2019). In order to cure parasite diseases, this article examines the therapeutic advancements made in these two healthcare systems. In conventional medicine, the development of antiparasitic drugs has improved dramatically. An entirely new strategy for combating malaria, one of the worst parasite illnesses, was made possible by the discovery of artemisinin and its derivatives. Current treatment guidelines for uncomplicated malaria call for the use of artemisinin-based combination treatments (ACTs) have drastically reduced the incidence of malaria deaths worldwide (Su and Miller, 2015).

In addition to malaria, conventional medicine has developed effective treatments for a number of parasitic infections. For instance, albendazole and mebendazole are often used to treat intestinal helminth infections like hookworm, roundworm, and whipworm. Ivermectin has been used to treat the parasite diseases onchocerciasis and lymphatic filariasis (Chai et al., 2021). Because of advancements in molecular diagnostics, parasite diseases can now be diagnosed more quickly and accurately. For example, polymerase chain reaction (PCR) and next-generation sequencing (NGS) techniques enable the highly sensitive and precise detection of parasites. This facilitates early detection, appropriate therapy, and monitoring of treatment results (Liu et al., 2023).

In traditional medical systems that are deeply rooted in indigenous cultures, plant-based therapies for parasite diseases have a long history. These systems have contributed significantly to the advancement of antiparasitic therapies. Because many plants naturally possess antiparasitic properties, they have been utilized to treat a variety of parasite infections (Yuan et al., 2016). For instance, the bark of the cinchona tree, a traditional malaria therapy, contains quinine, a potent anti-Plasmodium parasite. Neem, garlic, and Artemisia annua, among other healing herbs, have demonstrated antiparasitic activity against a variety of parasites. Traditional medicine systems also employ extra-natural compounds for their antiparasitic benefits (Odugbemi et al., 2006). Bee products like propolis and royal jelly, for example, have proven effective against some parasites. Moxibustion, acupuncture, and herbal baths are a few additional conventional methods that have been utilized to support the body's natural defense mechanisms and alleviate symptoms (Olas, 2022).

Because of their potential benefits, traditional and modern medical systems have been attempted to be combined. Integrative medicine combines evidence-based practices from the two systems to deliver complete and all-encompassing care. A collaborative investigation between traditional and conventional medical practitioners has shown promising results. Studies, for instance, have examined the synergistic effects of combining conventional herbal treatments with antiparasitic drugs. This all-encompassing approach could increase therapeutic efficacy, reduce drug resistance, and diminish side effects. Additionally, traditional medical procedures provide a wealth of opportunities for drug development (Yuan et al., 2016). Traditional antiparasitic drugs have often been modeled after naturally occurring compounds derived from medicinal plants. By merging information from conventional medicine, scientists can identify novel therapeutic targets and develop state-of-the-art therapy regimens. Therapeutic advancements for parasite infections have been accomplished in both traditional and conventional medical systems. Conventional medicine has made great achievements in the development of molecular diagnostics and antiparasitic drugs. The application of traditional medical systems, which are based on antiquated knowledge and natural remedies, has also helped in the management and treatment of parasitic diseases. These two strategies could be successfully combined (Yuan et al., 2016; Jayawardene et al., 2021).

## 3. Integrated Medicine System (Homeopathy and Allopathy)

Parasitic illnesses continue to pose major health problems on a global scale, affecting millions of individuals. Integrative medicine, which combines the core concepts and treatment techniques of different medical systems, offers a comprehensive approach to the treatment of parasitic illnesses. The therapy of parasitic infections has benefited from therapeutic advances made possible by the combination of homeopathy and allopathy, two well-known medical systems. Both allopathy and homeopathy are distinct medical disciplines with distinctive therapeutic modalities. Homeopathy, which is based on the principle that "like cures like," uses extremely diluted medications to promote the body's natural healing processes. Allopathy, or conventional medicine, focuses on treating specific ailments with drugs and other treatments (Ung et al., 2021).

In an integrated medical system, homeopathy and allopathy collaborate to deliver complete care. Homeopathic remedies can be given in conjunction with prescribed drugs to enhance treatment effects. This integration acknowledges the benefits of each system and aims to enhance patient care by combining the best components of each. The blending of homeopathy with allopathy has resulted in significant advancements in the treatment of parasitic illnesses. The use of homeopathic remedies can alleviate the symptoms of parasitic infections and boost the immune system (Bellavite, 2015). These all-natural remedies are selected using the idea of individualized care, which takes into account the unique symptoms and constitution of each patient. To target and remove parasites from the body right away, allopathic drugs are crucial. Numerous parasites can be successfully treated using antiparasitic drugs developed through allopathic research and development. For instance, medications like artemisinin-based combination therapies (ACTs) have significantly reduced malaria fatality rates (Yuan et al., 2016; Campbell and Soman-Faulkner, 2023).

Individualized treatment programs that take into consideration each patient's particular needs can be developed using both homeopathy and allopathy. Homeopathic treatments can be used to improve overall health, boost the body's natural defenses, and minimize the side effects of prescribed drugs. For effective treatment and eradication, however, allopathic medications precisely target the parasites. In order to undertake research and advance the treatment of parasitic illnesses, homeopathy and allopathy have collaborated (Bellavite, 2015). Integrated clinical trials and investigations have examined the efficacy and safety of combining homeopathic treatments with conventional antiparasitic drugs. These studies aim to identify synergistic effects and select the most effective treatment regimens for certain parasite infections (Kleijnen et al., 1991).

Procedures and recommendations for combining homeopathy with allopathy in the treatment of parasitic illnesses have also been produced through collaboration. These suggestions ensure that the integration fits with the guiding principles of both medical systems and is supported by data. They provide healthcare workers with a framework for providing interdisciplinary care while maintaining patient safety and improving treatment outcomes. Incorporating both allopathy and homeopathy into the treatment of parasitic illnesses results in a patient-centered approach that considers the unique needs and preferences of each individual (Mathie, 2003; Ghosh et al., 2014). This integrated approach provides holistic care by addressing the patient's overall health as well as the parasitic infection. By combining the advantages of both medical systems, healthcare practitioners may provide comprehensive treatment regimens that support the body's natural healing processes while specifically targeting and eliminating parasites. Combining homeopathy and allopathy in the treatment of parasitic illnesses has led to significant therapeutic advancements. This integrated medical approach combines the concentrated care of allopathy with the individualized approach of homeopathy (Jasemi et al., 2017; Chaughule and Barve, 2023).

## 4. Traditional Medicine in Multifaceted Therapy of Life-Threatening Human Diseases

More than two years have passed since the COVID-19 epidemic, which devastated economies, killed millions of people, and inflicted misery on a global scale. Although scientists from all around the world gathered and practically all countries experienced the disease in some way, a complete solution has not yet been discovered. Nevertheless, Success rates for the many antivirals and vaccines now in use are not uniform (Ng et al., 2022). The only way to lessen the disease's destructive consequences is to prevent it. Numerous vaccinations have been created and natural substances can alter the immune system. Communities everywhere have been encouraged to follow local health regulations during the ongoing COVID-19 pandemic so that no one gets sick and no one else gets sick. Nutrition-based therapies have been shown to be crucial for avoiding and treating viral infections, especially those that cause harm to the respiratory system (Nicholson, 2016).

More and more studies are being conducted on the effects of nutrition-based therapies for the prevention, diagnosis, and treatment of COVID-19, and this has led to a proliferation of publications on the use of traditional medicine, botanicals, and nutraceuticals (Soleymani et al., 2022). According to studies, those who are deficient in micronutrients may clearly see their immune being suppressed (Gombart et al., 2020). The T cell-mediated immune responses and the antibodies' adaptive responses have a major impact on how the immune system works. The host can effectively combat viral respiratory infections thanks to increased immunity (Nicholson, 2016).

As a vaccine and a specialized antiviral were still being sought after, and nothing was known about the unique virus itself, people all around the world were overloaded with information. It's unfortunate that not all information found online can be backed up by solid evidence. In March 2020, when the COVID-19 infection outbreak was at its height, data showed an uptick in the sale of elderberry and zinc supplements. These purchases had grown by 255% and 415%, respectively (Wieland et al., 2021). Verifying the information that its residents were exposed to was the responsibility of the governments and other relevant health agencies of each nation. Numerous businesses and organizations have received warnings for disseminating inaccurate information about how to treat and cure COVID-19 (Freckelton, 2020).

As 2022 draws to a close, research is still being done to develop the most effective COVID-19 vaccine and antivirals. It is even more important to create effective, accessible therapeutic methods to reduce the spread of these diseases, since many new diseases, some of which can be transmitted from animals to humans, have emerged in the recent two decades (Rizvi et al., 2023). Since ancient times, people have taken natural medicines in the form of vegetables and fruits. Today, some cuisines place a greater emphasis on the use of spices, condiments, and plant-based oils that contain a variety of therapeutic compounds and promote a longer and healthier life for the consumer. To expeditiously bring effective and long-lasting therapeutic solutions to market, it is necessary to research the use of conventional medicine and herbs to enhance the immune system (Rizvi et al., 2023). Due to their numerous powerful immunomodulatory, anti-inflammatory, and antiviral characteristics, natural products have a proven history of usage in a range of medical problems. Many natural supplements, when taken in pure and safe doses, have been demonstrated to improve clinical results by reducing virus susceptibility. As some medicinal natural items are known to have serious side effects, such as drug-drug and drug-food interactions, they should also be used cautiously and ideally only after consulting a healthcare professional (Rizvi et al., 2023). In this article, we will discuss the efficacy of several nutraceuticals and natural treatments, as well as the traditional medicinal practices of China and India, in treating a wide variety of illnesses and microbiological diseases, including COVID-19. Although nutraceuticals and other COVID-19 supportive care options may not be the sole approach to stop this epidemic, they may have a major impact on supportive and preventative measures in these unprecedented times. To determine the efficacy of various natural chemicals and to utilize their huge potential to treat a wide variety of illnesses and microbial infections, including COVID-19 and the sad emergence of new diseases in the future, more clinical trials are required (Rizvi et al., 2023).

Infectious diseases pose a threat to public health around the world. Our tireless work and research have led to the development of novel antiviral and antibiotic drugs that have allowed us to effectively treat the vast majority of ailments. Unfortunately, bacteria's ability to adapt and change over time is what has led to their resistance to antibiotics and antiviral drugs (Rizvi et al., 2023). The failure of microorganisms to respond to therapeutic drugs has increased the danger of complications, chronic infections, and preventable fatalities when treating infections. Therefore, the development of more effective, useful, and versatile medicines to prevent and treat both well-known and newly discovered diseases requires a multidisciplinary approach and teamwork (Rizvi et al., 2023). Recent research has shown that natural therapies can be effective in treating a wide range of medical conditions. The vast majority of active medicinal ingredients used today have their origins in nature. There is still untapped potential in natural products because not all natural resources have been investigated. To fully realize their potential and employ them as an alternative or primary therapy, this supports continuing financing for investigations and assessments of existing medical methods (Rizvi et al., 2023).

## 5. Inflammation: A Physiological Response against Diseases

Inflammation is caused by a wide variety of physiological responses to a variety of noxious stimuli, including infection, trauma, damage, toxins, and other imbalances (Nathan, 2002). An early inflammatory response is associated with the recruitment of leukocytes, mainly mast cells, and then macrophages from the circulation to the wounded regions (Nathan, 2002). Chronic inflammation, on the other hand, lasts for a long time and is the root cause of numerous diseases (Dunning, 2009).

## 5.1. Epigenetics of Inflammation

Macrophages are important regulators of inflammatory responses. Pathogen-associated molecular patterns (PAMPs) are short molecular sequences that are unique to each pathogen and are recognized by pattern-recognition receptors (PRRs) or sensors (such as Toll-like receptors, TLRs, and nitric oxide dismutase, or NOD proteins) after microbial invasion (PAMPs). Histamine and other pro-inflammatory cytokines including interleukin (IL)-1, tumor necrosis factor (TNF), and interleukin (IL)-6 are produced as a result of the activation of signaling pathways. The expression of inflammatory genes that encode cytokines, chemokines, and other inflammatory compounds is found to be regulated by pro-inflammatory transcription factors like the nuclear factor kappa B (NF-B) and activator protein (AP)-1, FOXP3, IRF, and STAT families. DNA methylation, histone modifications, and RNA-associated silencing by short non-coding RNAs are just some of the epigenetic processes that regulate transcription factors in addition to inflammatory genes (Foster and Medzhitov, 2009; Bayarsaihan, 2011). Subsequently, the body's systemic homeostasis drastically shifts to aid host defense.

## 5.2. DNA Methylation and Inflammation

Another crucial mechanism for controlling the expression of inflammatory genes is DNA methylation. Recent research has shown that LPS activates HDACs via TLR4-signaling to reduce the expression of the Thy-1 gene (Xing et al., 2015). When a condition like cystic fibrosis is present, the TLR2 gene experiences promoter hypomethylation, which increases the bronchial epithelial cells' pro-inflammatory response to bacterial peptidoglycan (Shuto et al., 2006). Methylation of DNA and acetylation of histone in intestinal epithelial cells maintain intestinal homeostasis (Takahashi et al., 2009). TNF and the related inflammation are controlled in part by epigenetic alterations, including DNA methylation and histone modifications (Sullivan et al., 2007). Changes in the epigenetic machinery caused by bacterial infections can alter the genome's state, influencing host defense or pathogen load (Bierne et al.,

2012). Maternal health, including infection by bacteria and viruses, influences changes in the expression of crucial developmental genes in the placenta, which are consequently linked to the development of the offspring, according to microarray studies in mice (Oskvig et al., 2012). Helicobacter pylori (HP) infection leads to inflammation and generates changes in the DNA methylation pattern in gastric epithelial cells, and this leads to a decrease in expression of the Runx3 locus in the gastric epithelial cells that are ultimately responsible for the disease (Niwa et al., 2010).

### 5.3. Histone Methylation in Inflammation

Histone methylation, which includes H3K4me3, H3K9me2, H3K9me3, and H3K27me3, is principally responsible for controlling the gene expression of CD4+ T cells and CD8+ T cells (Chang and Aune, 2007; Wei et al., 2009). According to studies, T cells' regulatory regions of gene loci undergo dynamic, intricate alterations in histone methylation when they divide into various subsets of effector T cells (Madrigal-Matute et al., 2013). When pathogens and pro-inflammatory cytokines are present, studies have revealed that Jmjd3, a member of the Jumonji family, is produced in macrophages, where it activates the polycomb-group (PcG) target genes and controls the levels of H3K27me3 and transcriptional activity in these genes. Aberrant DNA methylation occurs in certain of the PcG proteins that cause inflammation. PcG proteins attach to the target genes' regulatory areas and draw DNMTs there for more effective suppression. Additionally, pro-inflammatory genes are suppressed during sepsis by the NF-B/RelB pathway, which results in the induction of H3K9me3 (De Santa et al., 2007). Jmjd3 rewires the epigenome to remove histone marks, which controls differentiation and cell identity in macrophages and reduces inflammation. Continuous exposure to IL-4 activates Jmjd3 and causes the STAT6 promoter to release repressive H3K27me3 marks. In turn, Jmjd3 is positively regulated by activated STAT6 by binding to its promoter. Jmjd3's removal of H3K27 methylation markers causes certain inflammatory genes to express (Ishii et al., 2009). These data unequivocally show that histone methylation plays a dynamic function during the inflammatory response.

### 5.4. Histone Acetylation and Inflammation

When diverse agents like LPS, TNF, IL-1b, etc. produce inflammations, genes are activated by the acetylation of histone by HATs and suppressed by the activity of HDACs. However, additional intracellular kinase pathways including MAPKs and PI3K are also crucial. Many of these stimuli function by inducing pro-inflammatory transcription factors like NF-B and AP-1 (Adcock and Lee, 2006). HDACs are involved in the control of pro-inflammatory genes, according to recent research. In asthma, for example, corticosteroids shut off inflammatory genes by recruiting HDAC2 to the promoter region of the NF-B-activated inflammatory gene complex and thereby reducing HAT activity. A reduction in HDAC activity and HDAC2 expression has been observed in chronic obstructive pulmonary disease (COPD), a corticosteroid-resistant illness characterized by heightened inflammation and resistance to the effects of corticosteroids (Adcock et al., 2005). The cAMP response element binding protein p300 (CBP/p300) is able to acetylate histones in the promoter region of inflammatory genes thanks to its intrinsic HAT activity and its ability to recruit additional HATs (IL-1, IL-2, IL-8, and IL-12). The protein regulates gene expression by activating transcription. HDACs regulate the expression of both pro- and anti-inflammatory cytokines through the recruitment of co-repressor complexes and transcription factors such FOXP3, STATs, GATAs, ZEB1, and NF-B to gene promoters (Villagra et al., 2010). In response to cytokine therapy, the IKK of the IB kinase complex binds to NF-B promoters via polymerase II and CBP. There, it phosphorylates Ser10 on histone H3 and acetylates Lys9 on histone H3 (Ghosh and Karin, 2002; Yang et al., 2009). This also contributes to the subsequent acetylation of histone H3 on Lys14 by CBP (Yamamoto et al., 2003). By increasing the H3 phosphorylation marked promoters and promoting the recruitment to specific chromatin sites, the p38 protein plays a significant role in the activation of inflammatory and immunological responses (Saccani et al., 2002).

## 6. Targeted Drug Delivery and Nanotherapeutics

Parasitic illnesses continue to pose a serious threat to global health, necessitating the development of cutting-edge therapeutic approaches. Targeted drug delivery and nanotherapeutics have shown potential in the fight against parasitic diseases. This article highlights the therapeutic developments made feasible by the use of customized medication delivery systems and nanotherapeutics to combat parasitic infestations (Singh et al., 2017). Drugs are delivered directly to the infection site using targeted drug delivery systems, which increases therapeutic efficacy and minimizes side effects. When it comes to parasitic diseases, these systems have a number of advantages. They can improve drug stability, bioavailability, and drug concentration at the site of action (Wen et al., 2015).

When administered to infected tissues or cells via nano-sized carriers including liposomes, nanoparticles, and micelles, antiparasitic drugs have demonstrated promise. These containers can contain and protect the medication, enabling a controlled release and prolonged circulation throughout the body. Additionally, the changed surfaces of the carriers may enable specific interactions with the surfaces of parasites or infected cells, aiding the administration of customized treatment (Patra et al., 2018; Sun et al., 2019). For instance, liposomes or nanoparticles can be modified to contain ligands that specifically bind to receptors on the surface of Plasmodium parasites to cure malaria. This makes it possible to deliver antimalarial drugs specifically to the parasites, improving treatment efficiency and reducing systemic toxicity (Anamika et al., 2020; Memvanga and Nkanga, 2021).

The use of nanoparticles as therapeutic agents to treat disease is referred to as "nanotherapeutics." Nanoparticles offer unique properties, such as their small size, large surface area, and adjustable surface characteristics, which are suitable for combating parasite illnesses. The field of parasitology can benefit from nanotherapeutics in a number of ways. They can improve a medicine's solubility, stability, and bioavailability, improving drug delivery to parasites. Additionally, certain properties of nanoparticles can be altered to aid in their targeting and parasite absorption (Desai, 2012; Rudramurthy et al., 2016; Teleanu et al., 2018). Some nanoparticles have antiparasitic characteristics that naturally eliminate parasites or stop their reproduction. For instance, research has shown that silver nanoparticles have broad-spectrum antiparasitic effects against a range of parasites, including protozoa and helminths. Other nanoparticles, such as polymer-based nanocarriers, can be loaded with antiparasitic drugs and released only at the infection site to improve therapeutic efficacy (Yin et al., 2020; Patel et al., 2021; Sethi et al., 2022).

## Conclusion

Nanotherapeutics can also circumvent biological barriers that hinder the effectiveness of traditional medication delivery methods. For example, the blood-brain barrier might make it difficult for drugs to reach parasites that harm the central nervous system. Nanoparticles can get around this obstacle, making it possible to successfully treat many challenging parasite diseases. Despite the immense potential of targeted drug delivery and nanotherapeutics, there are still a number of challenges to be solved. Drug resistance is a risk for nanotherapeutics, a problem that is particularly troublesome in parasitic illnesses. Therefore, research must focus on developing novel drug delivery systems and combination therapies to fight resistance mechanisms. The safety profile of nanotherapeutics also has to be thoroughly investigated. Toxic or immunological reactions may result from complex interactions between nanoparticles and biological systems. Therefore, extensive preclinical and clinical research is needed to ensure their safety and effectiveness.

Future studies in this field will concentrate on developing multifunctional nanosystems that can deliver a variety of drugs or combination therapies. The development of stimuli-responsive drug delivery systems, which allow controlled medicine release that is triggered by specific conditions at the infection site, is another benefit of nanotechnology. For the treatment of parasitic diseases, promising therapeutic advancements include nanotherapeutics and targeted drug delivery systems. These techniques enhance the effectiveness of treatments, boost drug delivery to the desired location, and minimize side effects.

## References

Adcock, I. M., Ito, K., & Barnes, P. J. (2005). Histone deacetylation: an important mechanism in inflammatory lung diseases. *Journal of Chronic Obstructive Pulmonary Disease*, 2(4), 445–455.

Adcock, I. M., & Lee, K. Y. (2006). Abnormal histone acetylase and deacetylase expression and function in lung inflammation. *Inflammation Research*, 55, 311–321.

Anamika, J., Nikhar, V., Laxmikant, G., Priya, S., Sonal, V., & Vyas, S. P. (2020). Nanobiotechnological modules as molecular target tracker for the treatment and prevention of malaria: Options and opportunity. *Drug Delivery and Translational Research*, 10(4), 1095–1110.

Ballestar, E., Esteller, M., & Richardson, B. C. (2006). The epigenetic face of systemic lupus erythematosus. *The Journal of Immunology*, 176(12), 7143–7147.

Bayarsaihan, D. (2011). Epigenetic mechanisms in inflammation. *Journal of Dental Research*, 90(1), 9–17.

Baylin, S. B. (2005). DNA methylation and gene silencing in cancer. *Nature Clinical Practice Oncology*, 2(1), S4--S11.

Bellavite, P. (2015). Homeopathy and integrative medicine: Keeping an open mind. *Journal of Medicine and the Person*, 13(1), 1–6.

Berdasco, M., Ropero, S., Setien, F., Fraga, M. F., Lapunzina, P., Losson, R., Alaminos, M., Cheung, N.-K., Rahman, N., & Esteller, M. (2009). Epigenetic inactivation of the Sotos overgrowth syndrome gene histone methyltransferase NSD1 in human neuroblastoma and glioma. *Proceedings of the National Academy of Sciences*, 106(51), 21830–21835.

Bhavsar, P., Ahmad, T., & Adcock, I. M. (2008). The role of histone deacetylases in asthma and allergic diseases. *Journal of Allergy and Clinical Immunology*, *121*(3), 580–584.

Bierne, H., Hamon, M., & Cossart, P. (2012). Epigenetics and bacterial infections. *Cold Spring Harbor Perspectives in Medicine*, 2(12), a010272.

Campbell, S., & Soman-Faulkner, K. (2023). Antiparasitic Drugs. In *StatPearls*. StatPearls Publishing. http://www.ncbi.nlm.nih.gov/books/NBK544251/.

Chai, J. Y., Jung, B. K., & Hong, S. J. (2021). Albendazole and Mebendazole as Anti-Parasitic and Anti-Cancer Agents: An Update. *The Korean Journal of Parasitology*, 59(3), 189–225.

Chang, S., & Aune, T. M. (2007). Dynamic changes in histone-methylation'marks' across the locus encoding interferon-$γ$ during the differentiation of T Helper type 2 cells. *Nature Immunology*, 8(7), 723–731.

Chaughule, R. S., & Barve, R. S. (2023). Role of herbal medicines in the treatment of infectious diseases. *Vegetos*, 1–11. https://doi.org/10.1007/s42535-022-00549-2.

De Santa, F., Totaro, M. G., Prosperini, E., Notarbartolo, S., Testa, G., & Natoli, G. (2007). The histone H3 lysine-27 demethylase Jmjd3 links inflammation to inhibition of polycomb-mediated gene silencing. *Cell*, 130(6), 1083–1094.

Desai, N. (2012). Challenges in the development of nanoparticle-based therapeutics. *The AAPS Journal*, 14(2), 282–295.

Doi, A., Park, I.-H., Wen, B., Murakami, P., Aryee, M. J., Irizarry, R., Herb, B., Ladd-Acosta, C., Rho, J., Loewer, S., & others. (2009). Differential methylation of tissue- and cancer-specific CpG island shores distinguishes human induced pluripotent stem cells, embryonic stem cells and fibroblasts. *Nature Genetics*, 41(12), 1350–1353.

Dunning, T. (2009). Periodontal disease-the overlooked diabetes complication. *Nephrology Nursing Journal*, *36*(5), 489–495.

Egger, G., Liang, G., Aparicio, A., & Jones, P. A. (2004). Epigenetics in human disease and prospects for epigenetic therapy. *Nature*, 429(6990), 457–463.

Ehrlich, M. (2009). DNA hypomethylation in cancer cells. *Epigenomics*, 1(2), 239–259.

Esteller, M. (2011). Non-coding RNAs in human disease. *Nature Reviews Genetics*, 12(12), 861–874.

Fedoriw, A., Mugford, J., & Magnuson, T. (2012). Genomic imprinting and epigenetic control of development. *Cold Spring Harbor Perspectives in Biology*, *4*(7), a008136.

Foster, S. L., & Medzhitov, R. (2009). Gene-specific control of the TLR-induced inflammatory response. *Clinical Immunology*, 130(1), 7–15.

Fraga, M. F., Ballestar, E., Paz, M. F., Ropero, S., Setien, F., Ballestar, M. L., Heine-Suñer, D., Cigudosa, J. C., Urioste, M., Benitez, J., & others. (2005). Epigenetic differences arise during the lifetime of monozygotic twins. *Proceedings of the National Academy of Sciences*, 102(30), 10604–10609.

Freckelton, I. (2020). COVID-19: Fear, quackery, false representations and the law. *International Journal of Law and Psychiatry*, 101611. https://doi.org/10.1016/j.ijlp.2020.101611.

Ghosh, S., & Karin, M. (2002). Missing pieces in the NF-$κ$B puzzle. *Cell*, 109(2), S81--S96.

Ghosh, S., Saha, S., Koley, M., Kundu, M., Mondal, R., & Patra, S. (2014). Access to and utilization of the health services among the patients in a government homeopathic hospital in West Bengal, India: A cross-sectional study. *Journal of Evidence-Based Complementary and Alternative Medicine*, *19*(4), 247–252.

Glozak, M. A., & Seto, E. (2007). Histone deacetylases and cancer. *Oncogene*, 26(37), 5420–5432.

Gombart, A. F., Pierre, A., & Maggini, S. (2020). A review of micronutrients and the immune system--working in harmony to reduce the risk of infection. *Nutrients*, 12(1), 236.

Gopalakrishnan, S., Van Emburgh, B. O., & Robertson, K. D. (2008). DNA methylation in development and human disease. *Mutation Research/Fundamental and Molecular Mechanisms of Mutagenesis*, 647(1–2), 30–38.

Gray, S. G., & De Meyts, P. (2005). Role of histone and transcription factor acetylation in diabetes pathogenesis. *Diabetes/Metabolism Research and Reviews*, 21(5), 416–433.

Guo, C., Liu, L., Jia, Y., Zhao, X., Zhou, Q., & Wang, L. (2012). A novel variant of Oct3/4 gene in mouse embryonic stem cells. *Stem Cell Research*, *9*(2), 69–76.

Hansen, J. C., Ghosh, R. P., & Woodcock, C. L. (2010). Binding of the Rett syndrome protein, MeCP2, to methylated and unmethylated DNA and chromatin. *IUBMB Life*, 62(10), 732–738.

Hewagama, A., & Richardson, B. (2009). The genetics and epigenetics of autoimmune diseases. *Journal of Autoimmunity*, 33(1), 3–11.

Ho, S. M. (2010). Environmental epigenetics of asthma: an update. *Journal of Allergy and Clinical Immunology*, *126*(3), 453–465.

Ishii, M., Wen, H., Corsa, C. A. S., Liu, T., Coelho, A. L., Allen, R. M., Carson IV, W. F., Cavassani, K. A., Li, X., Lukacs, N. W., & others. (2009). Epigenetic regulation of the alternatively activated macrophage phenotype. *Blood, The Journal of the American Society of Hematology*, 114(15), 3244–3254.

Jasemi, M., Valizadeh, L., Zamanzadeh, V., & Keogh, B. (2017). A Conceptual Analysis of Holistic Care by Hybrid Model. *Indian Journal of Palliative Care*, 23(1), 71–80.

Jayawardene, K. L. T. D., Palombo, E. A., & Boag, P. R. (2021). Natural Products Are a Promising Source for Anthelmintic Drug Discovery. *Biomolecules*, 11(10), 1457.

Jin, B., Li, Y., & Robertson, K. D. (2011). DNA methylation: Superior or subordinate in the epigenetic hierarchy? *Genes & Cancer*, *2*(6), 607–617.

Jones, P. A., & Takai, D. (2001). The role of DNA methylation in mammalian epigenetics. *Science*, 293(5532), 1068–1070.

Kanwal, R., & Gupta, S. (2012). Epigenetic modifications in cancer. *Clinical Genetics*, 81(4), 303–311.

Keating, S. T., Plutzky, J., & El-Osta, A. (2016). Epigenetic changes in diabetes and cardiovascular risk. *Circulation Research*, 118(11), 1706–1722.

Kleijnen, J., Knipschild, P., & ter Riet, G. (1991). Clinical trials of homoeopathy. *British Medical Journal*, 302(6772), 316–323.

Liu, Q., Jin, X., Cheng, J., Zhou, H., Zhang, Y., & Dai, Y. (2023). Advances in the application of molecular diagnostic techniques for the detection of infectious disease pathogens (Review). *Molecular Medicine Reports*, 27(5), 104.

Lund, A. H., & van Lohuizen, M. (2004). Epigenetics and cancer. *Genes & Development*, *18*(19), 2315–2335.

Madrigal-Matute, J., Rotllan, N., Aranda, J. F., & Fernández-Hernando, C. (2013). MicroRNAs and atherosclerosis. *Current Atherosclerosis Reports*, 15, 1–8.

Mathie, R. T. (2003). The research evidence base for homeopathy: A fresh assessment of the literature. *Homeopathy: The Journal of the Faculty of Homeopathy*, *92*(2), 84–91.

Memvanga, P. B., & Nkanga, C. I. (2021). Liposomes for malaria management: The evolution from 1980 to 2020. *Malaria Journal*, 20. https://doi.org/10.1186/s12936-021-03858-0.

Nathan, C. (2002). Points of control in inflammation. *Nature*, 420(6917), 846–852.

Ng, T. I., Correia, I., Seagal, J., DeGoey, D. A., Schrimpf, M. R., Hardee, D. J., Noey, E. L., & Kati, W. M. (2022). Antiviral drug discovery for the treatment of COVID-19 infections. *Viruses*, 14(5), 961.

Nicholson, L. B. (2016). The immune system. *Essays in Biochemistry*, 60(3), 275–301.

Niwa, T., Tsukamoto, T., Toyoda, T., Mori, A., Tanaka, H., Maekita, T., Ichinose, M., Tatematsu, M., & Ushijima, T. (2010). Inflammatory processes triggered by *Helicobacter pylori* infection cause aberrant DNA methylation in gastric epithelial cells. *Cancer Research*, 70(4), 1430–1440.

Odugbemi, T. O., Akinsulire, O. R., Aibinu, I. E., & Fabeku, P. O. (2006). Medicinal plants useful for malaria therapy in Okeigbo, Ondo State, Southwest Nigeria. *African Journal of Traditional, Complementary, and Alternative Medicines*, 4(2), 191–198.

Olas, B. (2022). Bee Products as Interesting Natural Agents for the Prevention and Treatment of Common Cardiovascular Diseases. *Nutrients*, 14(11), 2267.

Oskvig, D. B., Elkahloun, A. G., Johnson, K. R., Phillips, T. M., & Herkenham, M. (2012). Maternal immune activation by LPS selectively alters specific gene expression profiles of interneuron migration and oxidative stress in the fetus without triggering a fetal immune response. *Brain, Behavior, and Immunity*, 26(4), 623–634.

Park, E., Kim, Y., Ryu, H., Kowall, N. W., Lee, J., & Ryu, H. (2014). Epigenetic mechanisms of Rubinstein--Taybi syndrome. *Neuromolecular Medicine*, 16, 16–24.

Patel, V., Chavda, V., & Shah, J. (2021). Nanotherapeutics in neuropathologies: Obstacles, challenges and recent advancements in cns targeted drug delivery systems. *Current Neuropharmacology*, 19(5), 693–710.

Patra, J. K., Das, G., Fraceto, L. F., Campos, E. V. R., Rodriguez-Torres, M. del P., Acosta-Torres, L. S., Diaz-Torres, L. A., Grillo, R., Swamy, M. J., Sharma, S., Habtemariam, S., & Shin, H. S. (2018). Nano based drug delivery systems: Recent developments and future prospects. *Journal of Nanobiotechnology*, 16(1), 71.

Pikaard, C. S. (2000). The epigenetics of nucleolar dominance. *Trends in Genetics*, 16(11), 495–500.

Portela, A., & Esteller, M. (2010). Epigenetic modifications and human disease. *Nature Biotechnology*, 28(10), 1057–1068.

Quintero-Ronderos, P., Montoya-Ortiz, G., & others. (2012). Epigenetics and autoimmune diseases. *Autoimmune Diseases*, 2012.

Reik, W., Santos, F., & Dean, W. (2003). Mammalian epigenomics: eprogramming the genome for development and therapy. *Theriogenology*, 59(1), 21–32.

Rizvi, S. A. A., Einstein, G. P., Tulp, O. L., Sainvil, F., & Branly, R. (2023). Introduction to traditional medicine and their role in prevention and treatment of emerging and Re-emerging diseases. *Journal of Traditional Medicine*, *X*(X), X–X.

Robertson, K. D. (2005). DNA methylation and human disease. *Nature Reviews Genetics*, 6(8), 597–610.

Rudramurthy, G. R., Swamy, M. K., Sinniah, U. R., & Ghasemzadeh, A. (2016). Nanoparticles: Alternatives Against Drug-Resistant Pathogenic Microbes. *Molecules*, *21*(7), 836.

Saccani, S., Pantano, S., & Natoli, G. (2002). p38-dependent marking of inflammatory genes for increased NF-$κ$B recruitment. *Nature Immunology*, *3*(1), 69–75.

Sadri-Vakili, G., & Cha, J. H. J. (2006). Mechanisms of disease: Histone modifications in Huntington's disease. *Nature Clinical Practice Neurology*, 2(6), 330–338.

Serban, G. (2019). Future prospects in the treatment of parasitic diseases: 2-Amino-1,3,4-Thiadiazoles in leishmaniasis. *Molecules*, 24(8), 1557.

Sethi, B., Kumar, V., Mahato, K., Coulter, D. W., & Mahato, R. I. (2022). Recent advances in drug delivery and targeting to the brain. *Journal of Controlled Release*, 350, 668–687.

Sharma, S., Kelly, T. K., & Jones, P. A. (2010). Epigenetics in cancer. *Carcinogenesis*, 31(1), 27–36.

Shuto, T., Furuta, T., Oba, M., Xu, H., Li, J.-D., Cheung, J., Gruenert, D. C., Uehara, A., Suico, M. A., Okiyoneda, T., & others. (2006). Promoter hypomethylation of Toll-like receptor-2 gene is associated with increased proinflammatory response towardbacterial peptidoglycan in cystic fibrosis bronchial epithelial cells. *The FASEB Journal*, 20(6), 782–784.

Singh, L., Kruger, H. G., Maguire, G. E. M., Govender, T., & Parboosing, R. (2017). The role of nanotechnology in the treatment of viral infections. *Therapeutic Advances in Infectious Disease*, 4(4), 105–131.

Soleymani, S., Naghizadeh, A., Karimi, M., Zarei, A., Mardi, R., Kordafshari, G., Esmaealzadeh, N., & Zargaran, A. (2022). COVID-19: General strategies for herbal therapies. *Journal of Evidence-Based Integrative Medicine*, 27, 2515690X211 053641.

Su, X., & Miller, L. H. (2015). The discovery of artemisinin and nobel prize in physiology or medicine. *Science China. Life Sciences*, 58(11), 1175–1179.

Sullivan, K. E., Reddy, A. B. M., Dietzmann, K., Suriano, A. R., Kocieda, V. P., Stewart, M., & Bhatia, M. (2007). Epigenetic regulation of tumor necrosis factor alpha. *Molecular and Cellular Biology*, 27(14), 5147–5160.

Sun, Y., Chen, D., Pan, Y., Qu, W., Hao, H., Wang, X., Liu, Z., & Xie, S. (2019). Nanoparticles for antiparasitic drug delivery. *Drug Delivery*, 26(1), 1206–1221.

Takahashi, K., Sugi, Y., Hosono, A., & Kaminogawa, S. (2009). Epigenetic regulation of TLR4 gene expression in intestinal epithelial cells for the maintenance of intestinal homeostasis. *The Journal of Immunology*, 183(10), 6522–6529.

Teleanu, D. M., Chircov, C., Grumezescu, A. M., Volceanov, A., & Teleanu, R. I. (2018). Blood-Brain Delivery Methods Using Nanotechnology. *Pharmaceutics*, 10(4), 269.

Ung, L., Stothard, J. R., Phalkey, R., Azman, A. S., Chodosh, J., Hanage, W. P., & Standley, C. J. (2021). Towards global control of parasitic diseases in the COVID-19 era: One Health and the future of multisectoral global health governance. *Advances in Parasitology*, 114, 1–26.

Urdinguio, R. G., Sanchez-Mut, J. V, & Esteller, M. (2009). Epigenetic mechanisms in neurological diseases: genes, syndromes, and therapies. *The Lancet Neurology*, 8(11), 1056–1072.

Varier, R. A., & Timmers, H. T. M. (2011). Histone lysine methylation and demethylation pathways in cancer. *Biochimica et Biophysica Acta (BBA)-Reviews on Cancer*, 1815(1), 75–89.

Villagra, A., Sotomayor, E. M., & Seto, E. (2010). Histone deacetylases and the immunological network: implications in cancer and inflammation. *Oncogene*, 29(2), 157–173.

Wei, G., Wei, L., Zhu, J., Zang, C., Hu-Li, J., Yao, Z., Cui, K., Kanno, Y., Roh, T. Y., Watford, W. T., & others. (2009). Global mapping of H3K4me3 and H3K27me3 reveals specificity and plasticity in lineage fate determination of differentiating CD4+ T cells. *Immunity*, 30(1), 155–167.

Wen, H., Jung, H., & Li, X. (2015). Drug delivery approaches in addressing clinical pharmacology-related issues: Opportunities and challenges. *The AAPS Journal*, 17(6), 1327–1340.

Wieland, L. S., Piechotta, V., Feinberg, T., Ludeman, E., Hutton, B., Kanji, S., Seely, D., & Garritty, C. (2021). Elderberry for prevention and treatment of viral respiratory illnesses: A systematic review. *BMC Complementary Medicine and Therapies*, 21(1), 1–15.

Xing, S., Nie, F., Xu, Q., Deng, Y., Li, W., Yang, Z., Zhao, X., Zhu, P., Wang, X., Gao, Y., & others. (2015). HDAC is essential for epigenetic regulation of Thy-1 gene expression during LPS/TLR4-mediated proliferation of lung fibroblasts. *Laboratory Investigation*, 95(10), 1105–1116.

Yamamoto, Y., Verma, U. N., Prajapati, S., Kwak, Y. T., & Gaynor, R. B. (2003). Histone H3 phosphorylation by IKK-$\alpha$ is critical for cytokine-induced gene expression. *Nature*, 423(6940), 655–659.

Yang, J., Park, Y., Zhang, H., Xu, X., Laine, G. A., Dellsperger, K. C., & Zhang, C. (2009). Feed-forward signaling of TNF-$\alpha$ and NF-$\kappa$B via IKK-$\beta$ pathway contributes to insulin resistance and coronary arteriolar dysfunction in type 2 diabetic mice. *American Journal of Physiology-Heart and Circulatory Physiology*, 296(6), H1850--H1858.

Yin, I. X., Zhang, J., Zhao, I. S., Mei, M. L., Li, Q., & Chu, C. H. (2020). The antibacterial mechanism of silver nanoparticles and its application in dentistry. *International Journal of Nanomedicine*, 15, 2555–2562.

Yuan, H., Ma, Q., Ye, L., & Piao, G. (2016). The traditional medicine and modern medicine from natural products. *Molecules*, 21(5), 559.

Zeng, J., Nagrajan, H. K., & Yi, S. V. (2014). Fundamental diversity of human CpG islands at multiple biological levels. *Epigenetics*, 9(4), 483–491.

Zhang, Z., & Zhang, R. (2015). Epigenetics in autoimmune diseases: Pathogenesis and prospects for therapy. *Autoimmunity Reviews*, 14(10), 854–863.

## Chapter 10

# Current Paradigms in Understanding Oncogenesis and Cancer: From Basics to Advanced Personalized Medicines and Targeted Nanotherapeutics

**Varruchi Sharma**[1]
**Sonal Datta**[2]
**Atul Sankhyan**[3]
**Anil Panwar**[4]
**Diwakar Aggarwal**[2]
**Sushil Kumar Upadhyay**[2]
**Manoj Singh**[2]
**Amit Joshi**[1]
**Poonam Bansal**[2]
**and Anil K Sharma**[5,*]

[1]Department of Biotechnology & Bioinformatics, Sri Guru Gobind Singh College, Chandigarh, India
[2]Department of Bio-Sciences and Technology, Maharishi Markandeshwar (Deemed to be University), Mullana-Ambala, (Haryana), India
[3]Department of Public Health Dentistry, HPGDCH, Shimla, India
[4]Department of Molecular Biology, Biotechnology & Bioinformatics, College of Basic Sciences & Humanities, CCS Haryana Agricultural University, Hisar, Haryana
[5]Department of Biotechnology, Amity University, Mohali, Punjab, India

In: Therapeutic Advances in Human Health and Diseases
Editors: Sushil Kumar Upadhyay, Manoj Singh and Anil Kumar Sharma
ISBN: 979-8-89113-304-4

## Abstract

Worldwide, cancer has been the leading cause of cancer-related deaths among women. At the early stages of diagnosis, the treatment choices are allegedly more effective in terms of curing the condition however, at the advanced stages, the therapy still presents significant clinical challenges. Prior reports of several targeted medicines have sparked interest in discovering new treatments that might increase the survival rate in cancer patients. There are several different types of cancer, which are classified based on the cell types and organs they attack. Concerning cancer, like most breast cancers, apparently has an active PI3K/AKT/mTOR (mammalian target of rapamycin) signaling pathway, which promotes uncontrollable cell proliferation and tumor formation. As a result, targeting this crucial route becomes a growing area of therapeutic interest, particularly in the management of cancer. With these facts in mind, the present review has focused on preclinical and clinical trials in which a number of PI3K/AKT/mTOR pathway inhibitors (acting at various levels) have been employed either alone or in combination with other drugs to treat cancer. Also, the review deals with an extensive understanding of mTOR's structural control and dysregulation, as well as first- and second-generation PI3K/AKT/mTOR pathway inhibitors, targeted therapy, and the significance of mTOR inhibitory medications in the management of cancer, are additional highlights.



**Keywords:** cancer, targeted therapy, P13K/AKT/mTOR, inhibitors, therapeutics, biomarkers, diagnosis


## 1. Introduction

Cancer is a disease in which normal cells start dividing uncontrollably and spread to other parts of the body. When a gene or several genes are mutated, cancerous cells are generated which then create cell clusters or tumors. Cancer is a leading cause of death worldwide. Symptoms include sudden weight loss or weight gain, chronic fatigue, changes in the skin like darkening or redness of the skin, sores that are not healing, unexplained pain, fever, bleeding, a lump under the skin, changes in bowel habits, and persistent cough (Saini et al., 2020). Causes include smoking cigarettes and cigars, eating food rich in sugar and fat, exposure to radiation or toxins, etc. Mostly cancer has four main stages: Stage I: The cancer is localized to a small area and has not spread to other parts of the body. Stage II: The cancer has grown, but it has not spread.

Stage III: The cancer has grown larger and has possibly spread to other parts. Stage IV: The cancer has spread to other organs or areas of your body. This is the advanced cancer stage. Treatment includes chemotherapy, radiation therapy, surgery, hormonal therapy, bone marrow transplant, and immunotherapy (Sharma et al., 2019b).

There are four general types of cancer: 1) Carcinoma is found in the skin or body tissues that line or cover other organs. 2) Sarcoma is found in connective or supportive tissues such as bones, muscles, cartilage, and blood vessels. 3) Leukemia is a cancer of white blood cells that starts in the tissue that makes blood cells, such as bone marrow 4) Lymphoma and myeloma are cancers of the immune system. There are more than 100 types of cancer, but the most common cancer is breast cancer, primarily affecting females. Lung cancer is the second most common cancer. There are two types of lung cancer: non-small cell cancer and small cell lung cancer. Prostate cancer affects males, Colorectal cancer affects the colon and rectum of the digestive system (Morgan et al., 2023), Blood cancers include leukemia and lymphoma, Lung cancer occurs due to excessive smoking, Skin cancer occurs in areas of the body that have been repeatedly exposed to sunlight, Sign of Bladder cancer includes blood in urine, difficulty in urination, Endometrial cancer is a type of cancer that affects the endometrium, which is the lining of the uterus (Ruchi Sharma et al., 2017; Jassim et al., 2023).

## 2. Common Types of Cancer

Breast cancer, leukemia, colorectal cancer, lymphoma, prostate cancer, melanoma, sarcoma, pancreatic cancer, multiple myeloma, kidney cancer, thyroid cancer, bladder cancer, carcinoma, uterine cancer, non-small cell lung cancer, oropharyngeal cancer are the most common types of cancer in which carcinomas covers the skin or in tissues that line or cover internal organs. (Chhikara et al., 2023). Sarcomas include connective or supportive tissues such as bone, cartilage, fat, muscle or blood vessels, etc. The third type of leukemia is cancer of the white blood cells (Sharma et al., 2010; Siegel et al., 2023).

In India, the new cancer cases for the year 2022 were approximately 1,461,427, which predicts an estimated chance of one in nine individuals developing cancer during their lifetime. In context to the world, it is estimated that 19.3 million new cancer cases were reported in the current year, and almost 10.0 million cancer deaths occurred in 2020 (Berenguer et al., 2023; Vogel et al., 2023).

When it comes to Breast cancer, is a type of cancer that develops from breast cells or tissues. Usually, breast cancer starts in the inner lining of milk ducts or the lobules that supply them with milk. A malignant tumor can spread to other parts of the body. Cancer that starts in the lobules is known as lobular carcinoma, while one that develops from the ducts is called ductal carcinoma (Stepan et al., 2023). Breast cancer is the most common malignancy among women all over the world. In recent studies, it has been observed that the same has surpassed the leading cause of global cancer incidence in 2020, with an estimated 2.3 million new cases, representing 11.7% of all cancer cases (Mehrotra et al., 2022). In many epidemiological studies, it was revealed that the global burden of breast cancer disease is likely to cross almost 2 million people to be invaded by the year 2030 (Yuan et al., 2023).

The symptoms of breast cancer disease include a lump in the breast, pain in the armpits or breast that does not seem to be related to the woman's menstrual period, pitting or redness of the skin of the breast, rash around one of the nipples, an area of thickened tissue in a breast, discharge in the nipples, change in appearance of the breast (Yuan et al., 2023), changes in size or the shape of the breast, skin of the breast started to peel, scale or flake. Women who carry the BRCA1 and BRCA2 genes have a considerably higher risk of developing breast and/or ovarian cancer (Khadwal et al., 2020). P53 is another gene that is associated with an increased risk of breast cancer (Kingsbury 2007). Women with a history of certain types of benign (non-cancerous) breast lumps are more prone to developing cancer in the coming time of their life. Those with denser breast tissue are also more likely to develop breast cancer (Cerma et al., 2023). Moreover, women who experienced early onset of periods or later onset of menopause have an elevated risk of breast cancer (Raghav et al., 2022). Post-menopausal women who are obese or overweight may also be at a higher risk. Additionally, the risk of breast cancer rises with the amount of alcohol a woman regularly consumes (Tian et al., 2023b). Undergoing X-rays and CT scans may raise a woman's risk of developing breast cancer. Hormone replacement therapy (HRT) can also slightly increase women's risk of breast cancer. Furthermore, women with cosmetic breast implants who develop breast cancer may have a higher risk of premature death from the disease compared to other females (Sharma et al., 2021a, Sharma et al., 2022).

The primary breast cancer treatment options may include radiotherapy (Breast radiation therapy, Chest wall radiation therapy, Breast boost, Lymph nodes radiation therapy, Breast brachytherapy, Surgery (Lumpectomy, Mastectomy, Sentinel node biopsy Axillary lymph node dissection Breast reconstruction surgery), Biological therapy (Trastuzumab, Lapatinib, Bevacizumab) Hormone therapy (Tamoxifen, Aromatase inhibitors), Chemotherapy (Ely and Vioral 2007; Sharma et al., 2021c).

A new study has confirmed the existence of four main subtypes of breast cancer: Luminal A, luminal B, HER2, and basal-like. Luminal A - the least aggressive and most common subtype - accounts for 42% to 59% of all breast cancers (Cerma et al., 2023). Luminal B typically occurs in younger women and accounts for about 10% of all breast cancers. Basal-like subtype typically occurs in younger women and African American women, and HER-2 the enriched subtype is characterized by high-grade tumors and poor outcomes (Sham et al., 2023). Luminal A and luminal B are known as estrogen receptor (ER)-positive, since they contain estrogen receptors that bind to the hormone estrogen, which helps the tumor cells grow (Singh 2023). Luminal A cancers have the best outcomes, while luminal B cancers grow slightly faster than luminal A and have a slightly less positive outcome (Ruchi Sharma et al., 2017). HER2-positive: This sub-type of cancer contains a protein called human epidermal growth factor receptor 2 (HER2), that causes the cancer cells to grow. This type of cancer tends to grow more quickly and may have a poor outcome, though it can often be treated successfully with drugs such as Herceptin, which targets the HER2 protein to prevent cell growth. Basal-like: This sub-type of cancer is also known as 'triple-negative', meaning its cells have no estrogen or progesterone hormone receptors and have normal amounts of HER2. This type of cancer is more common in women who carry a mutation in their BRCA1 gene and younger and African American women. These cancers tend to grow quickly, don't respond as well to many of the available treatments and have poor outcomes (Sehrawat et al., 2021).

As reported in the journal Diabetologia, Postmenopausal women who survived breast cancer are more likely to develop diabetes, compared to other women of their age who did not have breast cancer. Breast cancer survivors undergoing chemotherapy were especially at risk of developing diabetes (Sharma et al., 2021b, Sharma et al., 2021).

ESPL1 has been known as a candidate oncogene in luminal B cancers. Its expression may help improve prognostication. Inhibiting ESPL1 may represent a promising therapeutic approach for these poor prognosis tumors. Compared to normal breast samples, ESPL1 was over-expressed in 52% of luminal tumors, and much more frequently in luminal B (83%) than luminal A tumors (29%) (Sharma et al., 2021).

Most genetic forms of breast cancer are caused by mutations in the BRCA1 and BRCA2 genes, whose primary function is the DNA repair of double-strand breaks. A wide range of variants were identified in the BRCA1 and BRCA2 genes. Two pathological variants were detected in the breast cancer patient group: a mutation in BRCA2 at the chromosomal position chr13:32890665, which affected the first position of the 5' splice region following exon 2; and a mutation in BRCA1 at chr17:41219635, causing an in-frame triple nucleotide deletion of valine 1688 (8.3%) (Balabanski et al., 2014).

Single Nucleotide Polymorphisms (SNPs) in genes involved in the DNA Base Excision Repair (BER) pathway are associated with cancer risk in carriers of mutations in the high-penetrance susceptibility genes BRCA1 and BRCA2, given the relation of synthetic lethality that exists between one of the components of the BER pathway, PARP1 (poly ADP ribose polymerase), and both BRCA1 and BRCA2. DNA glycosylases involved in the first steps of the BER pathway are associated with cancer risk in BRCA1/2 mutation carriers. (Osorio et al., 2014).

Runx2 is best known as an essential factor in osteoblast differentiation and bone development. In the mammary gland, Runx2 is known to be expressed and participate in the regulation of mammary-specific genes. Differential and temporal expression of gene Runx2 is observed during mammary epithelial differentiation. RUNX2 has been linked to metastatic cancer in some established breast cell lines; retention of expression is associated with a more invasive phenotype. mTOR (mammalian Target of Rapamycin) also known as FK506-binding protein 12-rapamycin-associated protein 1 (FRAP1). This protein is encoded by the mTOR gene (Liao et al. 2011). mTOR regulates cell metabolism, cell growth, cell proliferation, cell motility, cell survival, protein synthesis, and transcription. mTOR regulates the phosphorylation of proteins and monitors nutrient availability, cellular energy levels, oxygen levels, and mitogenic signals (Tian, et al. 2023a).

## 3. PI3K/Akt/mTOR Signaling in Normal Cells

mTOR is a regulator of several cell processes in normal cells with the assistance of other protein, including PI3-kinase, Akt, and PTEN, and plays an essential role in mTOR signaling (Heras-Sandoval et al., 2014). PI3-kinase is an enzyme that helps in the phosphorylation of some cell membrane components. When these components become phosphorylated, they bind to another protein known as Akt. After binding, Akt becomes phosphorylated and activated, which triggers the activation of many signaling pathways that regulate cell survival, growth, and proliferation. mTOR promotes cell growth and proliferation by stimulating protein synthesis when activated by Akt. mTOR receives the signal from Akt and monitors the cell's environment in the presence of growth factors and nutrients (Kumar et al., 2020). mTOR can promote angiogenesis and increase nutrient uptake if the cell needs additional resources. mTOR can also increase the activity of Akt and enhance the other downstream effects of this protein. PTEN removes the phosphate groups added to membrane phospholipids by PI3-kinase and thus prevents the activation of Akt and its downstream pathways (Raghav et al., 2020a).

Serine/threonine protein kinase, known as the mammalian target of rapamycin (mTOR) controls cell growth, proliferation, and metabolism via signaling through the protein complexes mTORC1 and mTORC2. Evolutionarily, mTOR complex 1/2 (mTORC1/2) is conserved from yeast to mammals. Mammalian targets of rapamycin (mTOR) inhibitors were introduced, which was a significant advancement in the treatment of many malignancies (Sharma et al. 2018), including breast cancer. The serine/threonine-specific protein kinase that these inhibitors are known to block is a member of the phosphatidylinositol-3 kinase (PI3K) related kinase (PIKK) family. The PI3K/AKT/mTOR pathway can be ontogenically activated by a number of different methods, frequently including the mutation and/or amplification of RTK-encoding genes (Sharma 2021).

The microbe *Streptomyces hygroscopius* is well known for its anticancer, antifungal, and immunosuppressive activities, and is said to create the macrolide rapamycin. Rapamycin derivatives, such as rapalogs, were further developed as first-generation mTOR inhibitors with therapeutic benefits similar to rapamycin in various preclinical settings, but with increased hydrophilicity and the ability to be administered orally and intravenously (Singh et al., 2022). Due to partial mTOR inhibition, rapalogs were not enough to achieve widespread and effective anticancer effects. In addition, rapalogs' inhibition of mTORC1 failed to stop a negative feedback loop that phosphorylates and activates AKT (Sharma et al. 2021). These restrictions led to the development of the second generation of ATP-competitive mTORC1/mTORC2 dual inhibitors (Sharma et al., 2020b). In contrast to rapalogs, which only target mTORC1, they inhibit the kinase-dependent actions of mTORC1 and mTORC2, preventing the feedback stimulation of PI3K/AKT signaling. Additionally, it has been discovered that a few naturally occurring substances can inhibit mTOR signaling. The PI3K/AKT/mTOR pathway's function in the pathogenesis of breast cancer, as well as preclinical and *in vitro* results regarding PI3K/AKT/mTOR inhibitors, have been discussed in light of the aforementioned facts in order to create these inhibitors as prospective biomarkers against breast cancer (Chaudhary et al., 2020).

## 4. Structure Preview into mTOR and Pathway

mTORC1 and mTORC2 are the two structurally and functionally different complexes of mTOR that play significant roles in the pathway at various levels.

### 4.1. mTORC1

mTORC1 comprises mainly following five main components: Raptor (the regulatory-associated protein of mTOR), mammalian lethal with Sec13 protein 8 (mLST8), proline-rich AKT substrate 40 kDa (PRAS40), Deptor (DEP-domain-containing mTOR-interacting protein) and mTOR. Raptor enrolls substrates for mTOR regulating the complex formation. mTOR is the catalytic subunit of mTORC1. Both PRAS40 and Deptor negatively regulate mTORC1. Enrollment of both PRAS40 and DEPTOR to mTORC1 upholds the reticence of the complex when there is a reduction in mTORC1 activity (Sharma et al., 2020b). PRAS40 directly inhibits mTORC1 kinase activity by binding to the substrate. Activation leads to phosphorylation of PRAS40 and Deptor by mTORC1, which shows a reduced physical interaction with mTORC1 and further encourages mTORC1 signaling. mTORC1 is a nutrient and energy sensor and is also reported to be involved in the regulation of biogenesis, lipid synthesis, autophagy, and mitochondrial metabolism. Also, various amino acids, serum, insulin, and other growth factors are known to forbid the activity of mTORC1 (Figure 1).

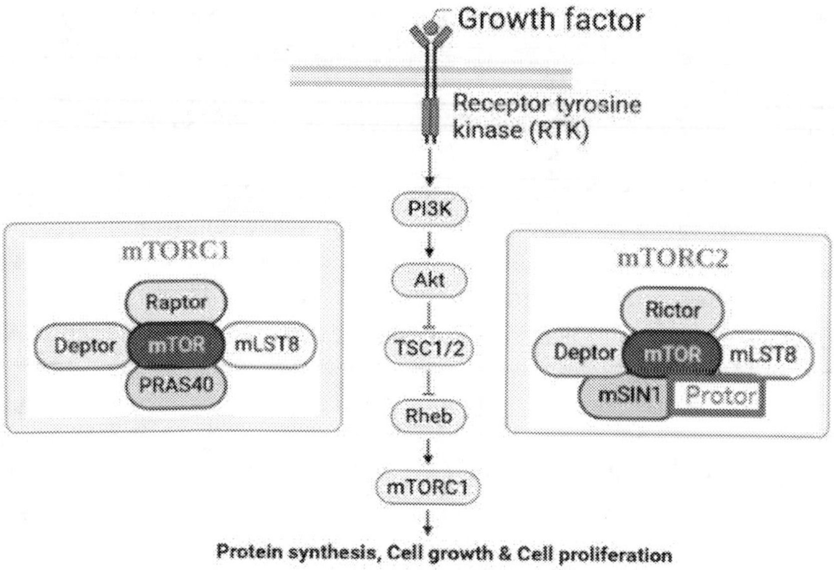


**Figure 1.** Overview of the mTOR Pathway and its Structure.

## 4.2. mTORC2

mTORC2 complex consists of the following six proteins: mTOR, mSIN1, Rapamycin-insensitive companion of mTOR (Rictor), mLST8, Protor-1 and Deptor. Some of the main components: mTOR, Deptor, and mLST8 are commonly pooled between mTORC1/C2 complexes. Rictor and mSIN1 are known to alleviate each other. Rictor and Protor-1 show common interactions. As in mTORC1, Deptor regulates mTORC2 activity negatively. mLST8 plays a critical role in the functioning of mTORC2, as the hit of this protein strongly or cuts the complex stability and activity. mTORC2 is an important regulator of the cytoskeleton through its stimulation of paxillin, Rac1, Cdc42, F-actin stress fibers, and RhoA (Sharma et al., 2023). mTORC2 phosphorylates the serine/threonine protein kinase Akt/PKB at serine residue S473, thereby disturbing survival and metabolism (Figure 1).

The mTOR domain structure consists of six main functional domains (1) HEAT domain (Huntington elongation factor 3, which is a subunit of protein phosphatase 2A and TOR1), and protein-protein interactions are facilitated by the same; (2) FAT (FRAP-ATM-TRAPP) domain; (3) FRB (FKBP12-rapamycin binding) domain plays as the primary inhibitory agent of rapamycin on Raptor-bound mTOR; (4) PIKK (PI3-kinase-related kinase) domain; (5) RD (Repressor domain); and (6) the carboxy-terminal FATC domain (Sharma et al., 2017) (Figure 1).

Twenty tandem HEAT repeats make up the N terminus of mTOR, and the kinase domain (also known as the catalytic domain) is located at the C terminus. Between HEAT repeats and the kinase domain are the FRB and FAT domains. The first 1350 residues of mTOR are made up of HEAT repeats, while the 650 residues that make up the FAT domain contain several TPRs (tetratricopeptide repeats). Tetratricopeptide repeats, and HEAT both extend the superhelical domains necessary for protein-protein interactions. The FAT domain has 28 alpha helices, which are organized in repetitions and create a solenoid with a "C" shape surrounding the kinase domain. There is a 100-residue structure called the FRB domain between the FAT and kinase domains. Binding to RICTOR and RAPTOR requires the FRB domain. The kinase domain comprises 550 residues and comprises two different lobes that bind to ATP: the N- and C-terminal lobes. The binding location for mLST8 is the C-terminal lobe. There are 35 residues in the FATC domain, which is found at the C-terminus. The loss of the repressor domain, which is located between the kinase and FATC domains, activates mTOR (Sharma et al., 2022c).

## 5. PI3K/AKT/mTOR Pathway

The cellular pathway PI3K/AKT/mTOR is a major regulator of cell metabolism, growth, proliferation, and survival. Angiogenesis, tumor growth, and other biological activities are the first to activate the route. Growth factors activate mTORC2, whereas the PI3K/AKT complex suppresses mTORC1, and the TSC1/TSC2 complex stimulates mTORC1. Through S6K activation and phosphorylation, followed by 4EBP1 inactivation, mTORC1 further controls ribosome assembly and protein synthesis (Sharma et al., 2020b).

mTORC1 regulates several proteins, including HIF-1 α (hypoxia-inducible factor 1α), CLIP-170 (cytoplasm linker protein-170), eEF2 (eukaryotic elongation factor 2) kinase, lipin, ODC (ornithine decarboxylase), PKCδ and PKCε, PP2A (protein phosphatase 2A), p21Cip1 and p27Kip1 cyclin-dependent kinase inhibitors, glycogen synthase, retinoblastoma protein, and activator of transcription-3. mTORC2 regulates the activity of the small GTPases Rac and Rho by phosphorylating PKC-, AKT, and paxillin (a focal adhesion-associated adaptor protein) (Sharma et al., 2020b).

mTOR is an important regulator of cell metabolism, growth, and proliferation. Various growth factors, ATP, amino acids, and oxygen levels regulate the PI3K/AKT/mTOR Pathway. The phosphorylation of AKT activates the mTORC1 signaling. Class I PI3K produces the second messenger, PtdIns (3,4,5) P3, which further binds to the pleckstrin-homology (PH) domain of AKT and PDK1. Due to the binding of PtdIns (3,4,5) P3 to the PH domain of AKT, the kinase is brought to the cell membrane, which is formed by phosphorylation of mTORC2 at Ser473 position and activation by phosphorylation of PDK1 at Thr308 position. PTEN controls AKT activation negatively by transforming PtdIns (3,4,5) P3 to PtdIns(4,5) P2; therefore, there is reduced recruitment of AKT to the cell membrane (Raghav et al., 2020b). GSK3, FOXO transcription factors TSC2, and several downstream substrates are known to activate AKT. When TSC2 is being phosphorylated, the complex formation of TSC1/TSC2 is discontinued, which induces the small GTPase Rheb into the GTP-bound active state and further leads to the activation of mTORC1 at Ser2448 (Sharma et al., 2022b). Upon phosphorylation and inhibition of PRAS40 by AKT, mTORC1 is negatively regulated by turning around its activation by Rheb. Both S6K1 and 4EBP1 get phosphorylated by mTORC1, which is activated by interrelating raptor and a TOR signaling (TOS) motif in S6K and 4EBP. S6K1 is further activated by TOR-insensitive signaling pathways such as PDK1, MAPK, and SAPK (stress-activated protein kinase). Despite this, the phosphorylation of S6K1 is important for its activation through mTORC1 and the phosphorylation sites of S6K1 are known to be hindered by mTOR inhibitors. Activated mTORC1 phosphorylates S6K1 and further phosphorylates 40S ribosomal protein S6 along with increasing translation of mRNAs with a 5′-terminal oligo-poly-pyrimidine (Sharma et al., 2020b). The targets of S6K1 include elongation factors, ribosomal proteins, and insulin growth factor2. 4EBP1 binds to eIF4E (eukaryotic translation initiation factor 4E) and deactivates it; therefore, the protein translation initiation is reduced. mTORC1 phosphorylates 4EBP1 at multiple sites for dissociation of eIF4E from 4EBP1 and therefore alleviates the inhibition of 4EBP1 on eIF4E-dependent translation beginning (Sharma et al., 2020b).

## 6. Diverse Classes of PI3K/AKT/mTOR Inhibitors and Their Therapeutic Potential

A new class of Class 1 PI3K-specific inhibitors, NVP-BKM120 has activity against PI3K and mTOR. According to reports, BKM120 caused the blocking of NF-B expression and PI3K/AKT signaling, which activated caspase-9 and caspase-3/7, further altering the expression of genes involved in apoptosis. Through the stimulation of cell death, BKM120 partially reverses the MDR phenotype in chemo-resistant breast cancer (Francipane et al., 2016). This effect was further mediated by suppressing the PI3K/AKT/NF-B axis. In a mouse model of breast cancer, the expression of phosphoinositide 3-kinase (PI3K) and the mitogen-activated protein kinase (MAPK) pathway were evaluated. NVP-BKM120, a pan-class IA PI3K inhibitor, caused the tumor to double in size after 5 to 26 days of treatment. NVP-BKM120 also inhibited angiogenesis, tumor cell growth, and activation of AKT (Bahrami et al., 2018).

Inhibiting PI3K led to DNA damage, poly-ADP-ribosylation (PAR), and -H2AX, but it also reduced the creation of Rad51 foci, indicating a critical function for PI3K activity in Rad51 recruitment. Olaparib, a PARP inhibitor, was found to only slightly slow tumor growth; however, the combination of NVP-BKM120 and olaparib significantly slowed tumor growth in xenotransplants from human BRCA1-related tumors and in the mouse model, delaying tumor doubling by more than 50 days. This finding suggests that combined PI3K and PARP inhibition can effectively treat BRCA1-related tumors (Eskiler and Ozturk 2022).

Further research revealed that NVP-BEZ235, a brand-new and orally accessible dual PI3K/mTOR inhibitor, has inhibitory effects on the PI3K/AKT/mTOR proteins p-p-mTOR, AKT, and p-70S6K. Additionally, this inhibitor prevented breast cancer cells from proliferating and caused apoptosis and autophagy (Martín Liberal et al., 2012).

It was shown that the traditional Chinese medicine herb jolkinolide B (extracted from the root of Euphorbia fischeriana Steud) significantly inhibited the PI3K/AKT/mTOR signaling pathway while inducing apoptosis in MDA-MB-231 cells. Additionally, it caused the Bcl-2/Bax ratio to decrease, which in turn promoted the release of cytochrome c from mitochondria and the activation of caspase-3. MCF-7 cells were subcutaneously injected into naked mice to examine the anticancer effects of jolkinolide B (JB) (Zhang et al., 2022). JB inhibited MCF-7 cell development, which was thereafter halted in the S phase. The findings demonstrated that when naked mice were injected with MCF-7 cells, tumor weight and volume were considerably altered. JB therapy also resulted in overexpression of PTEN and p-eIF4E and downregulation of p-PI3K, mTOR, cyclinD1, cyclinE, and p-Akt. N-Hydroxyphthalimide (NHPI) is a compound that inhibits the proliferation of human breast cancer BT-20 cells and has been shown to be effective (Raghav et al., 2022). In BT-20 human breast cancer cells, LoVo human colon adenocarcinoma cells, and HT-29 cells, NHPI inhibited the mTOR signaling pathway and showed anticancer efficacy (Wang et al., 2016a). After being exposed to NHPI (0–40 M) for 48 hours, the proliferation of BT-20, HT-29, and LoVo cells was reduced in a concentration-dependent manner. However, when treated with NHPI, the proliferation of human MCF-10A normal breast epithelial cells was unaffected. After being treated with NHPI, the BT-20, LoVo, and HT-29 cell lines showed morphological alterations in which the cells shrank and took on a round shape, whereas the MCF-10A cells from normal human breast epithelial tissue did not (Sharma et al., 2022a).

According to these findings, NHPI inhibited the growth of LoVo, BT-20, and HT-29 cells. NHPI caused cell cycle arrest in the G2/M phase by inhibiting the expression of cyclins CDC2 and B1 (Wang et al., 2016a). Both BT-20 and LoVo cells were arrested in the G2/M phase after being exposed to increased concentrations of NHPI for 24 hours. Comparatively, to the control, the proportion of cells arrested in the G2/M phase rose, which was accompanied by a reduction in the number of cells in the S phase of the cell cycle (Vr 2020) (Reshetnikova et al., 2007).

The levels of expression of important cell cycle regulators were studied to further comprehend the mechanism underlying the G2/M phase cell cycle arrest brought on by NHPI. When BT-20 and LoVo cells were exposed to NHPI for 24 hours, it was observed that the expression of the cellular proteins cyclin B1 and cdc2 was inhibited in a concentration-dependent manner (Grguric-Sipka et al., 2003). After 48 hours of NHPI treatment, BT-20 cells had a higher percentage of apoptotic cells. When BT-20 cells were exposed to NHPI for 24 hours, there was a decrease in the anti-apoptotic proteins survivin and Bcl-xL, activation of caspase 9 and caspase 3, and an increase in PARP cleavage (Grguric-Sipka et al., 2003).

In BT-20 and LoVo cells, NHPI also reduced the phosphorylation of mTORC1 substrates S6K1 and 4E-BP1 and S6K1 (S6) in a concentration-dependent manner. PI3K-mediated Akt phosphorylation at Thr308 was constrained by NHPI. Additionally, BT-20 cells treated with NHPI for 6 hours in a concentration-dependent manner resulted in the nuclear translocation of eIF4E (Grguric-Sipka et al., 2003).

These findings showed that NHPI decreased tumor growth in human breast xenografts by reducing mTORC1/mTORC2 signaling. Treatment with 40 mg/kg NHPI considerably reduced the tumor's weight and volume. Compared to vehicle controls, the tumor weight in BT-20 xenografts was decreased by 45%. According to these findings, NHPI exhibits strong anticancer efficacy in BT-20 xenografts (Sharma et al., 2019c).

To induce G1 arrest and autophagy in human breast cancer MCF-7 cells, ZSTK474 is a selective and novel class I phosphatidylinositol 3-kinase inhibitor. ZSTK474 successfully slowed the growth of human cancer xenografts *in vivo*. ZSTK474 also lowered the expression of nuclear cyclin D1 and Ki67 and repressed the expression of phospho-Akt, indicating PI3K inhibition. ZSTK474 therapy did not, however, lead to an increase in TUNEL-positive apoptotic cells. The use of ZSTK474 also resulted in marked G (0)/G (1) arrest being brought on (Kong et al., 2010).

ZSTK474 was identified to inhibit PI3K in nanomolar doses. According to molecular modeling studies, ZSTK474 acts as an ATP-competitive inhibitor by attaching to the ATP-binding pocket of PI3K. Lineweaver-Burk plot analysis showed that ZSTK474 acted as an ATP-competitive inhibitor for all PI3K isoforms (Kong and Yamori 2007). The activity of mTOR was also suppressed by ZSTK474 at a higher dose (100 M). ZSTK474 also inhibited the proliferation of human MCF-7 breast cancer cells (Chen et al., 2012).

Flow cytometric analysis showed that treatment with ZSTK474 also caused cell cycle arrest at the G1 phase. Several experiments, including transmission electron microscopy (TEM), monodansylcadaverine (MDC) staining, tandem mRFP-GFP-LC3 fluorescence microscopy, western blot, etc. showed that ZSTK474 could activate autophagy in MCF-7 cells (Wang et al., 2016b). The action of triggering autophagy may also block class I PI3K and the mTOR downstream regulators. Phase 1 clinical trials are being conducted with ZSTK474 to treat cancer (Wang et al., 2016b).

A best probable and specific inhibitor of PI3K and PI3K, AZD8835. In a mouse SKOV-3 xenograft tumor model with the H1047R PI3K mutation, AZD8835 completely inhibited tumor growth (93% tumor growth suppression) and pharmacodynamically modulated AKT phosphorylation when chronic oral dosing at 25 mg/kg b.i.d. was used (Barlaam et al., 2015). Furthermore, intermittent high-dose scheduling of AZD8835 demonstrated that more extensive exposures resulted in more potent pathway blockage and caused apoptosis (Barlaam et al., 2015). Compared to single drugs, the tumor regression rate was raised by 59 and 54%, respectively, when AZD8835 was coupled with fulvestrant or palbociclib. Proapoptotic and antiproliferative effects were both displayed by AZD8835. Clinical trials for AZD8835 are currently in phase I (Wen et al., 2020).

Pomolic acid (PA) is a triterpenoid and an active substance that comes from the Japanese euscaphis. Pomolic acid specifically targeted the p38-

MAPK and mTOR signaling cascades, which reduced HIF1/VEGF-mediated angiogenesis (Park et al., 2018). In contrast to MCF-7 and MDA-MB-231 cells, PA was found to have no effect on the production of HIF1 or VEGF when EGF was used to stimulate it. Additionally, PA reduced HIF1/VEGF expression in HUVEC and slowed *in vitro* EGF-induced angiogenesis (Park et al., 2016). It was found that the control PA exerted over HIF1, and VEGF expression was related to the resistance HIF1, and VEGF showed an EGF-induced mechanism. Pomolic acid also acted as a suppressant for both p38-MAPK and mTOR phosphorylation that EGF brought on. PA slowed down the translation of the HIF1 protein that EGF triggered by inhibiting the p38-MAPK and mTOR kinase signaling pathways (Park et al., 2018).

## 7. Targeted Therapies

Loss of *ARID1A* expression presents resistance to some drugs that help in inhibiting the HER2/PI3K/mTOR signaling cascade. Activation of annexin A1 (ANXA1) expression by the loss of ARIDIA is important for drug resistance via its AKT activation. It was found that in patients with HER2+ breast cancer, ANXA1 high expression is related to the resistance to adjuvant trastuzumab therapy. Therefore, activated ANXA1 serves as a prognostic biomarker for the designed treatment (Berns et al., 2016).

p70S6K1 is a serine-threonine kinase that regulates protein translation and is a marker for mTOR activity. Treatment of MCF-7 and HER2 breast cancer cells with increasing concentrations of lapatinib for >10 months caused a drastic decrease in the phosphorylation of p70S6K1 at ERK1/2-regulated sites (Thr (421)/Ser (424)). Lapatinib-resistant MCF-7/HER2-Lap10 cells exhibited a lapatinib-insensitive p70S6K1 hyperphosphorylation (Berns et al., 2016). The cotreatment with rapamycin suppressed p70S6K1 hyperactivation and synergistically resensitized MCF-7/HER2-Lap10 cells to lapatinib. p70S6K1 (mTOR effector p70 S6 kinase 1) is a biomarker for the biological effects of the dual-HER1/HER2 tyrosine kinase (Vazquez-Martin et al., 2008).

The *FBXW7* gene is a p53-dependent tumor suppressor gene in human tumors that undertakes deletion and/or mutation. Depletion of *FBXW7* increases the mTor and phosphorylated mTor levels (p-mTor) and also urges to suppress mTor target S6-kinase (PS6K). The genetic status of *FBXW7* and *PTEN* genes was examined on a panel of 53 breast cancer cell lines in one study (Cuella-Martin 2018). It was found that 23 out of 53 breast cancer cell lines showed the loss of FBXW7 as well and no such loss is observed in *PTEN.* Fourteen lines showed loss of *PTEN single copy*, suggesting that *FBXW7* and *PTEN* express some functional duplicity in the tumor development. Additionally, treatment with rapamycin of a set of 10 breast cancer cell lines at different concentrations of 200nM and 400nM. Cells with deletion or mutation of *FBXW7 or PTEN* showed significant sensitivity to killing by rapamycin. FBXW7 loss may also act as a significant biomarker for human tumors in the treatment with inhibitors of the mTOR pathway (Jemaa et al., 2012).

The assessment of the effect of the following; aromatase inhibitor, a novel Src inhibitor, AZD0530, and anastrozole investigated in this study either alone or in combination treatment plan. Both these two drugs together lead to a significant increase in p27 levels. Showed some indicated pathway expression in the tumors persistent to AZD0530 monotherapy. MCF-7Arom5 and MCF-Ca cell lines on treatment with different concentrations of the compound in single or both like anastrozole, 1 μmol/L AZD0530 (Chen, et al., 2008). Treatment with 100 μmol/L anastrozole considerably affected the cell cycle progression, a significant reduction from 52% to 22% in S-phase cells also a considerable increase in the % G0-G1. AZD0530 1 μmol/L alone (Src inhibitor), showed a minute effect on the cell cycle, with a slight fall in the % S-phase cells detected from 52% to 45%. In both cases, drugs caused G1 arrest within the time of 48 hours. Anastrozole alone had an effect on the phosphorylation of dMAPK but in little, however, AZD0530 increased pMAPK which was inhibited by cotreatment with anastrozole. As expected, AZD0530 caused a decrease in pSrc; however, anastrozole unexpectedly within 48 hours increased pSrc (Chen et al., 2009), whereas upon treatment, both anastrozole and AZD0530 caused inhibition in Src. The treatment combined with anastrozole and AZD0530 meaningfully inhibited Src, Akt, and MAPK activities even without causing any serious effect in total in the kinase levels. Whereas *in vivo* it has been observed that Anastrozole and AZD0530 affected breast cancer growth (Simpkins et al., 2018).

GDC-0980 is a selective, novel, and orally bioavailable class I PI3K/mTOR kinase inhibitor. GDC-0980 potently inhibits signal transduction downstream of both PI3K and mTOR, as measured by pharmacodynamic (PD) biomarkers. GDC-0980 was potent across a broad panel of cancer cell lines, with the greatest potency in breast, prostate, and lung cancers and less activity in pancreatic cancers and melanoma, consistent with KRAS and BRAF acting as resistance markers (Wallin et al., 2011). Treatment of cancer cell lines with GDC-0980 demonstrated G1 cell-cycle arrest and induced apoptosis in certain cancer cell lines. Low doses of GDC-0980 inhibited tumor growth in xenograft models, including those with activated PI3K, and loss of LKB1 or PTEN, and induced an exposure-related decrease in PD biomarkers (Sutherlin et al., 2011).

The sigma-2 receptor has been identified as a potential biomarker of proliferating cells in solid tumors. The mechanisms of sigma-2 ligand-induced cell death was studied in the human melanoma cell line MDA-MB-435 and the mouse breast cancer cell line EMT-6 (Wheeler et al., 2000). MDA-MB-435 and EMT-6 cells were treated with sigma-2 ligands. The three main sigma-2 ligands (SV119, WC-26, and RHM-138) induced caspase-3 activation, DNA fragmentation, and PARP-1 cleavage (Haller et al., 2012). The caspase inhibitor (Z-VAD-FMK) partially blocked DNA fragmentation and cytotoxicity. It was demonstrated that sigma-2 ligand-induced caspase activation and apoptosis are partly responsible for cell death. WC-26, RHM-138, SV119 and siramesine reduced the expression levels of the downstream effectors of mammalian target of rapamycin (mTOR) (Matter-Reissmann et al., 2002), 4EBP1 and p70S6K and increased the production and processing of microtubule-associated protein light chain 3, an autophagosome marker suggesting that sigma-2 ligands inhibited mTOR pathway by inducing autophagy. All these four main sigma-2 ligands reduced the cyclin D1 expression in a time-dependent manner (Wood and Newcomb 2000). Moreover, RHM-138 decreased mainly cyclin E2 while WC-26 and SV119 decreased mainly cyclin B1, E2 and phosphorylation of retinoblastoma protein (pRb) and siramesine decreased mainly cyclin B1 and pRb (Woo et al., 2003).

A combination of Epidermal growth factor receptor (EGFR) and cyclooxygenase-2 (COX-2) inhibitors can effectively act as a reducing agent for cell growth in estrogen-dependent breast cancer cells. MCF-7 and SKBR-3 breast cancer cells were treated with either nimotuzumab or in combination with celecoxib (Wang et al., 2012). Both the cell lines showed sensitivity to celecoxib, but on the other hand, it's sensitive to the treatment with nimotuzumab. These drugs in combination, showed synergistic effects on cell killing resulting in SKBR-3 cells, in both cell lines there is an observation in the suppression of p-mTOR, p-EGFR, p-Akt and amplified in breast cancer 1 (AIB1) and in in MCF-7 expression of E-cadherin observed after treatment (Prosperi 2006). E-cadherin and AIB1 can be considered potential biomarkers to predict response in ER-positive breast cancer cells treated with EGFR and COX-2 inhibitors (Sharma et al., 2020a).

The effect of combined treatment with PCI-24781, a histone deacetylase inhibitor, and tamoxifen on Akt was evaluated in breast cancer cells. Both histone deacetylase and estrogen receptor inhibition down-regulate AKT protein and activity with cell death initiation. ER-positive MCF7 cell treatment was performed with tamoxifen and PCI-24781 and resulted in a dose-dependent significant increase in cell death with a gradual increase in the PCI-24781 concentration. The increased concentrations of PCI-24781 reduced Akt expression and activity ($P^{S473}$) and phosphorylation of downstream targets (FoxO1-$P^{S256}$ and mTOR-$P^{S2448}$) (Yang et al., 2021). Treatment of breast cancer cells with tamoxifen or PCI-24781 alone can lead to a modest decrease in ER, PRb, and Cyclin D1 expression whereas the combination of these two drugs can lead to a substantial reduction in ER, PRb, and Cyclin D1 levels. Thus, histone deacetylase regulation of AKT mRNA is a key mediator of the therapeutic combination of tamoxifen or PCI-24781 and may represent a novel biomarker for predicting response to this regimen (Raha et al., 2015).

ARQ 092 and ARQ 751 are potent and highly selective allosteric pan AKT inhibitors. PIK3CA/PIK3R1 and AKT1-E17K mutations can be used as predictive and potent biomarkers for patient selection in clinical studies for both ARQ 092 and ARQ 751 (Yu et al., 2015). The two ARQ 092 and ARQ 751 show a potential binding to the mutant forms (WT and E17K) of AKT1 and phosphorylated AKT at the threonine 308 and serine 473 amino acid residues as well as its substrate PRAS40 at threonine 246 in cancer cells. These inhibitors inhibited AKT activation by dephosphorylating the membrane-associated active form and preventing the inactive form from localizing into the plasma membrane (Ram et al., 2020).

p27KIP1 expression level can be used as a biomarker to predict response to rapalogs for breast cancer. In rapamycin activity and p27KIP1 expression, a correlation was evaluated in breast cancer cells and tumor xenograft models (Chen et al., 2010). The cells from the tissues expressing low levels of p27KIP1 exhibited resistance to rapamycin while those isolated from the breast tumor tissues expressing high levels of p27KIP1 were sensitive to rapamycin. There was a significant decrease in phosphorylated p70S6K1 and phosphorylated 4EBP1 by Rapamycin in both samples. HER3 and p95HER2 (p95) are predictive and potential biomarkers of clinical outcomes on trastuzumab therapy (Chen et al., 2010). In trastuzumab-treated metastatic HER2-positive breast cancer (MBC) patients, patients with tumors that expressed elevated levels of p95 (p95-high) experienced less favorable outcomes compared to the subgroup of patients with tumors that expressed low p95 levels (p95-low) (Lipton et al., 2013).

AR expression can be an independent predictive biomarker for response to NVP-BEZ235. NVP-BEZ235 inhibition in tumor cell proliferation was observed with the high dosage in a subset of breast cancer cell lines (Wang et al., 2014). Mutations or amplification *(PIK3CA/HER2)* in breast cancer cells, NVP-BEZ235 induces cell death, while all of the *PTEN*-dependent cell lines either deleted, mutated, or silenced are insensitive to NVP-BEZ235 (Sharma et al., 2019a). Dihydrotestosterone (DHT) and NVP-BEZ235 in combination inhibited tumor growth more effectively than either drug alone, along this also reduced tumor size to below that at their starting point. NVP-BEZ235 inhibits the activity of the PI3K/AKT/mTOR pathway at high doses. NVP-BEZ235, at low doses, decreases androgen receptor (AR) activity and suppresses androgen receptor (AR) expression in $AR^{+}/ER^{+}$ breast cancer. NVP-BEZ235–induced androgen receptor (AR) suppression decreased PTEN and KLLN expression in $AR^{+}/ER^{+}$ breast cancer cells. NVP-BEZ235 showed a suppression in AKT phosphorylation at higher concentrations; resulting to which it actually at low doses increasing the levels of AKT phosphorylation (Ser473) (Wang et al., 2014).

Hypoxia-inducible factor 1 (HIF-1) can be explored as a potential biomarker of response to therapeutic targets. The potential role of transcription factor hypoxia-inducible factor 1 (HIF-1) and its regulation by human epidermal growth factor receptor-2 (HER2) was investigated. Long-term letrozole-treated (LTLTCa) cells have higher expression of HIF-1α protein than MCF-7Ca cells (Patiar and Harris 2006). The regulation of HIF-1α expression in LTLTCa cells is regulated by the HER2-activated PI3K/Akt/mTOR pathway (Gonsalves and Kalra 2010). Lapatinib is a HER2 kinase inhibitor through which expression is not affected but decreases HER2 activation of the downstream kinase pathway. Trastuzumab is a monoclonal antibody of HER2 which reduces its expression and activation of downstream kinase pathways (Collins et al., 2021). Trastuzumab significantly reduced HER2 protein expression. On the other hand, lapatinib and trastuzumab inhibited activation of the MAPK and PI3K/Akt pathways. Both inhibitors also significantly decreased HIF-1α protein expression in LTLTCa cells. MAPK and PI3K/Akt/mTOR pathways are activated by HER2 and are known to regulate HIF-1α expression and activity (Ding et al., 2022). HIF-1α siRNA treatment also significantly decreased LTLTCa cell viability in the presence of increasing concentrations of letrozole (Kazi et al., 2013). HER2-activated PI3K/Akt pathway increases HIF-1α protein synthesis in LTLTCa cells. HIF-1α up-regulates expression of BCRP and other genes and leads to letrozole resistance and stem cell characteristics of LTLTCa cells (Kazi et al., 2015).

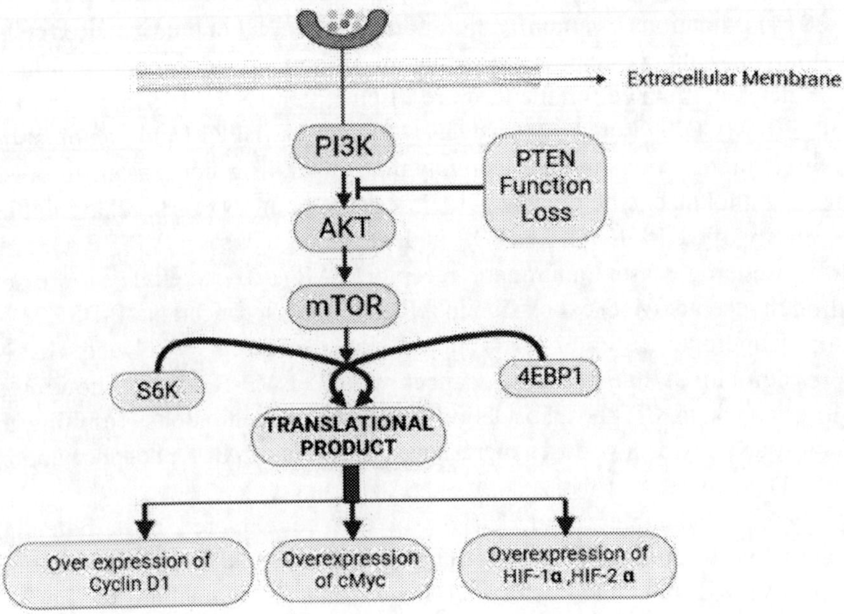


**Figure 2.** Mechanism of action for PI3K/AKT/mTOR inhibitors.

In Breast Cancer, Receptor Tyrosine kinase (RTK) incorporation establishes sensitivity to PI3Kα-selective Inhibitors. RTKs over-expression (also including c-MET, FGFR, HER3, and EGFR) re-established ERK phosphorylation and the feasibility of the cell concealed by BYL719 (Cremers 2019). This further suggested the proper and authenticated function of RTKs in cell proliferation & signaling. More concisely, the over-activation of c-MET and EGFR shows resistance, on the other hand, the over-activation of IGF-1R and/or HER2 showed some sensitivity to BYL719 in breast cancer cells (Cremers and Nguyen 2019). The efficacy/ safety profile of RTKs could be potentially developed as a predictive biomarker for the effectiveness of PI3Kα inhibitors.

Another inhibitor, DYRK2, whose uprooted expression encouraged Thr631 phosphorylation for the degradation of mTOR. Also, for the Everolimus sensitivity, Tyrosine phosphorylation-regulated kinase 2 could be a prognostic marker. The general action mechanism of the PI3K/AKT/mTOR inhibitors has been proposed in Figure 2.

## 8. Nanotherapeutics in Cancer

As discussed in previous sections, conventional cancer treatment methods are surgery, radiation therapy, and chemotherapy. The advancement in biomedical science research established the more target-specific mode of treatments for cancer, such as hormone therapy and immunotherapy. The major challenges in cancer treatment are the complex heterogenicity of tumor cells and the presence of cancer stem cells. The organ-specific tumor cell heterogeneity and a distinct tumor microenvironment could lead to therapeutic failure (Dagogo-Jack and Shaw 2018). Furthermore, approved cancer drugs have several limitations, such as short half-life, low efficacy, off-target effects, and most importantly, cytotoxicity (Tannock 1998). Nanotechnology is consistently evolving, and nanotherapeutics have immense potential to overcome these limitations. Nanotherapeutics have prolonged half-lives, improved drug solubility, minimized off-target effects, and low cell toxicity (Bertrand et al., 2014). The evolving potential of nanotherapeutics in cancer therapy is primarily attributed to their uniquely appealing features: their ability for enhanced permeability and retention effect (Blumcke et al.) (Matsumura and Maeda 1986) (Gerlowski and Jain 1986). Furthermore, nanoparticles can target the tumor and its microenvironment through active targeting, wherein tumor cells have an active drug uptake, and by passive targeting, which allows the localization of drugs in the tumor (Bertrand et al., 2014).

Doxorubicin was the first FDA-approved chemotherapeutic nano-drug approved in 1995. Doxil is doxorubicin HCl encapsulated in stealth liposomes, which could prolong drug circulation and specific delivery at the tumor site (Barenholz 2012). Nanotherapeutics has come a long way in the last two decades, and our knowledge and their applications are rapidly expanding. The nanotherapeutics can also facilitate targeted drug delivery, which could increase drug utilization at the target/cancer site and reduce toxicity. Ferroptosis is a recently discovered essential type of regulated cell death mainly characterized by iron overload and lipid peroxidation. Recently nanoparticles conjugated with chemicals or biological drugs have demonstrated the enhanced efficiency of existing inducers of ferroptosis and cancer therapy (Chen et al., 2023). Currently, several nanotherapeutics are in the preclinical and clinical stages for the treatment of various cancers, such as polymeric nanoparticles, micelles, nanobodies, magnetic nanoparticles, liposomes, niosomes, gold-nanoparticles, dendrimers, and carbon-nanotubes (Shi et al., 2017). Nanotherapeutics and other targeted therapies could overcome some of the intrinsic limitations of conventional cancer treatment.

And in the future, it holds immense potential for efficient and efficacious treatment of many diseases (Rajpoot et al., 2021).

## 9. Microbiome and Precision Medicine in Cancer

Almost one trillion microbes that harbor the human body play a positive role in maintaining the health of the individual. These diverse microbes are abundant in our body, especially in the oral cavity, gut region, and skin. The microbiome composition is influenced by various factors such as diet, environment, host genetics, etc. The distribution of microbial populations is quite distinct in healthy and diseased individuals. Upon alteration or dysbiosis of the microbiome, the person becomes prone to dreadful diseases including cancer (Rajpoot et al., 2018). Cancer is the outcome of an overexpression of many signature genes involved in cancer progression. Recent advancements in biotechnology techniques such as next-generation sequencing and metagenomics have already paved the way for a broader understanding of the microbial population present which further highlights the distinguishing features of the microbiome during healthy and disease states (Markus et al., 2023). The emergence of medical biotechnology is set to target the microbiome for therapeutic purposes by which personalized medicine can be made for treating various cancers and other chronic diseases (Sharma et al., 2021b). Individualized probiotic and prebiotic supplements, dietary interventions, and microbial transplantation can now reshape the microbiome, presenting a reasonable therapeutic strategy in an era of personalized medicine (Sheikh et al., 2020; Hanssen et al., 2021).

## 10. Conclusion

Today biotechnology has made it feasible that a patient should take those medicines to which they do not respond but take precisely appropriate medication according to the microbial flora present unique to each individual. Needless to say, biotechnology has set significantly high standards to cure ailing individuals, bringing newer paradigms to manage the health and well-being of an individual. Therefore, the need of the hour is to look into the modern therapeutic tools and advancements available to find an amicable solution to diagnose, treat, and manage cancer.

## References

Bahrami, A., Khazaei, M., Hasanzadeh, M., ShahidSales, S., Joudi Mashhad, M., Farazestanian, M., Sadeghnia, H. R., Rezayi, M., Maftouh, M., and Hassanian, S. M. (2018). Therapeutic potential of targeting PI3K/AKT pathway in treatment of colorectal cancer: rational and progress. *Journal of Cellular Biochemistry*, 119, 2460-2469.

Barenholz, Y. (2012). Doxil®--the first FDA-approved nano-drug: lessons learned. *Journal of Control Release*, 160, 117-134.

Barlaam, B., Cosulich, S., Delouvrié, B., Ellston, R., Fitzek, M., Germain, H., Green, S., Hancox, U., Harris, C. S., and Hudson, K. (2015). Discovery of 1-(4-(5-(5-amino-6-(5-tert-butyl-1, 3, 4-oxadiazol-2-yl) pyrazin-2-yl)-1-ethyl-1, 2, 4-triazol-3-yl) piperidin-1-yl)-3-hydroxypropan-1-one (AZD8835): A potent and selective inhibitor of PI3Kα and PI3Kδ for the treatment of cancers. *Bioorganic and Medicinal Chemistry Letters*, 25, 5155-5162.

Berenguer, C. V., Pereira, F., Câmara, J. S., and Pereira, J. A. (2023). Underlying features of prostate cancer—Statistics, risk factors, and emerging methods for its diagnosis. *Current Oncology*, 30, 2300-2321.

Berns, K., Sonnenblick, A., Gennissen, A., Brohée, S., Hijmans, E. M., Evers, B., Fumagalli, D., Desmedt, C., Loibl, S., and Denkert, C. (2016). Loss of ARID1A activates ANXA1, which serves as a predictive biomarker for trastuzumab resistance. *Clinical Cancer Research*, 22, 5238-5248.

Bertrand, N., Wu, J., Xu, X., Kamaly, N., and Farokhzad, O. C. (2014). Cancer nanotechnology: the impact of passive and active targeting in the era of modern cancer biology. *Advanced Drug Delivery Reviews*, 66, 2-25.

Blumcke, I., Thom, M., Aronica, E., Armstrong, D. D., Vinters, H. V., Palmini, A., Jacques, T. S., Avanzini, G., Barkovich, A. J., Battaglia, G., Becker, A., Cepeda, C., Cendes, F., Colombo, N., Crino, P., Cross, J. H., Delalande, O., Dubeau, F., Duncan, J., Guerrini, R., Kahane, P., Mathern, G., Najm, I., Ozkara, C., Raybaud, C., Represa, A., Roper, S. N., Salamon, N., Schulze-Bonhage, A., Tassi, L., Vezzani, A., and Spreafico, R. (2011). The clinicopathologic spectrum of focal cortical dysplasias: a consensus classification proposed by an ad hoc Task Force of the ILAE Diagnostic Methods Commission. *Epilepsia*, 52, 158-174.

Cerma, K., Piacentini, F., Moscetti, L., Barbolini, M., Canino, F., Tornincasa, A., Caggia, F., Cerri, S., Molinaro, A., and Dominici, M. (2023). Targeting pi3k/akt/mtor pathway in breast cancer: From biology to clinical challenges. *Biomedicines*, 11, 109.

Chaudhary, M., Dan, S., Sharma, V., and Sharma, A. K. (2020). Current perspective on dominant negative mutations: Trends, scope and relevance. *Biointerface Research in Applied Chemistry*, 11(4), 12020-12036.

Chen, G., Yang, N., Wang, X., Zheng, S. Y., Chen, Y., Tong, L. J., Li, Y. X., Meng, L. H., and Ding, J. (2010). Identification of p27/KIP1 expression level as a candidate biomarker of response to rapalogs therapy in human cancer. *Journal of Molecular Medicine*, 88, 941-952.

Chen, Y. T., Tan, K. A., Pang, L. Y., and Argyle, D. J. (2012). The class I PI3K/Akt pathway is critical for cancer cell survival in dogs and offers an opportunity for therapeutic intervention. *BMC Veterinary Research*, 8, 1-15.

Chen, Y., Guggisberg, N., Jorda, M., Gonzalez-Angulo, A., Hennessy, B., Mills, G. B., Tan, C. K., and Slingerland, J. M. (2009). Combined Src and aromatase inhibition impairs human breast cancer growth *in vivo* and bypass pathways are activated in AZD0530-resistant tumors. *Clinical Cancer Research*, 15, 3396-3405.

Chen, Y., Tan, C. K., and Slingerland, J. (2008). The Src inhibitor AZD0530 cooperates with Anastrozole to inhibit human breast cancer growth *in vitro* and *in vivo*. *Cancer Research*, 68, 1470-1470.

Chen, Z., Wang, W., Abdul Razak, S. R., Han, T., Ahmad, N. H., and Li, X. (2023). Ferroptosis as a potential target for cancer therapy. *Cell Death and Disease*, 14, 460.

Chhikara, B. S., and Parang, K. (2023). Global Cancer Statistics 2022: the trends projection analysis. *Chemical Biology Letters*, 10, 451-451.

Collins, D. M., Madden, S. F., Gaynor, N., AlSultan, D., Le Gal, M., Eustace, A. J., Gately, K. A., Hughes, C., Davies, A. M., and Mahgoub, T. (2021). Effects of HER family–targeting tyrosine kinase inhibitors on antibody-dependent cell-mediated cytotoxicity in HER2-expressing breast cancer. *Clinical Cancer Research*, 27, 807-818.

Cremers, C. G. (2019). A network-level investigation of signalling crosstalk and drug response in aggressive breast cancer. Monash University.

Cremers, C. G., and Nguyen, L. K. (2019). Network rewiring, adaptive resistance and combating strategies in breast cancer. *Cancer Drug Resistance*, 2, 1106.

Cuella-Martin, R. (2018). Molecular regulation of p53-dependent tumour suppressor responses by the p53 binding protein 1. University of Oxford.

Dagogo-Jack, I., and Shaw, A. T. (2018). heterogeneity and resistance to cancer therapies. *Nature Reviews Clinical Oncology*, 15, 81-94.

Ding, X., Sharko, A. C., McDermott, M. S., Schools, G. P., Chumanevich, A., Ji, H., Li, J., Zhang, L., Mack, Z. T., and Sikirzhytski, V. (2022). Inhibition of CDK8/19 Mediator kinase potentiates HER2-targeting drugs and bypasses resistance to these agents *in vitro* and *in vivo*. *Proceedings of the National Academy of Sciences*, 119, e2201073119.

Ely, S., and Vioral, A. N. (2007). Breast cancer overview. *Plastic and Aesthetic Nursing*, 27, 128-133.

Eskiler, G. G., and Ozturk, M. (2022). Therapeutic potential of the PI3K inhibitor LY294002 and PARP inhibitor Talazoparib combination in BRCA-deficient triple negative breast cancer cells. *Cellular Signalling*, 91, 110229.

Francipane, M. G., and Lagasse, E. (2016). Therapeutic potential of mTOR inhibitors for targeting cancer stem cells. *British Journal of Clinical Pharmacology*, 82, 1180-1188.

Gerlowski, L. E., and Jain, R. K. (1986). Microvascular permeability of normal and neoplastic tissues. *Microvascular Research*, 31, 288-305.

Gonsalves, C. S., and Kalra, V. K. (2010). Hypoxia-mediated expression of 5-lipoxygenase–activating protein involves HIF-1α and NF-κB and microRNAs 135a and 199a-5p. *The Journal of Immunology*, 184, 3878-3888.

Grguric-Sipka, S. R., Vilaplana, R. A., Pérez, J. M., Fuertes, M. A., Alonso, C., Alvarez, Y., Sabo, T. J., and González-Vílchez, F. (2003). Synthesis, characterization, interaction with DNA and cytotoxicity of the new potential antitumour drug cis-K [Ru (eddp) Cl2]. *Journal of Inorganic Biochemistry*, 97, 215-220.

Haller, J. L., Panyutin, I., Chaudhry, A., Zeng, C., Mach, R. H., and Frank, J. A. (2012). Sigma-2 receptor as potential indicator of stem cell differentiation. *Molecular Imaging and Biology*, 14, 325-335.

Hanssen, N. M., de Vos, W. M., and Nieuwdorp, M. (2021). Fecal microbiota transplantation in human metabolic diseases: from a murky past to a bright future? *Cell Metabolism*, 33, 1098-1110.

Heras-Sandoval, D., Pérez-Rojas, J. M., Hernández-Damián, J., and Pedraza-Chaverri, J. (2014). The role of PI3K/AKT/mTOR pathway in the modulation of autophagy and the clearance of protein aggregates in neurodegeneration. *Cellular Signalling*, 26, 2694-2701.

Jassim, G. A., Doherty, S., Whitford, D. L., and Khashan, A. S. (2023). Psychological interventions for women with non-metastatic breast cancer. *Cochrane Database of Systematic Reviews*, 5, CD008729.

Jemaa, M., Vitale, I., Kepp, O., Berardinelli, F., Galluzzi, L., Senovilla, L., Marino, G., Malik, S. A., Rello-Varona, S., and Lissa, D. (2012). Selective killing of p53-deficient cancer cells by SP600125. *EMBO Molecular Medicine*, 4, 500-514.

Kazi, A. A., and Baltimore, M. U. (2015). Investigating the regulation and potential role of nonhypoxic hypoxia inducible factor 1 (HIF 1) in aromatase inhibitor resistant breast cancer. *Breast Cancer Research*, 16(1), R15.

Kazi, A. A., Shah, P., Schech, A., Sabnis, G., Chumsri, S., and Brodie, A. (2013). Inhibiiton of non-hypoxic HIF-1 expression in letrozole-resistant breast cancer cells reduces their cancer stem cell characteristics. *Cancer Research*, 73, 95-95.

Khadwal, S., Singh, R., Singh, K., Sharma, V., and Sharma, A. K. (2020). Probing into the edible vaccines: Newer paradigms, scope and relevance. *Plant Archives*, 20, 5483-5495.

Kingsbury, K. (2007). The changing face of breast cancer. *Time*, 170(43), 36-40.

Kong, D.-x., and Yamori, T. (2010). ZSTK474, a novel phosphatidylinositol 3-kinase inhibitor identified using the JFCR39 drug discovery system. *Acta Pharmacologica Sinica*, 31, 1189-1197.

Kong, D., and Yamori, T. (2007). ZSTK474 is an ATP-competitive inhibitor of class I phosphatidylinositol 3 kinase isoforms. *Cancer Science*, 98, 1638-1642.

Kumar, S. A., Indu, S., Gautami, D., and VarRuchi, S. (2020). Oral squamous cell carcinoma (OSCC) in humans: Etiological Factors, diagnostic and therapeutic relevance. *Research Journal of Biotechnology*, 15, 10.

Liao, Y.-M., Kim, C., and Yen, Y. (2011). Mammalian target of rapamycin and head and neck squamous cell carcinoma. *Head and Neck Oncology*, 3, 1-7.

Lipton, A., Goodman, L., Leitzel, K., Cook, J., Sperinde, J., Haddad, M., Köstler, W. J., Huang, W., Weidler, J. M., and Ali, S. (2013). HER3, p95HER2, and HER2 protein expression levels define multiple subtypes of HER2-positive metastatic breast cancer. *Breast Cancer Research and Treatment*, 141, 43-53.

Markus, V., Paul, A. A., Teralı, K., Özer, N., Marks, R. S., Golberg, K., and Kushmaro, A. (2023). Conversations in the Gut: The Role of Quorum Sensing in Normobiosis. *International Journal of Molecular Sciences*, 24, 3722.

Martín Liberal, J., Lagares-Tena, L., Sáinz-Jaspeado, M., Mateo-Lozano, S., García del Muro, X., and Tirado, O. M. (2012). Targeted therapies in sarcomas: challenging the challenge. *Sarcoma*, 2012.

Matsumura, Y., and Maeda, H. (1986). A new concept for macromolecular therapeutics in cancer chemotherapy: mechanism of tumoritropic accumulation of proteins and the antitumor agent smancs. *Cancer Research*, 46, 6387-6392.

Matter-Reissmann, U. B., Forte, P., Schneider, M. K., Filgueira, L., Groscurth, P., and Seebach, J. D. (2002). Xenogeneic human NK cytotoxicity against porcine endothelial cells is perforin/granzyme B dependent and not inhibited by Bcl-2 overexpression. *Xenotransplantation*, 9, 325-337.

Mehrotra, R., and Yadav, K. (2022). Breast cancer in India: Present scenario and the challenges ahead. *World Journal of Clinical Oncology*, 13, 209-218.

Morgan, E., Arnold, M., Gini, A., Lorenzoni, V., Cabasag, C., Laversanne, M., Vignat, J., Ferlay, J., Murphy, N., and Bray, F. (2023). Global burden of colorectal cancer in 2020 and 2040: Incidence and mortality estimates from GLOBOCAN. *Gut*, 72, 338-344.

Park, J. H., Jang, K. M., An, H. J., Kim, J. Y., Gwon, M. G., Gu, H., Park, B., and Park, K. K. (2018). Pomolic acid ameliorates fibroblast activation and renal interstitial fibrosis through inhibition of SMAD-STAT signaling pathways. *Molecules*, 23, 2236.

Park, J. H., Yoon, J., and Park, B. (2016). Pomolic acid suppresses HIF1α/VEGF-mediated angiogenesis by targeting p38-MAPK and mTOR signaling cascades. *Phytomedicine*, 23, 1716-1726.

Patiar, S., and Harris, A. L. (2006). Role of hypoxia-inducible factor-1α as a cancer therapy target. *Endocrine-Related Cancer*, 13, S61-S75.

Prosperi, J. R. (2006). *In vitro* and *in vivo* characterization of the estrogen dependent human breast cancer cell line, MCF-7, over-expressing cyclooxygenase-2. The Ohio State University.

Raghav, M., Sharma, V., Chaudhary, M., Tuli, H. S., Saini, A. K., and Sharma, A. K. (2020a). Essence of PTEN: a broad-spectrum therapeutic target in cancer. *Biointerface Research in Applied Chemistry*, 11(2), 9587-9603.

Raghav, M., Sharma, V., Chaudhary, M., Tuli, H. S., Saini, A. K., and Sharma, A. K. (2020b). Essence of PTEN: a Broad-Spectrum Therapeutic Target in Cancer. *Biointerface Research in Applied Chemistry*, 11, 9587-9603.

Raghav, M., Sharma, V., Gupta, S., and Kaushal, A. (2022). In-silico designing of a potent ligand molecule against PTEN (Phosphatase and tensin homolog) implicated in Breast Cancer. *Journal of experimental Biology and Agricultural Sciences*, 10, 1016-1023.

Raghav, M., Sharma, V., Bansal, P., Punj, V., and Sharma, A. K. (2022). Phosphatase and Tensin Homolog (PTEN) as a negative regulator of PI3K and AKT pathway. *Indian Journal of Natural Sciences*, 13, 45155-45163.

Raha, P., Thomas, S., Thurn, K. T., Park, J., and Munster, P. N. (2015). Combined histone deacetylase inhibition and tamoxifen induces apoptosis in tamoxifen-resistant breast cancer models, by reversing Bcl-2 overexpression. *Breast Cancer Research*, 17, 1-16.

Rajpoot, M., Bhattacharya, R., Sharma, S., Gupta, S., Sharma, V., and Sharma, A. K. (2021). Melamine contamination and associated health risks: Gut microbiota does make a difference. *Biotechnology and Applied Biochemistry*, 68, 1271-1280.

Rajpoot, M., Sharma, A. K., Sharma, A., and Gupta, G. K. (2018). Understanding the microbiome: emerging biomarkers for exploiting the microbiota for personalized medicine against cancer. *Seminars in Cancer Biology*, 52(1), 1-8.

Ram, G., Sharma, V., Sheikh, I., Sankhyan, A., Aggarwal, D., and Sharma, A. (2020). Anti-cancer potential of natural products: recent trends, scope and relevance. *Letters in Applied NanoBioScience*, 9, 902-907.

Reshetnikova, G., Troyanovsky, S., and Rimm, D. L. (2007). Definition of a direct extracellular interaction between Met and E-cadherin. *Cell Biology International*, 31, 366-373.

Ruchi Sharma, V., Kumar Gupta, G., Sharma, A. K., Batra, N., Sharma, D. K., Joshi, A., and Sharma, A. K. (2017). PI3K/Akt/mTOR intracellular pathway and breast cancer: factors, mechanism and regulation. *Current Pharmaceutical Design*, 23, 1633-1638.

Saini, A., Kumar, M., Bhatt, S., Saini, V., and Malik, A. (2020). Cancer causes and treatments. *International Journal of Pharmaceutical Sciences and Research*, 11, 3121-3134.

Sehrawat, N., Yadav, M., Singh, M., Kumar, V., Sharma, V. R., and Sharma, A. K. (2021). Probiotics in microbiome ecological balance providing a therapeutic window against cancer. *Seminars in Cancer Biology*, 70, 24-36.

Sham, N. F. R., Hasani, N. A. H., Hasan, N., Karim, M. K. A., Fuad, S. B. S. A., Hasbullah H. H., and Ibahim, M. J. (2023). Acquired radioresistance in EMT6 mouse mammary carcinoma cell line is mediated by CTLA-4 and PD-1 through JAK/STAT/PI3K pathway. *Scientific Reports*, 13, 3108.

Sharma, A. K., Sharma, V. R., Gupta, G. K., Ashraf, G. M., and Kamal, M. A. (2019a). Advanced glycation end products (AGEs), glutathione and breast cancer: Factors, mechanism and therapeutic interventions. *Current Drug Metabolism*, 20, 65-71.

Sharma, V. (2021). Bioinformatics and its applications in environmental science and health and its applications in other disciplines. *Sambodhi*, 4(1), 88-93.

Sharma, V. (2022). PI3Kinase/AKT/mTOR Pathway in breast cancer; pathogenesis and prevention with mTOR inhibitors. *Proceedings of the International Virtual Seminar on Recent Trends in Life Sciences and Biotechnology*, 7, 184-191.

Sharma, V., Panwar, A., Sankhyan, A., Ram, G., and Sharma, A. K. (2022a). Exploring the potential of chromones as inhibitors of novel coronavirus infection based on molecular docking and molecular dynamics simulation studies. *Biotechnology and Applied Biochemistry*, 13.

Sharma, V., Panwar, A., Sharma, A., Punj, V., Saini, R. V., Saini, A. K., and Sharma, A. K. (2022b). A comparative molecular dynamic simulation study on potent ligands targeting mTOR/FRB domain for breast cancer therapy. *Biotechnology and applied Biochemistry*, 69, 1339-1347.

Sharma, V., Panwar, A., and Sharma, A. K. (2020a). Molecular dynamic simulation study on chromones and flavonoids for the in silico designing of a potential ligand inhibiting mTOR pathway in breast cancer. *Current Pharmacology Reports*, 6, 373-379.

Sharma, V., Panwar, A., and Sharma, A. K. (2021a). P13K/AKT/mTOR novel biomarkers for breast cancer. *GEN Open*, 1, 83-91.

Sharma, V., Saini, P., Sheikh, I., Upadhyay, S. K., Sharma, U., Sharma, B., and Sharma, A. K. (2017). Role of plant secondary metabolites as potential antimalarial drugs. *The Systematic Reviews in Pharmacy*, 8, 13-18.

Sharma, V., Sankhyan, A., Varshney, A., Choudhary, R., and Sharma, A. K. (2020b). Current paradigms to explore the gut microbiota linkage to neurological disorders. *Neurology*, 8, 68-79.

Sharma, V., Sehrawat, N., Sharma, A., Yadav, M., Verma, P., and Sharma, A. K. (2022c). Multifaceted antiviral therapeutic potential of dietary flavonoids: Emerging trends and future perspectives. *Biotechnology and Applied Biochemistry*, 69, 2028-2045.

Sharma, V., Sharma, A., Punj, V., and Priya, P. (2019b). Recent nanotechnological interventions targeting PI3K/Akt/mTOR pathway: A focus on breast cancer. *Seminars in Cancer Biology*, 59, 133-146.

Sharma, V., and Sharma, A. K. (2021). An in-silico approach for designing a potential antagonistic molecule targeting β 2-adrenoreceptor having therapeutic significance. *Letters in Applied NanoBioScience*, 10, 2063-2069.

Sharma, V., Sharma, A. K., Panwar, A., Sheikh, I., Sharma, A., Dhir, S., Dhama, K., and Thakur, R. (2022). In-silico designing of an inhibitor against mTOR FRB domain: Therapeutic implications against breast cancer. *Journal of Experimental Biology and Agricultural Science*, 10(5), 1016-1023.

Sharma, V., Sharma, A. K., Yadav, M., Sehrawat, N., Kumar, V., Kumar, S., Gupta, A., Sharma, P., and Chakrabarti, S. (2023). Prediction models based on miRNA-disease relationship: Diagnostic relevance to multiple diseases including COVID-19. *Current Pharmaceutical Biotechnology*, 24, 1213-1227.

Sharma, V., Sharma, N., Sheikh, I., Kumar, V., Sehrawat, N., Yadav, M., Ram, G., Sankhyan, A., and Sharma, A. K. (2021b). Probiotics and prebiotics having broad spectrum anticancer therapeutic potential: recent trends and future perspectives. *Current Pharmacology Reports*, 7, 67-79.

Sharma, V. R., Sharma, D. K., Sharma, A. K., Mishra, N., and Batra, N. (2010). New and potential therapies for the treatment of breast cancer: An update for oncologists. *Breast Cancer*, 2, 3.

Sharma, V. R., Singh, M., Kumar, V., Yadav, M., Sehrawat, N., Sharma, D. K., and Sharma. A. K. (2021c). Microbiome dysbiosis in cancer: Exploring therapeutic strategies to counter the disease. *Seminars in Cancer Biology*, 70, 61-70.

Sheikh, I., Sharma, V., Tuli, H. S., Aggarwal, D., Sankhyan, A., Vyas, P., Sharma, A. K., and Bishayee, A. (2020). Cancer chemoprevention by flavonoids, dietary polyphenols and terpenoids. *Biointerface Research in Applied Chemistry*, 11, 8502-8537.

Shi, J., Kantoff, P. W., Wooster, R., and Farokhzad, O. C. (2017). Cancer nanomedicine: progress, challenges and opportunities. *Nature Reviews Cancer*, 17, 20-37.

Siegel, R. L., Miller, K. D., Wagle, N. S., and Jemal, A. (2023). Cancer statistics, 2023. *Ca Cancer J Clin*, 73, 17-48.

Simpkins, F., Jang, K., Yoon, H., Hew, K. E., Kim, M., Azzam, D. J., Sun, J., Zhao, D., Ince, T. A., and Liu, W. (2018). Dual Src and MEK inhibition decreases ovarian cancer growth and targets tumor initiating stem-like cells. *Clinical Cancer Research*, 24, 4874-4886.

Singh, H. (2023). Role of molecular targeted therapeutic drugs in treatment of breast cancer: a review article. *Global Medical Genetics*, 10, 079-086.

Singh, M., Kumar, V., Sehrawat, N., Yadav, M., Chaudhary, M., Upadhyay, S. K., Kumar, S., Sharma, V., Kumar, S., and Dilbaghi, N. (2022). Current paradigms in epigenetic anticancer therapeutics and future challenges. *Seminars in Cancer Biology*, 83, 422-440.

Stepan, K. O., Mazul, A. L., Larson, J., Shah, P., Jackson, R. S., Pipkorn, P., Kang, S. Y., and Puram, S. V. (2023). Changing epidemiology of oral cavity cancer in the United States. *Otolaryngology–Head and Neck Surgery*, 168, 761-768.

Sutherlin, D. P., Bao, L., Berry, M., Castanedo, G., Chuckowree, I., Dotson, J., Folks, A., Friedman, L., Goldsmith, R., and Gunzner, J. (2011). Discovery of a potent, selective, and orally available class I phosphatidylinositol 3-kinase (PI3K)/mammalian target of rapamycin (mTOR) kinase inhibitor (GDC-0980) for the treatment of cancer. *Journal of Medicinal Chemistry*, 54, 7579-7587.

Tannock, I. F. (1998). Conventional cancer therapy: promise broken or promise delayed? *The Lancet*, 351(S2), S9-S16.

Tian, L. Y., Smit, D. J., and Jücker, M. (2023a). The role of PI3K/AKT/mTOR signaling in hepatocellular carcinoma metabolism. *International Journal of Molecular Sciences*, 24, 2652.

Tian, Y., Chen, Z. H., Wu, P., Zhang, D., Ma, Y., Liu, X. F., Wang, X., Ding, D., Cao, X. C., and Yu, Y. (2023b). mir497hg-derived mir-195 and mir-497 mediate tamoxifen resistance via pi3k/akt signaling in breast cancer. *Advanced Science*, 10, 2204819.

Varruchi, Sharma, N., and Sharma, A. K. (2018). In-silico designed and optimized lead inhibiting breast cancer mTOR FRB domain substrate recruitment mechanism. IN Patent, 201.

Vazquez-Martin, A., Oliveras-Ferraros, C., Colomer, R., Brunet, J., and Menendez, J. (2008). Low-scale phosphoproteome analyses identify the mTOR effector p70 S6 kinase 1 as a specific biomarker of the dual-HER1/HER2 tyrosine kinase inhibitor lapatinib (Tykerb®) in human breast carcinoma cells. *Annals of Oncology*, 19, 1097-1109.

Vogel, C. L., Cobleigh, M. A., Tripathy, D., Gutheil, J. C., Harris, L. N., Fehrenbacher, L., Slamon, D. J., Murphy, M., Novotny, W. F., and Burchmore, M. (2023). Efficacy and safety of trastuzumab as a single agent in first-line treatment of HER2-overexpressing metastatic breast cancer. *Journal of Clinical Oncology*, 41, 1638-1645.

Varruchi, S. (2020). Bioinformatics and its applications in environmental science and health and its applications in other disciplines. *Sambodhi Journal*, 4, 88-93.

Wallin, J. J., Edgar, K. A., Guan, J., Berry, M., Prior, W. W., Lee, L., Lesnick, J. D., Lewis, C., Nonomiya, J., and Pang, J. (2011). GDC-0980 is a novel class I PI3K/mTOR kinase inhibitor with robust activity in cancer models driven by the PI3K pathway. *Molecular Cancer Therapeutics*, 10, 2426-2436.

Wang, M., Zhou, A., An, T., Kong, L., Yu, C., Liu, J., Xia, C., Zhou, H., and Li, Y. (2016a). N-Hydroxyphthalimide exhibits antitumor activity by suppressing mTOR signaling pathway in BT-20 and LoVo cells. *Journal of Experimental and Clinical Cancer Research*, 35, 1-12.

Wang, R., Zhang, Q., Peng, X., Zhou, C., Zhong, Y., Chen, X., Qiu, Y., Jin, M., Gong, M., and Kong, D. (2016b). Stellettin B induces G1 arrest, apoptosis and autophagy in human non-small cell lung cancer A549 cells via blocking PI3K/Akt/mTOR pathway. *Scientific Reports*, 6, 27071.

Wang, Y. X., Gao, J. X., Wang, X. Y., Zhang, L., and Liu, C. M. (2012). Antiproliferative effects of selective cyclooxygenase-2 inhibitor modulated by nimotuzumab in estrogen-dependent breast cancer cells. *Tumor Biology*, 33, 957-966.

Wang, Y., Yu, Q., He, X., Romigh, T., Altemus, J., and Eng, C. (2014). Activation of AR sensitizes breast carcinomas to NVP-BEZ235's therapeutic effect mediated by PTEN and KLLN upregulation. *Molecular Cancer Therapeutics*, 13, 517-527.

Wen, X., Zhou, Y., Zeng, J., and Liu, X. (2020). Recent development of 1, 2, 4-triazole-containing compounds as anticancer agents. *Current Topics in Medicinal Chemistry*, 20, 1441-1460.

Wheeler, K., Wang, L., Wallen, C., Childers, S., Cline, J., Keng, P., and Mach, R. (2000). Sigma-2 receptors as a biomarker of proliferation in solid tumours. *British Journal of Cancer*, 82, 1223-1232.

Woo, J. H., Kim, Y. H., Choi, Y. J., Kim, D. G., Lee, K. S., Bae, J. H., Min, D. S., Chang, J. S., Jeong, Y. J., and Lee, Y. H. (2003). Molecular mechanisms of curcumin-induced cytotoxicity: induction of apoptosis through generation of reactive oxygen species, down-regulation of Bcl-X L and IAP, the release of cytochrome c and inhibition of Akt. *Carcinogenesis*, 24, 1199-1208.

Wood, D. E., and Newcomb, E. W. (2000). Cleavage of Bax enhances its cell death function. *Experimental Cell Research*, 256, 375-382.

Yang, T., Wang, P., Yin, X., Zhang, J., Huo, M., Gao, J., Li, G., Teng, X., Yu, H., and Huang, W. (2021). The histone deacetylase inhibitor PCI-24781 impairs calcium influx and inhibits proliferation and metastasis in breast cancer. *Theranostics*, 11, 2058.

Yu, Y., Savage, R. E., Eathiraj, S., Meade, J., Wick, M. J., Hall, T., Abbadessa, G., and Schwartz, B. (2015). Targeting AKT1-E17K and the PI3K/AKT pathway with an allosteric AKT inhibitor, ARQ 092. *PLoS One*, 10, e0140479.

Yuan, Y., Long, H., Zhou, Z., Fu, Y., and Jiang, B. (2023). PI3K–AKT-Targeting breast cancer treatments: Natural products and synthetic compounds. *Biomolecules*, 13, 93.

Zhang, Y. Y., Yan, Y., Zhang, J., Xia, C. Y., Lian, W. W., Wang, W. P., He, J., Zhang, W. K., and Xu, J. K. (2022). Jolkinolide B: A comprehensive review of its physicochemical properties, analytical methods, synthesis and pharmacological activity. *Phytochemistry*, 113448.

# Index

## A

## B

## C

## D

## E



## F

## G



## H

## L



## M

## N

## O



## P

## Q



## R

## S



## T

## U



## V



## W



## X